D1536872

Editorial Advisory Board

INTERNAL MEDICINE REVIEW

ARCO MEDICAL REVIEW SERIES

INTERNAL MEDICINE REVIEW

Second Edition

Robert E. Pieroni, M.D.
Professor of Internal Medicine
and
Professor of Family Medicine
College of Community Health Sciences
University of Alabama
Tuscaloosa

ARCO PUBLISHING, INC.
NEW YORK

Second Edition, First Printing

Published by Arco Publishing, Inc.
215 Park Avenue South, New York, N.Y. 10003

Copyright © 1978, 1983 by Arco Publishing, Inc.

Library of Congress Cataloging in Publication Data

Pieroni, Robert E.
  Internal medicine review.

  (Arco medical review series)
  1. Internal medicine—Examinations, questions, etc.
I. Title. II. Series. [DNLM: 1. Internal medicine—
Examination questions.   WB 18 P619i]
RC58.P48 1982   616'.0076   82-6777
ISBN 0-668-05488-3   AACR2

Printed in the United States of America

Contents

Chapters:

Chapters:

Preface

Internal medicine is a broad, expanding field with a large number of subspecialty areas. The present volume attempts to cover pertinent and important topics in these areas. It is obvious that in a text of this size, several major topics could only be covered briefly. Less common but nevertheless important entities are presented on occasion to provide the reader with a passing knowledge of these disease processes. Occasionally, certain important points are repeated in a different format for emphasis.

In addition to the standard internal medicine subspecialties, it was felt that other areas germane to the study of internal medicine should be included in this text. Therefore, sections on geriatrics, medical malpractice, dermatology, pharmacology, alterations in normal functions, signs and symptoms of disease, physical examination and history taking, and a special section on electrocardiography are included in the text. In addition, case histories and a pictorial section have been prepared with multiple-choice questions.

The format of the questions has purposely been varied to include multiple-choice questions, true-false questions, and other types. It is hoped that the specific questions and their mode of presentation will assist the reader in preparation for future examinations and improve skills in multiple-choice testing techniques.

The questions have been developed from a wide variety of sources including recent textbooks, monographs, as well as journals available in most health sciences libraries. Reference to these sources should be made for fuller exposition of the subject matter. Attempts have been made, whenever possible, to approximate or duplicate the original language of the authors in order to avoid discrepancies and distortions in interpretation. It should be repeated for emphasis that reference to the original sources will provide a more complete discussion of topics covered. This is especially pertinent since, as in all medicine, commentary on some of the topics could be considered controversial. The subject matter of internal medicine and other topics discussed in this text are constantly being revised and some answers have already or will in time become obsolete as new knowledge is gained.

Acknowledgments

I greatly appreciate the competent and skillful assistance of Maridy Bronstein and Cindy Trantham in the preparation of this manuscript. I dedicate this book to my family for their strong support, and to the students and residents of the College of Community Health Sciences, who made the effort enjoyable and worthwhile.

About the References in This Book

Two kinds of reference citation appear in this book, on the last line of each answer, on the right-hand side. Where the reference is to one of the textbooks listed at the end of the chapter, the citation will consist of a number combination that identifies the reference source and the page or pages where the information relating to the question and the correct answer may be found. For example, (8:497) refers you to page 497 of the eighth book on the list.

Where the reference is to a journal article, however, the complete citation appears to the right of the answer. For example, (*N Engl J Med*, 306:446, 1982) refers you to volume 306, page 446 of *The New England Journal of Medicine*, published in 1982.

CHAPTER 1

Pictorial Questions

Directions: For each of the following multiple-choice questions, select the ONE CORRECT answer.

Questions 1 to 17

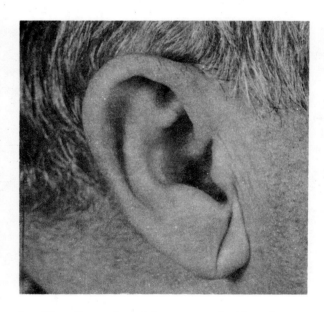

1. The diagonal earlobe crease in the above 65-year-old man has been associated with

   A. emphysema
   B. coronary heart disease
   C. gastrointestinal carcinoma
   D. diabetes mellitus
   E. multiple sclerosis

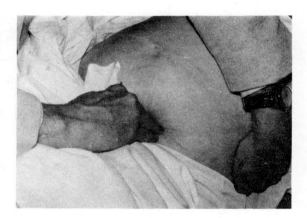

2. In the above 68-year-old female, the spleen tip is felt well below the umbilicus. The patient's CBC revealed an increase in all the formed elements of the blood. Which of the following is the most likely diagnosis?

   A. acute lymphocytic leukemia
   B. chronic lymphocytic leukemia
   C. polycythemia vera
   D. hypersplenism syndrome
   E. chronic myelocytic leukemia

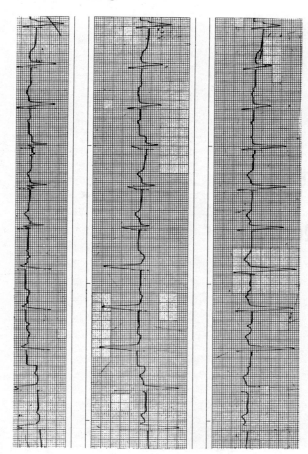

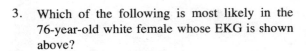

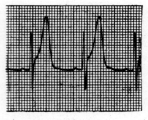

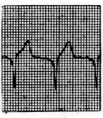

1   **2**

4. The above two V_2 tracings were obtained one day apart. Which of the following conditions did the patient most likely have?

    A. pericarditis
    B. early repolarization
    C. inferior MI
    D. anterior MI
    E. none of the above

3. Which of the following is most likely in the 76-year-old white female whose EKG is shown above?

    A. she has had an inferior MI
    B. she has had a true posterior MI
    C. she has had an anterior MI
    D. she has developed Mobitz II AV block
    E. none of the above

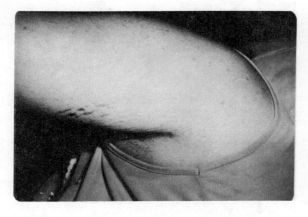

5. This 26-year-old female saw her physician because of recently developed facial acne. She was noted to be mildly hypertensive and displayed hirsutism and truncal obesity. Which of the following would be the most likely diagnosis in this patient?

    A. Addison's disease
    B. Stein-Leventhal syndrome
    C. Cushing's disease
    D. hypothyroidism
    E. acromegaly

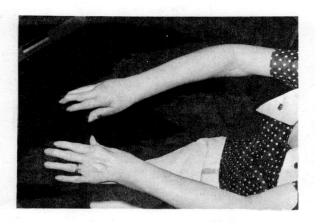

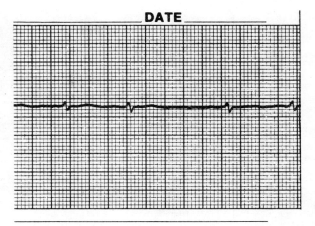

DATE

6. The 52-year-old female whose upper extremities are depicted above is unable to extend her arms. Which of the following disorders is she most likely to have?

A. gouty arthritis
B. systemic lupus erythematosus
C. polymyalgia rheumatica
D. rheumatoid arthritis
E. polyarteritis nodosa

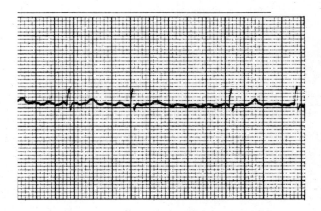

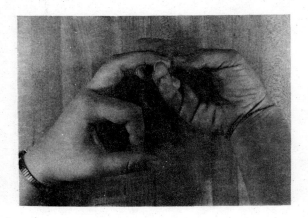

7. Which pathologic reflex is the examiner attempting to elicit in the above picture?

A. Babinski's sign
B. Hoffman's sign
C. Chvostek's sign
D. Homan's sign
E. Collins' sign

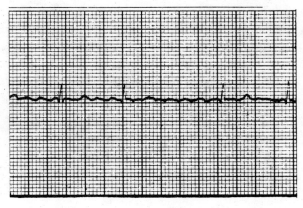

8. Which of the following disorders is most likely to be associated with the above rhythm strip?

A. hypothyroidism
B. hyperthyroidism
C. hypoparathyroidism
D. hyperparathyroidism
E. Cushing's disease

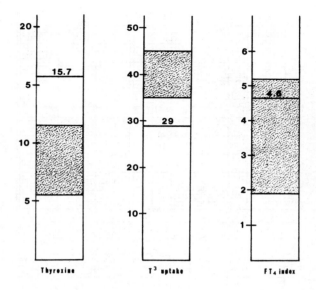

9. The above thyroid profile was obtained in a 25-year-old female with acute hepatitis B infection. The most likely diagnosis in this patient is

    A. Grave's disease
    B. autoimmune thyroiditis
    C. subacute thyroiditis
    D. T_3 hypothyroidism
    E. none of the above

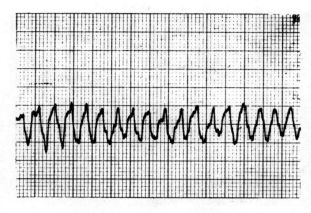

11. Use of which of the following would be appropriate therapy in the patient with the above rhythm strip?

    A. lidocaine
    B. bretylium
    C. digoxin
    D. KCl
    E. none of the above

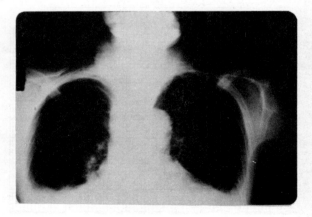

10. The female whose chest x-ray is shown above would be most likely to exhibit

    A. hyperresonance throughout the lung fields
    B. An S_3 gallop
    C. acid fast bacilli in her sputum
    D. erythema nodosum
    E. a paradoxical pulse

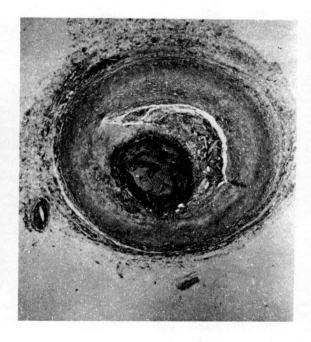

12. The above microscopic section of a coronary artery was obtained from a 58-year-old male who sustained a fatal myocardial infarction. Which of the following would be *least* likely in this patient?

A. he was a heavy cigarette smoker
B. he had high HDL levels
C. he was hypertensive
D. he was diabetic
E. he had a type A personality

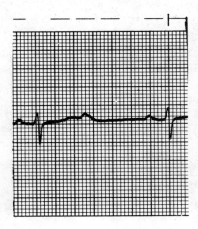

13. In the tracing shown above, the patient's heart rate is _____ beats per minute.

   A. 34
   B. 43
   C. 50
   D. 60
   E. 75

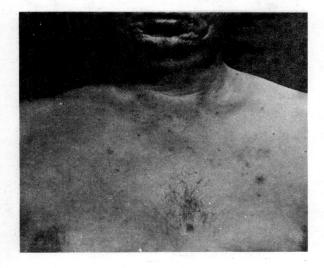

14. The 45-year-old male depicted above, in addition to numerous erythematous skin lesions, has

peripheral edema, a distended abdomen, and palmar erythema. Which of the following is the most likely diagnosis in this patient?

A. congestive heart failure
B. Laennec's cirrhosis
C. polyarteritis nodosa
D. chronic obstructive pulmonary disease
E. disseminated carcinoma

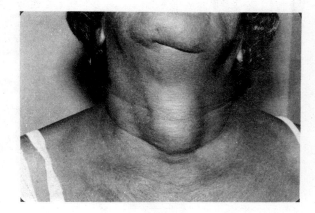

15. The above elderly female with a multinodular goiter was found to be euthyroid. After a radiographic dye procedure she developed thyrotoxicosis. This is known as the

A. Hope-Forbes effect
B. Willis-Ward effect
C. Jod-Basebow effect
D. Perry-Graves effect
E. none of the above

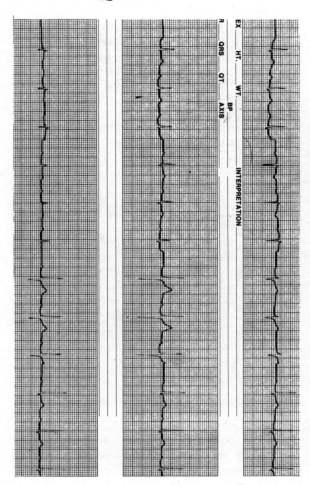

C.   a major manifestation of rheumatic fever
D.   a minor manifestation of rheumatic fever
E.   a major manifestation of subacute bacterial endocarditis

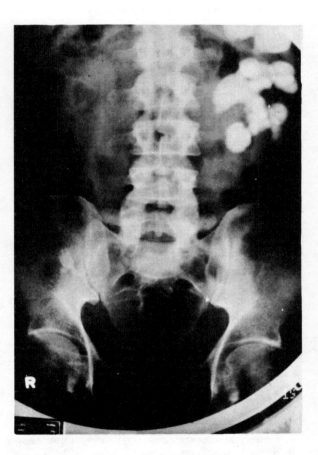

16.   A 16-year-old female developed arthritis, carditis, and erythema marginatum. The patient's EKG tracing is shown above. Findings on this tracing would be most likely to represent

A.   a major manifestation of juvenile rheumatoid arthritis
B.   a minor manifestation of juvenile rheumatoid arthritis

17.   Chronic urinary tract infections have been present in the patient depicted above. Urinalysis reveals a PH of 8. Which of the following organisms would be most likely to be cultured from the urine?

A.   *Staphylococcus*
B.   *Klebsiella*
C.   *Proteus*
D.   *Pseudomonas*
E.   *E. coli*

Questions 18 and 19

Questions 20 and 21

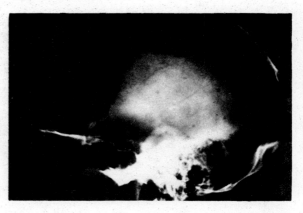

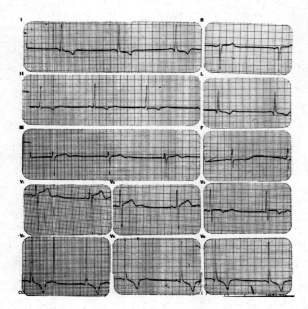

18. The above EKG was obtained in a 49-year-old black female. The most likely diagnosis is

    A. sick sinus syndrome
    B. complete heart block
    C. anterior myocardial infarction
    D. inferior myocardial infarction
    E. none of the above

19. Which of the following antihypertensive medications would be *least* likely to result in this patient's bradycardia?

    A. alpha methyldopa
    B. apresoline
    C. propranolol
    D. reserpine
    E. metoprolol

20. The above skull film was done on a 74-year-old white male complaining of headaches. For the past several years, he had been using increasing doses of aspirin for "arthritis" involving his hips. Recently he noted increasing pain in his thighs, which began to feel warm to the touch. He became progressively hard of hearing, which he attributed to "old age." The patient most likely has

    A. hyperparathyroidism
    B. Paget's disease
    C. metastatic carcinoma
    D. hypoparathyroidism
    E. none of the above

21. Which of the following is *not* true of the patient's disease?

    A. the initial event histologically is increased bone resorption mediated by such cells as osteoclasts, with later replacement of normal marrow by vascular, fibrous connective tissue
    B. some areas of bone may display evidence of both excessive resorption and chaotic new bone formation
    C. in the early stages, bone resorption predominates and bones are very vascular
    D. resorption involves both the organic and mineral phases of the bone
    E. the bone displays decreased density with cortical thinning

Questions 22 and 23

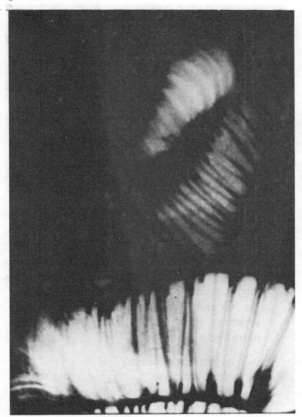

22. The above abdominal film is that of a middle-aged male with a prosthetic heart valve who had noted increased colicky abdominal pain and diarrhea over a two-day period. He then developed shock, severe abdominal tenderness, rigidity, leucocytosis, and fever. The patient most likely has developed

    A. acute appendicitis
    B. ulcerative colitis
    C. mesenteric vascular occlusion
    D. gallstone ileus
    E. none of the above

23. The most likely explanation for this patient's ischemic small bowel is

    A. embolism
    B. atherosclerotic narrowing
    C. nonocclusive ischemia
    D. venous thrombi
    E. none of the above

Questions 24 and 25

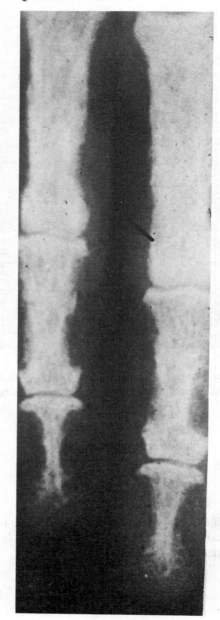

24. The patient whose finger films are depicted above has also been noted to have hypercalcemia. Which of the following would the patient be *least* likely to manifest?

    A. nephrocalcinosis
    B. diarrhea
    C. elevated urine calcium
    D. low to normal serum phosphate
    E. "band keratopathy"

25. In this disorder, about what percentage of cases are caused by a single adenoma?

   A. 2
   B. 15–20
   C. 40
   D. 50–60
   E. 80

Questions 26 to 30

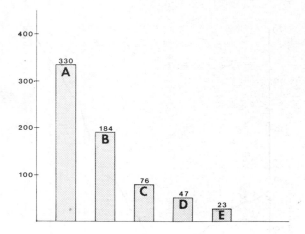

The leading causes of death in the United States for the year 1979 are shown above. Rates are given per 100,000 population. Match the following disorders with the appropriate lettered causes of mortality

26. accidents

27. malignant neoplasm

28. chronic obstructive pulmonary diseases and related conditions

29. cerebrovascular disease

30. diseases of the heart

Questions 31 to 35

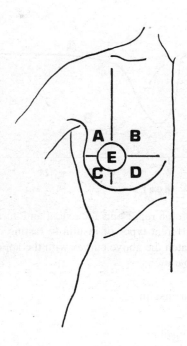

Match the above areas of the breast with the following frequencies with which breast carcinoma may develop in these anatomic locations

31. 5%

32. 10%

33. 15%

34. 25%

35. 45%

Questions 36 and 37

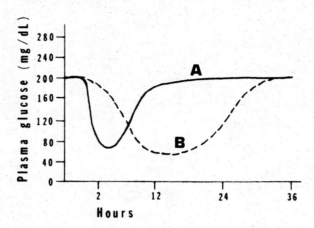

The above graph represents the extent and duration of action of different types of insulin in fasting diabetic patients. Match the above curves with the appropriate insulin preparations

36. regular insulin

37. NPH insulin

Questions 38 to 40

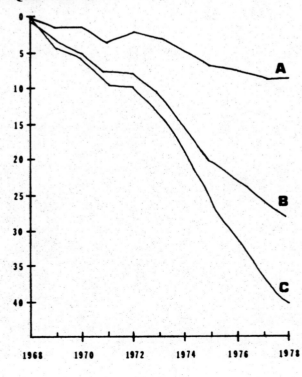

Match the lettered mortality trends with the specific causes listed below

38. stroke

39. major cardiovascular and coronary heart disease

40 all other causes

Questions 41 to 44

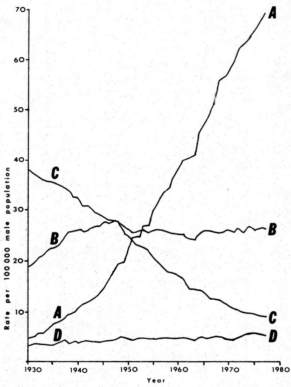

Match the above lettered mortality rates with the appropriate numbered type of carcinoma

41. lung

42. esophagus

43. colon

44. stomach

Answers and Commentary

Answers 1 to 3

1. **B.** An association between the presence of a diagonal earlobe crease and coronary heart disease has been supported by clinical data as well as by angiographic and post-mortem findings. However, recent studies in certain ethnic groups, including Japanese males and American Indians, have not supported this association.
(*Ann Intern Med*, 93:512, 1980)

2. **C.** Classically, polycythemia vera is characterized by splenomegaly as well as an elevated production of erythrocytes, granulocytes, and platelets. In general, the elevated hemoglobin concentration dominates this disorder.
(8:1576)

3. **E.** This patient developed complete heart block, which necessitated insertion of a permanent pacemaker. Pacemaker blips can be seen preceding QRS complexes.
(6:226)

4. **D.** In tracing 1, the height of the T wave is abnormal. Usually T waves are not above 10 mm in any of the precordial leads. Tall T waves may be found in patients with hyperkalemia, psychoses, cerebrovascular accidents, and some forms of ventricular overloading. They may also be found in patients with myocardial ischemia with or without infarction. The subsequent development of a Q wave in tracing 2 indicates that the patient sustained an anterior MI, which was found to be confined to the anterior septal region.
(6:22, 23)

5. **C.** Striae are shown on the upper arm of this female with Cushing's syndrome. Subjects with hypercortisolism may also have diabetes mellitus, hypercholesterolemia, and hypokalemic alkalosis. Disordered protein metabolism may result in skin fragility with ecchymoses and striae.
(8:780, 781)

6. **D.** The patient has symetrical fusiform swelling of PIP joints, with synovitis also involving her wrists and MCP joints. Some interossei muscle wasting is evident in the left hand. These findings, in addition to flexion contractures of her arms, are consistent with rheumatoid arthritis.
(7:318, 319)

7. **B.** For proper elicitation of Hoffmann's sign, the subject's wrist should be relaxed and dorsiflexed with fingers in a flexed position. The patient's middle finger is flicked by the examiner's thumb tip. A flicking adduction of the thumb, index finger, or both, represents a positive sign. Unlike Babinski's sign, Hoffmann's sign my occasionally be observed in normal subjects.
(4:108)

8. **B.** The rhythm strip shows an irregular rhythm characteristic of atrial fibrillation. In subjects with this dysrhythmia, hyperthyroidism should always be considered.
(4:243)

9. **E.** The patient is euthyroid. Acute hepatitis can result in an elevation of thyroxine- or thyronine-binding globulin (TBG), which can lead to increased T_4 with reduction of T_3 uptake. The free T_4 index remains normal, however.
(2:1696, 1697)

10. **B.** The x-ray shows blunting of the costophrenic angles. Bilateral pleural effusions are most likely to develop in patients with congestive heart failure, in which a third sound gallop is a characteristic finding.
(4:256)

11. **E.** The rhythm strip depicts ventricular fibrillation, a catastrophic event. It may be recognized by the absence of properly formed ventricular complexes. As in the above rhythm strip, the baseline undulates unevenly, and no clear-cut QRS deflections are formed. Treatment consists of immediate electrical defibrillation.
(6:123)

12. **B.** An atheromatous plaque and a thrombus are depicted in the coronary artery. All the factors listed have been associated with increased risk for develop-

ment of atherosclerosis, with the exception of high HDL levels. Actually, elevated HDL levels appear to exert a protective effect against development of atherosclerotic cardiovascular disease. (1:3)

13. **B.** The cardiac rate can be obtained by dividing the number of large blocks between successive QRS complexes into 300. In the above tracing seven large blocks occur between the QRS complexes, giving a rate of about 43. Borderline first-degree AV block is present, a finding frequently seen with slow heart rates. (6:11)

14. **B.** The patient, a chronic alcoholic, has Laennec's cirrhosis. Multiple spider nevi are depicted. These nevi usually involve the upper half of the body.(3:397)

15. **C.** Euthyroid subjects with multinodular goiters may develop iodide-induced thyrotoxicosis, the Jod-Basebow effect. They should avoid pharmacologic doses of iodide and should be cautiously monitored if radiographic dye procedures are to be performed. (7:202)

16. **D.** The tracing shows considerable first-degree AV block. A prolongation of the PR interval is considered a minor manifestation of rheumatic fever. Other minor manifestations include leucocytosis, elevated sedimentation rate, fever, and arthralgia. The presence of erythema marginatum is considered a major manifestation. (6:202)

17. **C.** The patient has a large staghorn calculus, involving the left kidney, and infected urolithiasis. This refers to a condition in which struvite (magnesium-ammonium-phosphate) stones develop in the presence of infection with a urea-splitting organism. In such subjects, urinary pH is greater than 7.5, which contributes to formation of hydroxyapatite and struvite crystals. Although all the organisms listed may produce urease, *Proteus* species are most frequently associated with struvite stones. (9:921)

Answers 18 and 19

18. **E.** The patient has long-standing severe hypertension requiring several medications. Prominent voltage and T-wave inversions, especially in the lateral leads, are consistent with a diagnosis of LVH with strain pattern. (6:52–53)

19. **B.** Apresoline results in arteriolar dilation with reflex tachycardia. All the other medications listed can result in bradycardia. (5:96)

Answers 20 and 21

20. **B.** The patient described most likely has Paget's disease of the bone. (2:1861)

21. **E.** In Paget's disease, bone is usually enlarged, with irregularly widened cortex in a coarse, striated pattern. There is increased density, which is occasionally focal in distribution. All other statements are true of this disease. (2:1860)

Answers 22 and 23

22. **C.** The film is most consistent with mesenteric vascular occlusion, a type of intestinal obstruction in which no mechanical occlusion of the intestine exists, but rather ischemia is the primary feature. (2:1438)

23. **A.** About 75% of cases of mesenteric vascular occlusion are the result of occlusion of the superior mesenteric artery by emboli or atherosclerotic narrowing. In this patient with a prosthetic valve, embolism was the most likely cause. (3:699)

Answers 24 and 25

24. **B.** The films are those of a patient with hyperparathyroidism. All the conditions listed with the exception of diarrhea are found in this disorder. In addition, thirst, nausea, anorexia, and vomiting are prominent symptoms. There is often a past history of peptic ulcer disease with obstruction or even hemorrhage. Constipation, asthenia, anemia, and weight loss may occur, and hypertension is commonly found. (3:698)

25. **E.** About 80% of cases of primary hyperparathyroidism are caused by a single adenoma. (3:699)

Answers 26 to 30

26. **D.** (*Mon Vital Stats Report*, vol. 28, No. 12, 1980)

27. **B.** (*Mon Vital Stats Report*, vol. 28, No. 12, 1980)

28. **E.** (*Mon Vital Stats Report*, vol. 28, No. 12, 1980)

29. **C.** (*Mon Vital Stats Report*, vol. 28, No. 12, 1980)

30. **A.** (*Mon Vital Stats Report*, vol. 28, No. 12, 1980)

Answers 31 to 35

31.	**D.**	(3:419)
32.	**C.**	(3:419)
33.	**B.**	(3:419)
34.	**E.**	(3:419)
35.	**A.**	(3:419)

Answers 36 and 37

36.	**A.**	(3:760)
37.	**B.**	(3:760)

Answers 38 to 40

38.	**C.**	(1:2)
39.	**B.**	(1:2)
40.	**A.**	(1:2)

Answers 41 to 44

41.	**A.**	(*Cancer J for Clinicians*, 31:19, 1981)
42.	**D.**	(*Cancer J for Clinicians*, 31:19, 1981)
43.	**B.**	(*Cancer J for Clinicians*, 31:19, 1981)
44.	**C.**	(*Cancer J for Clinicians*, 31:19, 1981)

Textbook References for Chapter 1

1. *Arteriosclerosis: Report of the Working Group on Arteriosclerosis of the National Heart, Lung, and Blood Institute: Summary, Conclusions, and Recommendations*, vol. 1 (1981): Prepared by the Working Group on Arteriosclerosis of the National Heart, Lung, and Blood Institute, National Institutes of Health, U.S. Government Printing Office, Washington, D.C.

2. Isselbacher, K.J., Editor (1980): *Harrison's Principles of Internal Medicine*, Ninth Edition, McGraw-Hill Book Company, New York.

3. Krupp, M.A. and Chatton, M.J. (1980): *Current Medical Diagnosis and Treatment, 1980*, Lange Medical Publications, Los Altos, California.

4. Delp, M.H. and Manning, R.T., Editors (1981): *Major's Physical Diagnosis: An Introduction to the Clinical Process*, Ninth Edition, W.B. Saunders Company, Philadelphia.

5. Freitag, J.J. and Miller, L.W., Editors (1980): *Manual of Medical Therapeutics*, Twenty-third Edition, Little, Brown and Company, Boston.

6. Marriott, H.J.L. (1977): *Practical Electrocardiography*, Sixth Edition, Williams & Wilkins Company, Baltimore.

7. Fishman, M.C., Hoffman, A.R., Klausner, R.D., et al (1981): *Medicine*, J.B. Lippincott Company, Philadelphia.

8. Harvey, A.M., Johns, R.J., McKusick, V.A., et al, Editors (1980): *The Principles and Practice of Medicine*, Twentieth Edition, Appleton-Century-Crofts, New York.

9. Earley, L.E. and Gottschalk, C.W., Editors (1979): *Strauss and Welt's Diseases of the Kidney*, Third Edition, Little, Brown and Company, Boston.

CHAPTER 2

Geriatrics

Directions: Indicate whether each of the following statements is true or false.

Questions 1 to 8

1. Severe depressive illness in the aged is rarely accompanied by suicidal ideation.

2. Neuroglycopenia may occur at "normal" blood glucose levels of 100–150 mg% in elderly patients.

3. With aging, the normal electrocardiogram reveals considerable change.

4. Pain is the most common presenting clinical symptom in peripheral vascular disease.

5. The capacity of the pituitary to secrete growth hormone in response to several stimuli is unaffected in the elderly.

6. Most subjects who develop tuberculosis are newly infected.

7. In subjects with strokes, should there be a question of increased intracranial pressure, the best procedure to perform is a lumbar puncture.

8. The liver enlarges with age.

Questions 9 to 13

Directions: For each of the following statements, select
A. if the question is associated with A only
B. if the question is associated with B only
C. if the question is associated with both A and B
D. if the question is associated with neither A nor B

9. Which of the following describe sleep in the elderly?

   A. there is considerable level 4 sleep
   B. there are few brief arousals
   C. both
   D. neither

10. If disorders such as carcinomas and artherosclerosis were to be eradicated,

   A. more subjects would approximate their potential maximum span of life
   B. the maxium life span would be extended
   C. both
   D. neither

11. The routine use of fluorohydrocortisone in elderly hypoadrenocortical patients

   A. is not recommended
   B. may lead to hypotension
   C. both
   D. neither

12. Depression in the aged is

    A. uncommon
    B. often mistaken for dementia
    C. both
    D. neither

13. With aging, bile

    A. is increased in quantity
    B. has a lower cholesterol composition
    C. both
    D. neither

Directions: For each of the following multiple-choice questions, select the ONE CORRECT answer.

Questions 14 through 16

14. Elderly individuals account for nearly _____ percent of suicides that are reported.

    A. 0.1–0.2
    B. 1–2
    C. 5
    D. 10
    E. 25

15. About what percentage of subjects with primary hyperparathyroidism are over 60 years of age?

    A. 10
    B. 33
    C. 55
    D. 66
    E. 80

16. Which of the following remain relatively constant in the aging lung?

    A. total lung capacity
    B. residual volume
    C. vital capacity
    D. forced expiratory volume
    E. maximal breathing capacity

Directions: Use the key below to answer the following questions:
    A. **if A is greater than or more appropriate than B.**
    B. **if B is greater than or more appropriate than A**
    C. **if A and B are approximately equal**

Questions 17 to 20

17. Pruritus in the elderly usually appears on the lower

    A. legs
    B. arms

18. The most frequent cause of cancer death in adult males is

    A. carcinoma of the lung
    B. carcinoma of the prostate

19. The slower metabolism and excretion of barbiturates and other hypnotics in the elderly

    A. may lead to reduced attention span
    B. may cause agitation

20. In aged subjects with osteoporosis, the fracture site is more frequently the femur in

    A. males
    B. females

Directions: Indicate whether each of the following statements is true or false.

Questions 21 to 29

21. In the elderly, the presence of minimal hypercalcemia in an asymptomatic individual with high iPTH levels mandates surgery.

22. Severe hypokalemia may appear as acute brain syndrome.

23. Production of follicle-stimulating hormone (FSH) declines in postmenopausal females.

24. Arsenical keratoses are in themselves malignant.

25. There is a male climacterium analogous to the menopause

26. The maximal rate of oxygen utilization by human beings during exercise increases with advancing age.

27. The most reliable method for establishing the diagnosis of senile cardiac amyloidosis is rectal biopsy.

28. Since the female breast atrophies with age, tumors such as fibroadenomas may become less prominent.

29. The incidence of bleeding ulcers increases with age.

Directions: For each of the following incomplete statements, ONE or MORE of the numbered completions is correct. In each case, select:
   A.   if 1, 2, and 3 are correct
   B.   if 1 and 3 are correct
   C.   if 2 and 4 are correct
   D.   if only 4 is correct
   E.   if all statements are correct

Questions 30 to 33

30. Drugs that are removed from the body primarily by renal excretion include

    1. penicillin
    2. amantadine
    3. aminoglycosides
    4. digitoxin

31. Thyroid functions that decrease with age include

    1. basal metabolic rate
    2. circulating thyroid hormone
    3. ^{133}I uptake
    4. thyroxin turnover during acute febrile illness may be

32. Blood transfusions are indicated in elderly patients with chronic anemias associated with

    1. cardiac failure
    2. angina pectoris
    3. cerebral insufficiency
    4. infection

33. Early symptoms of prostatic hyperplasia include

    1. hesitancy
    2. frequency
    3. nocturia
    4. increase in the force of the stream

Directions: Use the key below to answer the following questions. If the function listed
   A.   decreases with age
   B.   increases with age
   C.   remains relatively constant with age

Questions 34 to 36

34. _____ pulmonary diffusing capacity, CO_2

35. _____ arterial carbon dioxide pressure

36. _____ functional residual volume

Directions: For each of the following statements, select
   A.   if the question is associated with A only
   B.   if the question is associated with B only
   C.   if the question is associated with both A and B
   D.   if the question is associated with neither A nor B

Questions 37 to 42

37. The prophylactic use of antiparkinsonism drugs with antipsychotic drugs in the elderly is inadvisable because of their

    A.   anticholinergic additive effects
    B.   possible implication in tardive dyskinesia
    C.   both
    D.   neither

38. In which of the following disorders are systemic symptoms present?

    A. rheumatoid arthritis
    B. degenerative joint diseases
    C. both
    D. neither

39. Which of the following is/are associated statistically with a higher incidence of endometrial carcinoma?

    A. early onset of menopause (below 40 years)
    B. late onset of menopause (past 50 years)
    C. both
    D. neither

40. If involuntary loss of urine becomes incapacitating, and especially when it is associated with chronic infection, evaluation is indicated by

    A. cystoscopy
    B. cystometry
    C. both
    D. neither

41. Which of the following conditions should be considered in every elderly patient with congestive heart failure?

    A. valvular heart disease
    B. rheumatic heart disease
    C. both
    D. neither

42. Between the third and ninth decades of life

    A. the ribs elevate
    B. the diaphragm flattens
    C. both
    D. neither

Directions: Indicate whether each of the following statements is true or false.

Questions 43 to 50

43. The entire prostate is excised in a prostatectomy.

44. In the past few decades, tuberculosis has become mainly a disorder of younger persons.

45. Most drugs have a decreased central nervous system effect in the elderly.

46. Atrial septal defect (ASD) is a congenital cardiac anomaly that is being less readily found among the elderly.

47. One possible explanation for the increase in cancer in the elderly is that reduction of host resistance occurs with age.

48. The incidence of tetanus in subjects over 60 is less than that of the rest of the population.

49. Vulvar carcinoma has a peak incidence in the geriatric years.

50. With advancing age, the percentage of body fat tends to decrease.

Directions: Use the key below to answer the following questions:
  A. if A is greater than or more appropriate than B
  B. if B is greater than or more appropriate than A
  C. if A and B are approximately equal

Questions 51 to 55

51. Heart rate is higher during

    A. treadmill testing of cardiac patients
    B. intercourse

52. Which of the following drugs is associated with a greater risk of producing severe and prolonged hypoglycemia in the elderly?

    A. chlorpropamide
    B. tolbutamide

53. Spider angiomas are more commonly seen in

    A. men
    B. women

54. Which of the following decreases by the greatest amount with age?

    A. total number of cells in the body
    B. total mass of cells in the body

55. Benign positional vertigo or transient vertigo after sudden head movements indicates

    A. vestibular system involvement
    B. transient ischemia

Directions: For each of the following multiple-choice questions, select the ONE CORRECT answer.

Questions 56 to 59

56. What percentage of persons over age 65 have at least one chronic disease?

    A. 17
    B. 32
    C. 49
    D. 63
    E. 86

57. Which of the following has achieved the status of a recognized mode of therapy for organic brain syndromes?

    A. cerebrovascular dilators
    B. anticoagulants
    C. hyperbaric oxygen therapy
    D. B and C only
    E. none of the above

58. In 1900 what was the approximate life expectancy at birth for white males?

    A. 37 years
    B. 42 years
    C. 48 years
    D. 57 years
    E. 62 years

59. What percentage of individuals 65 and older currently are in long-term care facilities?

    A. 5
    B. 10

C. 20
D. 33
E. 50

Directions: Indicate whether each of the following statements is true or false.

Questions 60 to 68

60. Although females are still likely to outlive males, this advantage has narrowed.

61. Insulin release is delayed in older subjects.

62. Disease is more important than age in causing depression or mental illness.

63. Age must be considered the most potent risk factor for cardiovascular disease.

64. Studies of the coumarin anticoagulant warfarin have demonstrated decreased drug sensitivity in the elderly.

65. Periodontal disease is widespread among the aged.

66. The cerebral ventricles decrease in size with age.

67. There is an increase in intracellular water with age.

68. Degenerative joint disease develops in a minority of individuals.

Directions: Use the key below to answer the following questions. If the crystal is indicative of:
    A. gout
    B. pseudogout

Questions 69 to 70

69. _____ calcium pyrophosphate dihydrate

70. _____ monosodium urate monhydrate

Answers and Commentary

1. **False.** Severe depressive illness in the aged is frequently accompanied by suicidal ideation. Such thoughts may be relatively passive wishes for death or may be the beginning of an active plan to commit suicide. Therefore, they must be taken seriously. (6:111)

2. **True.** Antidiabetic agents should be used with care by the elderly patient. Elderly patients seem to tolerate glucose levels of 150–250 mg% better than the lower range, where irreversible brain damage may occur. A hypoglycemic patient may become confused and sleepy, with slurred speech, which may be mistaken for dementia. (3:16)

3. **False.** With aging, the normal electrocardiogram reveals little change. However, pathologic cardiac alterations accumulate with time and are revealed on the EKG. These alterations should not be considered normal signs of aging. (6:43)

4. **True.** In approaching a patient from the clinical aspect, pain is the most common presenting symptom in peripheral vascular disease. This pain may be either persistent or intermittent. (4:91)

5. **False.** The ability of the pituitary to secrete growth hormone in response to stimuli is diminished in the elderly. However, the clinical significance of this finding is not evident. (2:67)

6. **False.** Most persons who currently develop tuberculosis were previously infected, and bacteria may have remained dormant in tissues until activated. (6:59–60)

7. **False.** It is usually best to avoid lumbar puncture in stroke patients with increased intracranial puncture, since herniation is a possibility. (2:59)

8. **False.** With age, the liver actually shrinks. A post-mortem study indicated that the average peak liver weight was 1929 gm in the fourth decade and decreased to 1000 gm by the tenth decade of life. The most prominent decline occurred after the sixth decade. (6:47)

9. **D.** In infants, deep levels 3 and 4 sleep predominate. Arousal is rare throughout the sleep cycle. Levels 3 and 4 become less prominent with age, and brief arousals more common. In the elderly, there is little level 4 sleep and many brief arousals may occur. (6:52)

10. **A.** If disorders such as carcinoma and atherosclerosis were eradicated, more subjects would approximate their potential maximum span of life, but maximum life span would not be extended. (5:6)

11. **A.** The routine use of fluorohydrocortisone in elderly hypoadrenocortical patients is not recommended, since it may provoke fluid retention, lead to hypertension, and worsen heart failure. (2:87–88)

12. **B.** Depression is common in the elderly, affecting from 10 to 30%. It is frequently mistaken for dementia, especially if physicians and family members consider it "natural" in the aged. (5:72)

13. **D.** With age, less bile is produced but the consistency and the cholesterol composition increase. (1:208)

14. **E.** Elderly individuals account for nearly one fourth of suicides—between 5000 and 8000 a year. Many of these suicides can be prevented by prompt treatment of psychiatric disturbances, especially depression, and by encouraging older people to stay active and involved. (5:9)

15. **B.** The diagnosis of primary hyperparathyroidism in subjects with equivocal serum calcium levels has been facilitated in recent years by availability of assays of serum immunoreactive parathyroid hormone. (iPTH). (2:87)

19

16. **A.** Residual volume and functional residual volume increase in the aging lung. Expiratory reserve volume, inspiratory reserve volume, and forced expiratory volume decrease with age, as do vital and maximal breathing capacity. (1:206)

17. **A.** In the elderly, pruritus usually appears on the limbs, particularly on the lower legs. In severe xerosis, a typical pattern of reticulated erythema and rhomboidal scaling has been aptly described as erythema craquele. (2:143)

18. **A.** Carcinoma of the prostate is exceeded only by carcinoma of the lung as the most frequent cause of cancer deaths in adult males. (2:113)

19. **C.** The slower metabolism and excretion of barbiturates and other hypnotics in the elderly may also lead to apathy and torpor. In paradoxical situations, agitation and emotional lability may be evident. (3:16)

20. **A.** By the seventh and eighth decades of life, males catch up statistically with females in the frequency of osteoporosis. The femur is the more common fracture site in males, whereas vertebral fractures are more common in females. (2:10)

21. **False.** In these individuals, anesthetic and surgical risks and the concomitant presence of nonparathyroid disease (such as heart failure or pulmonary disease) represent greater threats than hyperparathyroidism. (2:87)

22. **True.** Severe hypokalemia may also result in anorexia and muscle weakness. The hypotension and dehydration can quickly led to oligemia, cerebrovascular insufficiency, and thrombosis, as the increased blood viscosity results in a declining flow through the arteriosclerotic vascular beds. (3:16)

23. **False.** The production of FSH by the brain actually increases in postmenopausal females, secondary to failure of ovarian function. FSH excess is felt to be responsible for menopausal symptoms. (6:48)

24. **False.** Arsenical keratoses are not in themselves malignant, but inorganic arsenic that may have been ingested a number of years previously is carcinogenic. (2:139)

25. **False.** Although there doesn't appear to be a male climacterium analogous to the menopause, alterations that affect sexual function do develop. (5:9)

26. **False.** The maximal rate of oxygen utilization by human beings during exercise, which is a measure of the maximal ability to perform physiologic work, diminishes with advancing age. (6:21)

27. **False.** A few elderly patients with advanced senile cardiac amyloidosis will exhibit vascular amyloid in the small arteries and veins of the GI tract, liver, kidney, and other organs. The frequency of such peripheral vascular involvement is such, however, that rectal biopsy is an unreliable method for establishing the diagnosis of senile cardiac amyloidosis. (4:78)

28. **False.** As the female breast atrophies with age, tumors such as fibroadenomas may become more prominent and can be mistaken for carcinomas. (1:205)

29. **False.** With age, the incidence of bleeding ulcers does not increase; however, the mortality from bleeding does rise with age. (2:77)

30. **A.** Since renal function decreases with age, dosage adjustment must be considered in the aged for drugs removed from the body primarily by renal excretion. (4:18)

31. **B.** Circulating thyroid hormone remains relatively constant throughout life. Thyroxin turnover during acute febrile illness is similar in the young and old. (1:209)

32. **E.** Blood transfusions may also be indicated in elderly patients with chronic anemias who have hematocrits below 25% and a hemoglobin concentration below 8 gm/100 ml. (2:67)

33. **A.** Diminution in the force of the stream is another early symptom of prostatic hyperplasia. Later in the course, obstructive symptoms such as postmicturitional dribbling, poor control, overflow incontinence, and irritated outlet may appear. Sepsis can develop in such patients. (4:231)

34. **A.** (1:207)

35. **C.** (1:207)

36. **B.** (1:207)

37. **C.** Antiparkinsonism drugs should be used in the elderly only for treatment of manifest symptoms. Intermittent use should replace indefinite use. (4:39)

38. **A.** In contrast to patients with inflammatory arthritis such as rheumatoid arthritis, subjects with degenerative joint disease do not develop systemic manifestations. (6:78)

39. **B.** Age at onset of menopause is relevant: late onset (past 50 years) has been associated statistically with a higher incidence of endometrial carcinoma. (2:102)

40. **C.** Such investigation is mandatory if surgery is being considered. As the competence of the proximal urethra declines with age, stress incontinence may develop, even to the point where patients must wear perineal pads at all times. (2:104)

41. **C.** Other causes of congestive heart failure in the elderly include systemic hypertension, pulmonary hypertension, pericardial disease, myocarditis, traumatic heart disease, and high-output failure states such as hyperthyroidism. (1:649)

42. **C.** Between the third and ninth decades, the ribs elevate whereas the diaphragm flattens, decreasing the capacity of the lungs to move air. (6:45)

43. **False.** The patient should be advised that the term "prostatectomy" is really a misnomer. The periurethral adenoma, not the entire prostate, is excised. (2:119)

44. **False.** In the past few decades, tuberculosis has become mainly a disorder of older subjects. This is not because TB has become more frequent among the aged, but because cases in younger subjects have diminished much more. (6:59)

45. **False.** There is an increased central nervous system effect in the elderly from many types of drugs, including antibiotics and digitalis. (1:647)

46. **False.** ASD is being more readily found among the elderly. Such patients may have been entirely free of cardiac problems before the first episode of CHF. Surgical closure of the defect may prove totally corrective in many instances. (2:41)

47. **True.** It is thought that many cancers arise and are destroyed early by the immune system in younger subjects, but that in the elderly, the immune system is not so effective. (2:110)

48. **False.** The incidence of tetanus in persons over 60 is more than four times higher than that of the rest of the population. For this reason, vaccination status should be ascertained in the elderly. For those who have received primary immunizations, booster doses of tetanus toxoid should be given every 10 years. (6:69)

49. **True.** Prompt biopsy for unexplained vulvar lesions in the elderly is advisable. No time should be lost in investigating lesions that are unresponsive to therapy, appear ulcerative, or otherwise look suspicious, though a whitish lesion is not necessarily precancerous. (2:102)

50. **False.** Assuming a constant body weight, as one ages from 18 to 85 years, body fat in men increases from 18 to 36%, and in women, from 33 to 48%. This indicates a declining lean cell mass and fluid volume, so the volume and pattern of distribution, blood levels, and excretory rates of drugs may all change. (3:16)

51. **A.** The heart rate is much higher during treadmill testing of cardiac patients than during sexual intercourse, and the death rate for treadmill testing is only 1 per 10,000 tests. (2:130)

52. **A.** Chlorpropamide is a longer-acting agent and approximately six times more potent than tolbutamide. (4:42)

53. **B.** Spider angiomas are central arterioles with projecting finger-like telangiectasia and are usually 2 to 3 mm in size. They are more commonly seen in woman and in patients with liver disease. (2:137)

54. **A.** The total number of body cells may diminish by 30% between youth and old age. However, the mass of these cells diminishes by a smaller percentage. (6:42)

55. **A.** Benign positional vertigo or transient vertigo after sudden head movements indicates some vestibular system involvement, probably old and nonprogressive, but not transient ischemia. (2:60)

56. **E.** These chronic diseases include cardiovascular and cerebrovascular problems, Alzheimer's and Parkinson's disease, arthritis, diabetes, psychiatric problems, and glaucoma. (3:16)

57. **E.** These, as well as certain psychotropic drugs, have all been tried as therapy for organic brain syndrome, but have generally given equivocal and controversial results. (4:109)

58. **C.** America has witnessed enormous gains in the average ages to which our citizens can expect to live. In 1900, life expectancy at birth for white males was about 48 years and for females, 51 years. For nonwhites, male life expectancy at birth was 32.5 years in 1900 and for females, 35.0 years. (6:119)

59. **A.** Contrary to what is commonly believed, only 5% of individuals 65 and older are now in long-term care facilities. (5:10)

60. **False.** Females are likely to outlive males. This advantage has actually widened over time (from about three years in 1900 to eight years currently). (6:120)

61. **True.** Additionally, the absolute amount of insulin secreted in response to a glucose load is decreased in apparently normal older individuals. (2:88)

62. **True.** Disease, significant social losses, and chronic personality characteristics appear to be more important than age itself in causing depression or mental illness. (6:108)

63. **True.** The incidence of cardiovascular mortality and morbidity increases with age, regardless of what interventions are undertaken. (2:47)

64. **False.** Studies of the coumarin anticoagulant warfarin have demonstrated increased drug sensitivity in the elderly, despite a pharmacokenetic similarity between young and old persons. (3:14)

65. **True.** The incidence of oral tumors also increases considerably with age. (6:86)

66. **False.** The enlargement of the cerebral ventricles with age is most marked in the lateral and third ventricles. (1:208)

67. **False.** With age, the number of metabolically active cells decreases, as does the amount of intracellular water. Water outside the cells, as well as plasma volume, however, stay relatively constant. (6:42)

68. **False.** Degenerative joint disease develops in nearly everyone. This results from the accumulated effect of wear and tear on the joints. (6:78)

69. **B.** (2:94)

70. **A.** (2:94)

Textbook References for Chapter 2

1. Taylor. R.B., Editor (1978): *Family Medicine: Principles and Practice*, Springer-Verlag, New York.

2. Reichel, W., Editor (1978): *The Geriatric Patient*, HP Publishing Company, New York.

3. Beber, C.R. and Lamy, P.P., Co-Chairmen (1978): *Medication Management and Education of the Elderly*, proceedings of a symposium, Washington, D.C., May 1, 1978, Excerpta Medica, New York.

4. Reichel, W. (1978): *Clinical Aspects of Aging*, Williams & Wilkins, Baltimore.

5. *A Report on Aging in America: Trials and Triumphs*, Research & Forecasts, Inc., Americana Healthcare Corporation, Monticello, Illinois, 1980.

6. *Working with Older People: A Guide to Practice: Volume II: Human Services*, Gerontological Society under contract with the Health Resources Administration, Department of Health, Education and Welfare, U.S. Government Printing Office, Washington, D.C. 1976.

CHAPTER 3

Patient Management

Questions 1 to 9

A 60-year-old chronic alcoholic is admitted to the hospital with an oral temperature of 102°, a pleuritic-type chest pain, anorexia, and weakness. For the past several weeks, the patient has had a cough productive of large amounts of purulent sputum. Physical examination revealed extremely poor dental hygiene with malodorous breath, extensive caries, and periodontal infection. Pulmonary findings consisted of signs of consolidation, rales, and cavernous breath sounds over the right lower lobe. Laboratory findings showed a polymorphonuclear leukocytosis with an increased percentage of immature forms, mild anemia and hypoalbuminemia. The chest X-ray revealed an area of consolidation containing a radiolucency in the superior segment of the right lower lobe.

1. The most likely diagnosis is

  A. pneumococcal pneumonia
  B. *Klebsiella* pneumonia
  C. bronchiectasis
  D. pulmonary tuberculosis
  E. lung abscess

2. The patient produced copious amounts of foul-smelling sputum. This is most consistent with

  A. a fungal infection
  B. an aerobic infection
  C. pulmonary tuberculosis
  D. an anaerobic infection
  E. none of the above

3. Concerning the pathogenesis of this condition, which of the following is true?

  A. the lower respiratory tract is normally sterile, even though it has been shown that oro- and nasopharyngeal contents are aspirated into dependent airways during sleep
  B. defense mechanisms may be overwhelmed by large numbers of microorganisms and/or unusually virulent bacteria
  C. local factors such as obstruction by food particles or necrosis from gastric fluid enhance the development of bacterial infection
  D. any event or underlying disorder that is associated with aspiration may lead to lung abscess
  E. all of the above

4. All of the following are true of lung abscess *except*

  A. improved techniques of anesthesia and surgery have virtually eliminated the problem of lung abscesses associated with general anesthesia and tonsillectomy

B. alcoholic stupor, drug overdosage, unconsciousness during seizures or strokes, defective swallowing, and prolonged debility impair protective reflexes and allow excess material from the oro- and nasopharynx and stomach to enter the tracheobronchial system

C. if aspiration occurs in a supine person, the anatomy of the airways favors movement into the right lung and then into either the posterior segment of the upper lobe or the superior segment of the lower lobe

D. the microorganisms that reach the lungs during aspiration will be the resident flora of the oro- and nasopharynx

E. a condition favoring aspiration and/or oral sepsis can be found in only a minority of patients with lung abscesses caused by anaerobic microorganisms

5. Which of the following is *incorrect*?

A. staphylococcal and *Klebsiella* pneumonias, and pneumonias caused by other microorganisms with necrotizing potential, are frequently associated with lung abscesses

B. tubercle bacilli are less likely to reach the upper lobes by bloodstream dissemination than through the airways

C. lung abscesses occur about three times more often in men than in women

D. infected cysts or bullae or an empyema with a bronchopleural fistula may resemble lung abscesses

E. since anaerobic organisms are universal inhabitants of the mouth, sputum obtained by transtracheal aspiration or transthoracic lung puncture or empyema fluid is preferred for cultural identification

6. In the treatment of lung abscesses,

A. penicillin is usually the drug of choice

in treating abscesses secondary to anaerobic infection and should be given in high doses (e.g., aqueous penicillin, 5 to 10 million units daily, intravenously)

B. *Bacteroides fragilis,* which is resistant *in vitro* to penicillin, may be found in up to 25% of patients; therefore, if the patient is seriously ill or fails to respond to penicillin, chloramphenicol, active against almost all anaerobes, is the preferred drug

C. clindamycin and metronidazole are very active against most anaerobes, including *Bacteroides fragilis*

D. in view of the partial resistance of anaerobic organisms and the tendency for signs and symptoms to recur if antimicrobial agents are discontinued prematurely, prolonged treatment for 4 to 6 weeks is necessary

E. all of the above

7. Which statement is *not* true of the treatment of lung abscesses?

A. the antibiotic regimen should be changed on the basis of changing flora in several sputum cultures

B. penicillin can be given intramuscularly or orally instead of intravenously after all signs of systemic toxicity (i.e., fever, leukocyte count) have subsided and when serial roentgenograms show appreciable clearing of the contiguous pneumonia, reduction in the size of the cavity, and absence of a fluid level within the cavity

C. serial roentgenograms of the chest should show gradual diminution of the cavity in subsequent months

D. delayed closure is common, and as long as resolution progresses, no further therapy is indicated

E. surgical intervention is seldom necessary

8. All of the following are true of the role of surgery in patients with lung abscess *except*

A. tube thoracostomy or some other form of surgical drainage may be needed to manage uncontrolled sepsis and systemic manifestations in patients with poorly draining acute lung abscesses

B. massive hemoptysis requires emergency surgery (i.e., thoracotomy and resection)

C. incomplete resolution of a chronic lung abscess is sufficient reason for resectional surgery

D. resection is indicated for severe or recurrent hemoptysis or recurrence of infection

E. resection is indicated for associated symptomatic bronchiectasis and suspicion of malignancy

9. After successful medical treatment of lung abscess, which of the following would be most appropriate in managing the patient described in the case study?

A. prophylactic penicillin for at least 2 years

B. prophylactic tetracycline for at least 2 years

C. proper dental care

D. bronchoscopy performed at yearly intervals

E. none of the above

Questions 10 to 25

As a medical consultant, you are asked to see a 58-year-old male with oliguria. The patient had a long history of peptic ulcer disease and recently had been admitted to the hospital because of hematemesis. On admission his systolic blood pressure was 60, he was tachycardic, and vomiting large amounts of bright red blood. He was rapidly transfused with multiple units of whole blood restoring his vital signs towards normal. His urine output, however, was low, and the scant amount of urine that was obtained was bloody. Urinalysis revealed the presence of proteinuria and the urine sodium concentration was 90 mEq/liter.

10. The most likely diagnosis is

A. chronic renal failure

B. acute glomerulonephritis

C. acute tubular necrosis

D. acute cortical necrosis

E. hepatorenal syndrome

11. All the following are true of acute renal failure *except*

A. the glomeruli are intact except when extremely severe and prolonged ischemia has produced renal cortical necrosis

B. even those cases which follow the administration of known tubular poisons are generally aggravated by vascular insufficiency and renal ischemia

C. acute renal failure is the most frequent cause of death in epidemic hemorrhagic fever

D. pregnancy appears in some way to protect against ischemic renal insults

E. tubular necrosis has been triggered by sudden defervescence following salicylate administration, and status epilepticus

12. Common causes of acute tubular necrosis include

A. marked hemolysis

B. hypotension following burns, rapid hemorrhage, or surgery

C. bacteremic shock

D. crushing injuries

E. all of the above

13. In renal tubular necrosis, all of the following are true *except*

A. in most patients, casts appear to be the cause of diminished urine flow rather than a result

B. following acute renal ischemia which usually initiates tubular necrosis, renal blood flow is decreased to approximately one-third to one-half normal during the first days of oliguria

C. there is some evidence that reduction in glomerular filtration is a vasoconstrictive response mediated through the macula densa and the juxtaglomerular apparatus

D. increased interstitial pressure secondary to edema probably reduces renal blood flow and filtration rate and collapses tubules

E. the presence of interstitial edema may be inferred from the increased weight of the kidneys during acute tubular necrosis

14. The clinical features of acute tubular necrosis include all the following *except*

A. although the urine specific gravity may be high owing to the presence of red blood cells and protein, its freezing point is close to that of plasma, and the sodium concentration is usually over 50 mEq/liter

B. traces of glucose may appear in the urine

C. complete anuria for more than 24 hr is infrequently encountered, though it is common to see less than 30 to 40 ml urine for several days

D. fever is uncommon after the first day or two

E. leukocytosis is uncommon and only occurs with infection

15. Generally, in acute tubular necrosis, oliguria lasts about how many days?

A. 1 to 2
B. 3 to 6
C. 7 to 9
D. 10 to 14
E. over 21

16. In acute renal failure,

A. serum amylase and lipase concentrations may be elevated as a result of renal failure per se, without implying active pancreatitis

B. increments of 50 mg/100 ml/day in blood urea nitrogen are not uncommon in previously healthy persons who have undergone severe crushing injuries or overwhelming infections

C. cardiovascular complications including hypertension may arise during the oliguric phase

D. although overhydration is the most important cause of pulmonary edema, signs of pulmonary congestion and cardiac failure may appear even in patients who have not gained weight, probably because water has been added to the extracellular fluid from the dissolution of tissue

E. all of the above

17. Which of the following is *not* true of the complications of acute renal failure?

A. diastolic hypertension becomes evident in about 25% of patients during the second week of oliguria

B. if pericarditis develops, it has a grave prognosis

C. serious electrocardiographic abnormalities rarely occur when the serum potassium level is below 7 mEq/liter but are almost always present at levels of about 9 mEq/liter

D. the rate of rise of serum potassium reflects the catabolic response of the patient to injury

E. arrhythmias are frequent and are not necessarily associated with potassium intoxication or removal

18. The most frequent complication of acute tubular necrosis and the most common cause of death is

A. cardiovascular complications
B. potassium loss
C. infection
D. neurologic manifestations
E. none of the above

19. Concerning neurologic complications of acute renal failure,

A. neurologic manifestations are common, the two most important being coma and convulsions

B. hyponatremia may be responsible for somnolence or seizures early in the course of the disorder and may be corrected by hypertonic saline solution, with proper regard for the complications of overhydration and heart failure

C. hypocalcemia may predispose to convulsions
D. seizures may be focal in nature or generalized
E. all of the above

20. In some patients, tubular necrosis is not associated with oliguria (or the period of diminished urine flow is so short as to pass unrecognized). In such patients,

A. the urine volume is not flexible or responsive to body needs and may be fixed at perhaps 800 to 1200 ml/day
B. the diagnosis is appreciated only when the blood urea nitrogen level is seen to rise at the rate of 15 to 20 mg/100 ml/day and when the patient becomes edematous owing to retention of fluids in excess of the excretory capacity of the kidneys
C. the urine, unlike that in most other edema-forming states, contains sodium in a concentration higher than 20 to 30 mEq/liter, and the concentration of total solutes does not differ significantly from that of plasma
D. all of the above
E. none of the above

21. During the early diuretic phase of recovery from acute renal failure,

A. hyperkalemia, congestive heart failure, and convulsions may complicate the clinical picture
B. pyelonephritis sometimes makes its appearance and when infection occurs, death is common
C. diuresis is usually associated with a striking weight loss, representing loss of fluid accumulated during the period of oliguria
D. the urinary concentration of sodium usually varies from 50 to 75 mEq/liter
E. all of the above

22. Which of the following is *not* true concerning most patients who have recovered from acute tubular necrosis?

A. anemia sometimes persists for weeks or

months, gradually disappearing without benefit of hematinics
B. muscle weakness and joint stiffness slowly improve
C. although azotemia generally disappears and renal function may be restored, renal blood flow and glomerular filtration rate usually do not return completely to normal
D. hypertension is a common sequel to the disorder
E. hypertension may complicate the unusual case of cortical necrosis in a patient who survives anuria

23. Early in the course of our patient's renal failure, his potassium rose to 8.5 mEq/liter. An electrocardiogram was ordered. Which of the following might be expected to occur as the potassium rises to very toxic levels?

A. the T wave becomes high and peaked
B. the P wave disappears
C. the QRS complex becomes broad and slurred
D. bradycardia and arrhythmias ensue, and the ventricular complexes finally resemble those of ventricular tachycardia
E. all of the above

24. All of the following may be used as adjunct measures in the treatment of hyperkalemia to lower serum potassium levels *except*

A. sodium polystyrene sulfonate (Kayexalate)
B. sodium bicarbonate or sodium lactate
C. infusions of hypertonic glucose solution with insulin
D. infusions of calcium
E. artificial dialysis

25. Which of the following is *not* true concerning the treatment of acute renal failure and its complications?

A. heart failure should be initially treated with digitalis in loading doses much lower than would usually be used
B. testosterone propionate or norethan-

drolone, 25 to 50 mg daily, may reduce nitrogen breakdown

C. after the diagnosis is established, an accurate estimate of the daily output may be obtained by catheterizing the patient using sterile precautions only once in 24 to 48 hr, thus dispensing with an in-lying bladder catheter

D. the prime indication for artificial dialysis in acute renal failure is uncontrollable hyperkalemia

E. mounting acidosis in the presence of congestive heart failure is a clear indication for dialysis

Questions 26 to 35

A 40-year-old female noted gradual onset of severe pain and tenderness involving first one then both sides of her lower neck. There was fullness and a sensation of pressure in the thyroid area. The pain radiated up the lateral aspects of the neck and into the jaw and ear. The patient had difficulty swallowing and choked over saliva. In addition she developed mild fever, sore throat, malaise, and fatigue. She was taking no medication and had been completely well until about three weeks previously, when she had what appeared to be a viral-type upper respiratory infection. On examination, the thyroid appeared enlarged and was extremely tender to palpation.

26. The most likely diagnosis

A. Reidel's thyroiditis
B. Graves' disease
C. Hashimoto's thyroiditis
D. subacute thyroiditis
E. none of the above

27. The disorder has also been referred to as

A. granulomatous thyroiditis
B. acute thyroiditis
C. De Quervain's thyroiditis
D. all of the above
E. none of the above

28. This disease is about how much as common as Graves' disease?

A. one-tenth

B. one-half
C. 2 times
D. 5 times
E. 10 times

29. All of the following are true of the disease *except*

A. may represent an immune response to a viral infection
B. may result from direct viral invasion of the thyroid
C. has occurred in outbreaks of mumps
D. there is an excellent correlation between the histologic abnormalities and the clinical picture
E. the disorder is painful and disabling, but does not last long

30. Which would be an unexpected histological finding in this patient?

A. enlarged thyroid with dense infiltration by polymorphonuclear cells, lymphocytes, and plasma cells
B. absence of fibrosis
C. many pyknotic thyroid follicular cells
D. the follicular structure is destroyed
E. small granulomas with giant cells

31. In subacute thyroiditis,

A. the patient sometimes develops symptoms and signs of mild hyperthyroidism
B. the clinical status is usually that of euthyroidism or rarely hypothyroidism
C. the disease tends to remit spontaneously or, because of therapy, to recur after a period of two to three weeks, and this cycle may recur several times
D. over the course of one to twelve months, the process finally subsides
E. all of the above

32. In the diagnosis of subacute thyroiditis,

A. the leukocyte count may be elevated to 15,000 to 20,000, or may be normal
B. the sedimentation rate is characteris-

tically high, and may reach 100 mm/hr (Westergren)

C. anemia is said to accompany the illness, although the cause is unknown

D. on scan, RAIU is suppressed in the involved portion of the gland, which may be one lobe or the entire thyroid, and the RAIU is often zero

E. all of the above

33. Which of the following would *not* be characteristic of this disorder?

A. fluorescent scanning shows the involved thyroid tissue to have lost all iodine stores

B. the T$_4$ and FTI may be elevated because of iodoprotein or excess thyroid hormone released during the acute phase of the illness, making the patient thyrotoxic

C. during recovery, the TSH and RAIU may be transiently elevated while T$_4$ is depressed, and then over a period of two to three months, all tests return to normal

D. antibody titers against thyroid antigens are higher than those in Hashimoto's thyroiditis, and the responses are sustained

E. the process can usually be differentiated from acute thyroiditis because of the localization to the thyroid, absence of signs of infection, characteristically high sedimentation rate, and depressed radioactive iodide uptake

34. Which of the following would be *least* useful in the patient's therapy?

A. aspirin, up to 6 g daily

B. desiccated thyroid, if the disease has gone on for more than a few days, because TSH stimulation may exacerbate the process

C. corticosteroids, if the illness does not subside with simple measures

D. surgery, in the rare event that a chronic, tender enlargement of the thyroid persists despite therapy and re-

quires surgical resection

E. radioactive iodine

35. What is the approximate chance that the patient will develop permanent hypothyroidism?

A. 0%
B. 10%
C. 25%
D. 50%
E. 100%

Questions 36 to 42

A 24-year-old white female attended a picnic at which chicken salad had been served. About 24 hr after eating, she noticed severe cramping abdominal pain, nausea, retching, and diarrhea. She began to sweat and noted increased salivation. She also developed a severe headache. Several of her companions complained of similar symptoms.

36. The most likely etiology of the patient's symptoms was

A. botulism
B. staphylococcal food poisoning
C. salmonella food poisoning
D. *Clostridium perfringens* food poisoning
E. enterococcal food poisoning

37. Foods may produce illness by

A. becoming contaminated with microorganisms
B. becoming contaminated with the products of microorganisms
C. being poisons themselves
D. containing noxious chemicals
E. all of the above

38. The most common bacterial food poisoning in the United States is due to

A. botulism
B. staphylococcus
C. salmonella
D. *Clostridium perfringens*
E. enterococcus

39. All of the following are true of staphylococcal food poisoning *except*

    A. if food is held at ambient temperature in a warm climate after preparation, later reheating or boiling will prevent illness
    B. studies indicate that enterotoxin probably has its primary site of action in the central nervous system, and that vomiting is a centrally induced response
    C. the period between ingestion and illness is short, one to six hr, occasionally a little longer
    D. since terminal heating may kill the organisms in food without inactivating enterotoxin, staphylococci may not be grown from food under suspicion
    E. animal assays for the detection of enterotoxin are being replaced by serologic methods based on gel diffusion after preliminary extraction and concentration

40. Which of the following is *not* true of staphylococcal food poisoning?

    A. the illness is caused by toxin formed in food before its ingestion
    B. the illness depends on the ingestion of living organisms
    C. staphylococci of human origin contaminating meat or confectionery constitute the source of most outbreaks
    D. about 10% of outbreaks are milkborne, and the organism is then usually of bovine origin
    E. staphylococcal strains which form enterotoxin are almost always coagulase-positive

41. Concerning staphylococcal food poisoning,

    A. diarrhea invariably occurs
    B. symptoms usually last over a day
    C. enterotoxin is produced at ordinary domestic refrigerator temperatures
    D. after eating contaminated food, symptoms will occur earlier than would be found with botulism
    E. bacteriophage typing for identifying the source of the responsible strain is

no longer used for epidemiology studies

42. The patient described may be best treated with

    A. a parasympathetic agent
    B. trivalent antitoxin
    C. antibiotics
    D. all of the above
    E. none of the above

Questions 43 to 48

A physician is asked to see a 41-year-old black male with a "fever of unknown origin." In addition to weight loss, the patient has developed severe hypertension (210/130). During a routine physical examination six months earlier, he had been normotensive. Other problems which had developed since this earlier examination include renal insufficiency (BUN 80, creatinine 7.2), diffuse adenopathy, muscle tenderness and wasting, migratory arthralgias, and the recent onset of foot drop. His CBC reveals a normocytic normochromic anemia (hematocrit 29) with a leukocytosis (15,000 with a shift to the left). His Westergren sedimentation rate is 92.

43. Which of the following is the most likely diagnosis?

    A. systemic lupus erythematosus
    B. polyarteritis nodosa
    C. rheumatoid arthritis
    D. carcinoma of the pancreas
    E. hepatorenal syndrome

44. Which of the following is true of this patient's condition?

    A. it is more common in females
    B. it is usually a disease of the aged
    C. this disorder has not been reported in infants
    D. this disorder predominantly affects the autonomic nervous system
    E. virtually any organ in the body may be involved, but most frequently affected are the kidneys and heart

45. During periods of the patient's disease activity, on pathological examination, one may find evidence of

    A. healing
    B. excessive fibrosis, which may be sufficiently extensive to form gross nodules
    C. intimal proliferation leading to thrombosis and arterial occlusion with infarction
    D. weakening and aneurysmal dilatation of the arterial wall which may rupture, or arterial dissection
    E. all of the above

46. In this patient, the prognosis would most likely be

    A. excellent with treatment
    B. favorable if he obtains a renal transplant
    C. favorable if his anemia is controlled
    D. poor
    E. excellent if there is no evidence of pulmonary involvement

47. The finding of a striking eosinophilia in a patient with this disorder would suggest involvement of the

    A. brain
    B. heart
    C. lungs
    D. muscle
    E. testes

48. Current therapy for this condition would include

    A. hydroxychloroquine sulfate (Plaquenil)
    B. gold therapy
    C. steroids in large doses
    D. total body irradiation
    E. immune serum globulin

Questions 49 to 58

A 34-year-old female is admitted to the hospital because of severe abdominal pain. The pain is colicky in nature, and associated with spasm without any localizing signs. She has had several operations for appendicitis and cholelithiasis but pathological findings did not support these diagnoses. The periodic attacks of intense abdominal colic are usually accompanied by nausea and vomiting, fever, tachycardia, and leukocytosis. More recently she has noted neuritic-type pain in the extremities with areas of hypesthesia and paresthesia. The patient has been under psychiatric care for multiple, vague, "neurotic" complaints even when she has been in remission from attacks of abdominal colic. On questioning, it was learned that several members of her family have had similar problems but no clear-cut diagnosis has ever been offered.

49. The most probable cause of the patient's complaints and findings is

    A. conversion reaction
    B. renal colic
    C. acute intermittent porphyria
    D. tertiary syphilis
    E. hemolytic crisis

50. During an earlier episode of abdominal pain, the patient was told to save her urine for laboratory evaluation. Inadvertently, the urine was left in contact with the sunlight for several hours. Which of the following might have been expected to occur?

    A. dissolution of renal stones
    B. color change (burgundy wine to black) due to homogentistic acid formation
    C. color change (burgundy wine to black) due to formation of uroporphyrin
    D. immobilization of spirochetes
    E. none of the above

51. Porphobilinogen may be quantitated by which modification of the Ehrlich reaction?

    A. Sulkowitz
    B. Watson-Schwartz
    C. Folin-Wu
    D. Benedict
    E. none of the above

52. All of the following are true of acute, intermittent porphyria *except*

A. during relapse, the presence of porphobilinogen is a constant feature
B. during remission, the porphobilinogen reaction is usually positive, but a negative test does not exclude the diagnosis of this type of porphyria
C. patients excrete excessive quantities of uroporphyrin (Types I and III), coproporphyrin (Types I and III), and other as yet unidentified porphyrins
D. the porphyrin content of the bone marrow is elevated
E. the liver regularly exhibits increased quantities of porphyrin, especially porphyrin precursors

53. Which of the following is *not* true of acute, intermittent porphyria?

A. the major chemical manifestations are best explained as resulting from overproduction of porphyrin precursors, secondary to induction of hepatic ALA synthetase
B. drugs such as barbiturates and estrogens which induce ALA synthetase must be avoided
C. the disorder is probably transmitted as a mendelian recessive characteristic
D. foot and wrist drop may occur
E. hypertension may accompany an attack; there may be temporary loss of vision, and convulsions have been described

54. Acute intermittent porphyria is characterized clinically by

A. periodic attacks of intense abdominal colic, usually accompanied by nausea and vomiting
B. obstinate constipation
C. neurotic or even psychotic behavior
D. neuromuscular disturbances
E. all of the above

55. In acute intermittent porphyria,

A. sensory changes are usually prominent
B. signs of the upper motor neuron changes are usually present

C. the mortality rate is low
D. the course of the disorder is extraordinarily varied
E. in general, the neuromuscular and psychotic symptoms are early manifestations

56. Which of the following may be (a) precipitating factor(s) in some patients with this disorder?

A. menstruation and pregnancy
B. infection
C. alcohol
D. lead
E. all of the above

57. The Watson-Schwartz test is positive

A. in erythropoietic porphyria
B. in porphyria cutanea tarda symptomatica
C. with porphyria cutanea tarda hereditaria during attacks
D. with porphyria cutanea tarda hereditaria between attacks
E. all of the above

58. The most effective treatment of an acute attack is to provide

A. ACTH
B. corticosteroids
C. a liberal intake of glucose
D. BAL
E. EDTA

Questions 59 to 66

A 44-year-old female has recently been embarrassed by periodic blushing episodes. She mentions that frequently after eating, ingesting alcohol, or when she is tired or excited she has attacks of flushing involving her head and neck. These attacks last for a variable amount of time but during prolonged attacks she has developed lacrimation and periorbital edema. She has also been troubled with diarrhea and during some of her attacks developed audible wheezing.

59. Of the following, which is the most likely diagnosis?

    A. psychoneurosis
    B. carcinoid syndrome
    C. calcitonin-secreting tumor
    D. Addison's disease
    E. hyperthyroidism

60. All of the following are true of this condition *except*

    A. serotonin is the sole mediator
    B. this condition is associated with slowly growing neoplasms of enterochromaffin cells
    C. the metastatic tumors associated with this condition usually arise from small primary tumors in the ileum
    D. the condition may be produced by neoplasms arising from the small intestine, organs derived from the embryonic foregut (e.g., bronchus, stomach, pancreas, and thyroid), and from ovarian or testicular teratomas
    E. there is an unusual proclivity for metastasis to the liver

61. Patients with this syndrome may have tumors which elaborate any of the following *except*

    A. serotonin
    B. histamine
    C. adrenocorticotropic hormone (ACTH)
    D. bradykinin
    E. aldosterone

62. Which of the following is *not* true of this disorder?

    A. primary carcinoid tumors of the appendix are common, but they rarely metastasize
    B. primary carcinoid tumors of the large intestine may metastasize but do not exhibit an endocrine function
    C. carcinoid tumors have an unusually fast rate of growth
    D. for much of the duration of the illness, morbidity may result largely from the endocrine function of the tumor

E. death results from cardiac or hepatic failure and from complications associated with tumor growth

63. Carcinoid syndrome

    A. is a cause of sustained hypertension
    B. commonly results in a rise in blood pressure during flushing
    C. may result in development of purple telangectasia, primarily on the face and neck and most marked in the malar area
    D. has not been associated with malabsorption
    E. may result in deposition of fibrous tissue on the endocardium of the valvular cusps and cardiac chambers; this occurs primarily in the left side of the heart

64. The diagnostic hallmark of this syndrome is

    A. overproduction of 5-hydroxyindoles with increased urinary excretion of 5-hydroxyindoleacetic acid
    B. increased blood serotonin levels
    C. increased blood bradykinin levels
    D. increased histamine in tumor tissue
    E. none of the above

65. Tumors from which of the following locations can produce the syndrome before metastatic disease occurs?

    A. ovarian teratoma
    B. testicular teratoma
    C. bronchus
    D. all of the above
    E. none of the above

66. Concerning treatment of this disorder,

    A. palliative resection of hepatic metastases is beneficial in carefully selected cases
    B. resection of large isolated hepatic metastases has led to relief of the symptoms of carcinoid syndrome and marked reductions in urinary 5-HIAA excretion for periods of several years

C. of numerous approaches to chemotherapy of the tumor, the most promising appears to be regional arterial perfusion with agents such as 5-fluorouracil

D. pharmacologic therapy directed at the humoral mediators of the syndrome is useful in some cases

E. all of the above

Questions 67 to 74

A 34-year-old male was brought to the emergency room in a deep coma. He was given intravenous glucose without effect. His friend admitted that the patient had been a habitual drinker, consuming considerable "moonshine" from various sources. His blood pressure was found to be elevated and his rectal temperature was 103°. A lumbar puncture was performed and revealed a slightly elevated pressure with increased protein, a mild pleocytosis and normal glucose. His CBC showed a hypochromic anemia and the technician reported considerable basophilic stippling. There was a slight reduction in platelets. Routine blood studies were normal except for increased uric acid and decreased albumin. Urinalysis revealed proteinuria.

67. Of the following, the most likely diagnosis is

   A. viral meningitis
   B. bacterial meningitis
   C. basilar skull fracture
   D. heavy metal poisoning
   E. thrombotic thrombocytopenia purpura

68. The probable cause of the patient's coma was

   A. cytomegalic virus (CMV) infection
   B. *Klebsiella* pneumonia with seeding to the meninges
   C. disseminated intravascular coagulation
   D. arsenic in the bootleg whiskey
   E. lead in the bootleg whiskey

69. The most serious toxic effect of lead poisoning results from its effect on the

   A. formed elements of the blood
   B. kidney

C. liver
D. brain and peripheral nervous system
E. bone

70. All of the following are true of chronic lead poisoning *except*

   A. pathologic findings include inflammation of the gastrointestinal mucosa and renal tubular degeneration
   B. there may be cellular infiltration around capillaries and arterioles
   C. cerebral edema and degeneration of nerve and muscle cells occur
   D. the liver has intranuclear inclusion bodies
   E. the kidneys have intranuclear inclusion bodies

71. Concerning the treatment of lead poisoning, all of the following are correct *except*

   A. lead in tissues such as in the central nervous system is rapidly removed by deleading agents
   B. adults with acute lead encephalopathy should be given dimercaprol and calcium disodium edetate (EDTA)
   C. toxicity from tetraethyl lead and tetramethyl lead does not respond to chelation therapy
   D. oral penicillamine can be used on an outpatient basis
   E. until recently, the death rates of patients with lead encephalopathy was about 25%; about half of those who survived had permanent mental deterioration

72. All of the following are compatible with lead intoxication *except*

   A. decreased urine coproporphyrin
   B. increased plasma or urine delta-amino-levulinic acid
   C. glycosuria or proteinuria
   D. hemoglobin below 10 g/100 ml
   E. the appearance of radiopaque material on a plain film of the abdomen and radiopaque lead lines in the wrists and knees

73. Lead poisoning may result in all of the following *except*

    A. lead line in the gums
    B. metallic taste
    C. abdominal colic
    D. encephalitis
    E. decrease in reticulocytes in most cases

74. The hematological changes secondary to lead intoxication may include all of the following *except*

    A. from 50 to 100 stippled cells per 100,000 erythrocytes
    B. decrease in hemoglobin and in total number of red blood cells below 4 million
    C. decrease in all forms of basophilic cells
    D. increase in percentage of mononuclears
    E. anisocytosis, poikilocytosis, and nucleated red cells present in the peripheral circulation

Questions 75 to 84

A 24-year-old laboratory technician who works in a state mental institution develops malaise, fever, fatigue, headaches, and vomiting. She also notices that her urine has become darker recently. On questioning, she recalls having stuck her finger with a needle several months ago.

75. The most likely diagnosis is

    A. infectious mononucleosis
    B. hepatitis A
    C. hepatitis B
    D. biliary cirrhosis
    E. chronic active hepatitis

76. Treatment will most likely involve

    A. hepatitis B vaccine
    B. neomycin, one g p.o. every four hr
    C. 20 to 30 g protein diet
    D. vitamin K-dependent clotting factors (Konyne)
    E. none of the above

77. Concerning hepatitis, which of the following statements is true?

    A. direct spread by nonparenteral route does not occur in hepatitis B
    B. skin rash and joint pains are more frequently associated with hepatitis A infection than with hepatitis B
    C. hepatitis A symptoms are usually more severe and last longer than hepatitis B symptoms
    D. chronic complications are seen more frequently in hepatitis A than in hepatitis B
    E. the frequency of chronic antigenemia is greatest in patients with mild or asymptomatic hepatitis B infection

78. For persons without serious underlying disease, the incidence of chronic antigenemia following acute hepatitis B infection has been shown to be

    A. less than 10%
    B. 15%
    C. 25%
    D. 40%
    E. 68%

79. In the United States and western Europe what percentage of asymptomatic adults are chronic carriers of hepatitis B antigen?

    A. 0.001 to 0.006%
    B. 0.01 to 0.06%
    C. 0.1 to 0.6%
    D. 1 to 6%
    E. 10 to 60%

80. All of the following are true of this patient's disorder *except*

    A. failure to detect hepatitis B antigen in a patient with acute hepatitis excludes the diagnosis of hepatitis B
    B. hepatitis B antigen may remain detectable for as long as three months after the onset of clinical symptoms
    C. following disappearance of hepatitis B antigen after acute hepatitis B infection, antibody to the hepatitis B antigen usually becomes detectable; this antibody usually persists for long periods and serves as a marker of previous hepatitis B infection

D. infection with type B virus is believed to confer lifelong immunity; however, susceptibility to type A hepatitis infection is not altered

E. in well-defined outbreaks of hepatitis B, very few secondary cases have appeared among close personal contacts (including prison cellmates) suggesting that the spread of hepatitis B by nonparenteral means may occur infrequently

81. Which statement is *not* true of hepatitis A?

A. water is the most common vehicle responsible for common source outbreaks

B. contaminated shellfish, particularly raw or partially cooked oysters or clams, are the most commonly identified vehicles of food-borne hepatitis

C. available data suggest that a significant percentage of patients who develop hepatitis after receiving blood transfusions are infected with hepatitis A virus

D. women who acquire viral hepatitis during pregnancy appear to have a greater risk of fulminant disease and death

E. immune serum globulin (ISG) is not effective in preventing infection

82. It has been convincingly demonstrated that hepatitis B may be transmitted by

A. stool
B. urine
C. saliva
D. all of the above
E. none of the above

83. Concerning hepatitis B,

A. an increased prevalence of antigenemia has been observed in spouses of chronic hepatitis B antigen carriers

B. analysis of surveillance data from the United States suggests that indirect transmission of hepatitis B by parenteral routes remains the most common means by which type B virus is spread

C. women who acquire acute hepatitis B while pregnant do not transmit the infection to their infant

D. all of the above
E. none of the above

84. Concerning the use of ISG in hepatitis A, all of the following are true *except*

A. should be administered to all close contacts of patients with hepatitis A, particularly household members and other intimate associates who are at high risk of acquiring the disease

B. should be given as soon as possible after the exposure has occurred

C. may be administered up through four to five weeks postexposure, provided symptoms of hepatitis have not yet appeared

D. the administration of ISG after exposure to hepatitis A acts to lessen the severity of clinical manifestations of disease rather than prevent infection

E. is of considerable value in the treatment of hepatitis A

Questions 85 to 92

A 27-year-old female visits her internist with a complaint of chest pain. She describes a waxing and waning of the pain throughout the day rather than discrete attacks of sharp chest pain. Occasionally the episodes of pain last only a few seconds. On physical examination, her physician detects a systolic click, a late systolic murmur, and frequent premature ventricular contractions. The murmur becomes prolonged by standing and during the Valsalva maneuver.

85. The most likely diagnosis would be

A. idiopathic hypertrophic subaortic stenosis
B. mitral valve prolapse syndrome
C. subacute bacterial endocarditis
D. marantic endocarditis
E. Marfan's syndrome

86. All of the following might be expected to be true of the patient's condition *except*

A. in addition to chest discomfort, the patient may complain of palpitations, syncope, light-headedness, or fatigue
B. it occurs more commonly among men
C. the syndrome includes a spectrum from the asymptomatic patient to those in heart failure from mitral regurgitation
D. all maneuvers that decrease left ventricular volume move the clicks or murmur toward the first heart sound while those maneuvers that increase left ventricular volume presumably have the opposite effect
E. the prolapse murmur tends to be prolonged, but not necessarily intensified, by standing, doing the Valsalva maneuver, or inhaling amyl nitrite

87. An unexpected electrocardiographic finding in this patient would be

A. ST-segment abnormalities and T wave inversions
B. shortened QT interval
C. prominent U waves
D. all of the above
E. none of the above

88. Which of the following is (are) true of this syndrome?

A. patients are usually aware of arrhythmias
B. during the patient's subjective experience of palpitations, arrhythmias are invariably recorded
C. false-positive treadmill exercise tests have been recorded
D. all of the above
E. none of the above

89. In this patient,

A. echocardiography probably would reveal abrupt posterior motion of the mitral valve echo toward the left atrium during systole
B. echocardiography can be used as the single hallmark for the diagnosis of this condition

C. angiography is a perfect tool for diagnosing this condition
D. all of the above
E. none of the above

90. That this syndrome may result from more than just a valvular abnormality and may involve the myocardium is suggested by the occurrence in some of these patients of

A. chest pain
B. cardiac arrhythmias
C. abnormal left ventricular contractile patterns and occasional cardiac decomposition
D. abnormal lactate production
E. all of the above

91. All of the following are true of this syndrome *except*

A. chordae tendineae are elongated, the mitral valve is edematous and thickened, and histopathological examination suggests a degenerative process
B. preliminary echocardiographic studies suggest that more than 1% of the population shows a recognizable pattern of this syndrome
C. endocarditis prophylaxis is recommended at the time of dental or surgical procedures
D. the chronic fatigue found in this condition responds dramatically to propranolol
E. there is a tendency for exercise-induced ventricular premature beats and ventricular tachycardia to be suppressed with propranolol therapy in doses up to 320 mg/day

92. Complications of this disorder include

A. endocarditis
B. severe life-threatening arrhythmia
C. valvular insufficiency with or without ruptured chordae tendineae
D. acute mitral regurgitation
E. all of the above

Questions 93 to 122

A 55-year-old male has noted the gradual appearance of a tremor of his right hand, and has more recently been affected in his left upper extremity. He has noticed that his handwriting has become tremulous; the handwriting also tends to fade out and becomes smaller as it continues. He has felt more easily fatigued in performing acts such as dressing. His wife states that she has noticed a change in his facial expression with weakness in his voice. Recently he seems to be dragging his legs when walking.

93.   The most likely diagnosis is

    A.   Huntington's chorea
    B.   multiple sclerosis
    C.   amyotrophic lateral sclerosis
    D.   Parkinson's disease
    E.   Wernicke's encephalopathy

94.   Diagnosis of this disorder is best made by

    A.   response to steroids
    B.   response to thiamine
    C.   history and physical examination
    D.   electromyography
    E.   CAT scanning

95.   All the following are true of this disorder *except*

    A.   true paralysis agitans occurs usually at 50 to 60 years of age but may develop after 40 years of age or beyond 60
    B.   a juvenile form has been described, occurring in the second decade of life
    C.   the postencephalitic variety is found at all ages but usually in young people of 15 years or more
    D.   men are much more commonly afflicted than women in the idiopathic variety, but in the postencephalitic type, the incidence is more evenly divided
    E.   blacks are more commonly affected

96.   A disorder which closely simulates features of classical paralysis agitans has been associated with the influenza pandemic following World War I. This postencephalitic parkinsonism is felt to be caused by encephalitis lethargica or von

    A.   Hippel-Landau's encephalitis
    B.   Recklinghausen's encephalitis
    C.   Economo's encephalitis
    D.   Willebrand's encephalitis
    E.   Streuben's encephalitis

97.   The cause of classic Parkinson's disease (paralysis agitans) is believed to be

    A.   viral
    B.   familial
    C.   toxic
    D.   idiopathic
    E.   hypoxic

98.   A parkinsonian syndrome has been described following intoxication with

    A.   manganese
    B.   lead
    C.   carbon monoxide
    D.   carbon disulfide
    E.   all of the above

99.   All of the following are true of the parkinsonian syndrome *except*

    A.   phenothiazine in very large doses may cause such a syndrome, but it is generally reversible
    B.   brain tumor frequently invades the basal ganglia area but is rarely responsible for a parkinsonian syndrome
    C.   there is good evidence that emotional strain is capable of producing a genuine disorder of this type
    D.   the appearance of parkinsonian features as a consequence of reserpine becomes explicable on the basis of the depletion of dopamine (and of other catecholamines) resulting from use of this agent
    E.   an elevation in acetylcholine (as with local application of acetylcholine itself, or following use of the experimental drug oxotremorine, or with anticho-

linesterase agents such as physostig-mine) can result in the appearance of parkinsonian features

100. In cases of parkinsonism, there is a striking reduction in what content of the striatum with a similar, although less striking, loss of homovanillic acid?

    A. acetylcholine
    B. dopamine
    C. histamine
    D. bradykinin
    E. none of the above

101. The disease process affects chiefly the

    A. substantia nigra and the pallidum
    B. striatum (caudate and putamen)
    C. thalamus
    D. cerebellum
    E. pons

102. The neostriatal cells are actually in a state of equilibrium under ordinary circumstances, modulated by the inhibitory dopaminergic system and by what facilitory changes?

    A. adrenergic
    B. serotonergic
    C. cholinergic
    D. all of the above
    E. none of the above

103. The relative specificity of derangement in the dopamine-influenced inhibition in parkinsonism in particular is underscored by the fact that in other diseases of the basal ganglia presenting with disorders of movement such as Huntington's chorea,

    A. dopamine and homovanillic acid concentrations are decreased
    B. dopamine and homovanillic acid concentrations are normal
    C. dopamine and homovanillic acid concentrations are increased
    D. dopamine concentrations are increased, but homovanillic acid concentrations are decreased
    E. dopamine concentrations are decreased, but homovanillic acid concentrations are increased

104. In the human, a distinct lessening of the clinical features of the parkinsonian state may be obtained by

    A. increasing the concentration of dopamine by adding L-dopa
    B. increasing the concentration of dopamine by preventing degradation of dopamine by the use of MAO inhibitors
    C. reducing the activity of the cholinergic apparatus by the use of anticholinergic drugs such as belladonna alkaloids and synthetic derivatives such as trihexyphenidyl HCl (Artane)
    D. all of the above
    E. none of the above

105. Which of the following is *not* true of the symptoms of Parkinson's disease?

    A. the development of the disorder is gradual and insidious in the majority of cases, the appearance of the disease being so slow as to escape detection in its earliest phases
    B. tremor is commonly the first symptom to attract attention
    C. slowness of movement is an early symptom but is not as frequently a source of complaint as tremor
    D. pain in one or both arms, particularly the shoulder, may be an early manifestation
    E. the manifestations of the disorder are usually unilateral throughout its course

106. On examination, the objective findings of Parkinson's disease vary with the stage of development of the disorder. Typically, all of the following are characteristic *except*

    A. in early cases, the face is immobile, the arm or arms fail to swing in walking, and the fingers move in the typical resting tremor
    B. in more advanced cases, the body is bent forward, the arms are slightly flexed, tremor is usually present in the fingers, and the gait is shuffling and often festinating

   C.   there may be moderate to severe rigidity of the musculature and relative weakness of the muscles; the voice is low and eventually almost inaudible, and saliva drains from the corners of the mouth
   D.   as the disease advances, the rigidity becomes greater but the tremor becomes less severe
   E.   death may be due to an intercurrent infection such as pneumonia

107. Which of the following is *not* true of the tremor of Parkinson's disease?

   A.   may be unilateral or bilateral
   B.   is distal, involving the fingers and hands much more often than the arms and forearms
   C.   is rhythmical, usually coarse, and occurs at a rate of four to seven/sec
   D.   in the hands, it is characterized by a posture of adduction of the thumb and fingers with a rhythmical rubbing of fingers and thumb, producing the so-called "pill-rolling tremor"
   E.   flexion and extension movements are seldom observed

108. Which of the following is *not* true of the tremor of Parkinson's disease?

   A.   the tremor is generally present at rest (static tremor) and disappears temporarily on movement
   B.   after the limb is moved and has come to rest, the tremor reappears
   C.   in many cases, the tremor not only persists during movement, but may at times be increased by it
   D.   the lips and face may be involved by tremor in advanced cases, and a coarse, rhythmical tremor of the head is common
   E.   tremor of the legs is more common than in the upper extremities

109. The tremors of Parkinson's disease disappear during

   A.   emotional stress
   B.   fatigue

   C.   anxiety
   D.   sleep
   E.   none of the above

110. In Parkinson's disease, rigidity, or resistance to passive motion, is present in all cases and may be expressed by

   A.   cogwheeling
   B.   decrease in associated movements
   C.   marche à petit pas with festinating gait
   D.   "freezing"
   E.   all of the above

111. Patients with Parkinson's disease would *not* be expected to manifest

   A.   an immobile or "masked" facies with infrequent blinking and smiling
   B.   handwriting that is tremulous and macrographic
   C.   a general paucity of movement usually referred to as akinesis, and loss of extraneous movements, such as crossing the legs, gesturing, crossing the arms, and many other such movements made by the normal person
   D.   slow movement of a limb on command, with an appreciable latency before it has been carried out
   E.   defective ocular convergence in both the idiopathic and postencephalitic cases

112. All of the following are true of Parkinson's disease, *except*

   A.   actual muscle weakness is common and usually marked
   B.   the reflexes are usually decreased
   C.   plantar responses are ordinarily extensor
   D.   the glabellar reflex is positive
   E.   a snout or rooting reflex is sometimes seen, and occasional patients exhibit forced grasping

113. Which of the following is (are) true of oculogyric crises in Parkinson's disease?

   A.   more common in the postencephalitic than in the idiopathic variety

B. they are attacks of forced involuntary upward deviation of the eyes, usually in conjugate fashion, which can be overcome by strong exertion of the will for short periods, only to recur with relaxation

C. such attacks are entirely unpredictable in occurrence

D. all of the above

E. none of the above

114. The postencephalitic form of Parkinson's disease is associated with all of the following *except*

A. occurs at any age but usually appears before the age of 40 years

B. a history of encephalitis may be obtained or suggested by symptoms such as fever, diplopia, and hypersomnolence, but in many cases, no such history is obtainable, the disease occurring seemingly without previous infection

C. progress of the disease is often more rapid than in idiopathic or true paralysis agitans and greasy skin and sialorrhea are perhaps more common

D. tremor is always more prominent than in idiopathic paralysis agitans and choreoathetosis is not encountered

E. palilalia (repetition of a word or phrase) and echolalia (repetition of words addressed to the patient) are frequent

115. Tremors due to other causes must be differentiated from that of paralysis agitans. Which of the following is true of nonparkinsonian tremor?

A. the tremor of senility is constant and tends to involve the jaw and tongue as well as the limbs; the usual features of parkinsonism, such as rigidity, are ordinarily lacking; evidence of dementia is common

B. general paresis may cause tremor of the hands which is usually associated with facial and lingual tremors; it

rarely reaches the degree of the parkinsonian tremor

C. the tremor of alcoholism is constant and often accompanied by facial tremors; it tends to be most prominent when the limbs are held up against gravity (particularly in the withdrawal state; the tremor may be very coarse, at times interspersed with abrupt myoclonic jerks and often associated with severe gastrointestinal symptoms; rigidity is not present, and other features of paralysis agitans are lacking

D. familial, or benign essential tremor is at times mistaken for paralysis agitans; it usually occurs in males and is ordinarily minimal at rest, becoming evident when the limbs are outstretched and often continuing or even worsening during voluntary movements; a nodding tremor of the head and a tremulous voice are often associated and characteristically, this type of tremor is remarkably reduced qualitatively with the ingestion of alcohol

E. all of the above

116. The wife of the patient described in the report was very concerned about the course of her husband's disease and the eventual outlook. As her husband's physician, which statement would you feel is *least* likely to be true?

A. the course of the disease is usually downward without hope of complete recovery

B. the progression is usually slow, and clinical plateaus may be achieved, particularly in the postencephalitic variety

C. death is often from an intercurrent disease such as pneumonia, usually years after the onset of symptoms

D. there is no known cure for paralysis agitans or for the various types of parkinsonism with the exception of drug withdrawal in cases due to phenothiazine intoxication

E. drug therapy is without benefit

117. In Parkinson's disease, drug therapy is at times of great benefit. As working principles, it is important to keep in mind that

    A. the dosage of any of the effective drugs varies from case to case
    B. tolerance to one drug is often developed and that change or "staggering" of drugs is necessary from time to time
    C. in changing from one drug to another in the treatment of paralysis agitans, it is essential that the dosage of the new drug be as closely equivalent as possible to that of the old in order to avoid a letdown
    D. such simple measures as rest and general hygiene must not be neglected
    E. all of the above

118. Prior to the introduction of L-dopa (L-dihydroxyphenylalanine), the most widely available drugs for use in Parkinson's disease consisted of the naturally occurring belladonna alkaloids, their synthetic equivalents, and antihistaminics. These drugs have been found most helpful in controlling

    A. rigidity
    B. tremor
    C. akinesia
    D. all of the above
    E. none of the above

119. Synthetic belladonna-like agents with anticholinergic properties which have been used in Parkinson's disease include all of the following *except*

    A. Artane (trihexyphenidyl)
    B. Cogentin (benzotropine methanesulfonate)
    C. Akineton (biperiden)
    D. Parsidol (ethopropazine hydrochloride)
    E. Symmetrel (amantadine hydrochloride)

120. If the patient had been treated with one of the synthetic belladonna-like agents, possible side effects that might be explained to him could include

    A. blurred vision
    B. dryness of the mouth
    C. gastrointestinal disorders
    D. abnormal mentation
    E. all of the above

121. L-Dopa has been introduced fairly recently in therapy of primary parkinsonism, postencephalitic parkinsonism, and most other forms of parkinsonism. Which statement is *not* true of this drug?

    A. it is also effective in iatrogenic parkinsonism caused by phenothiazines and related medication
    B. tolerance to the emetic action of levodopa gradually develops over a period of several months
    C. if the patient has been taking one of the centrally acting anticholinergic agents such as trihexyphenidyl hydrochloride, biperiden, or benztropine mesylate, such medication should be continued, at least during the initial phases of levodopa therapy, to help control anorexia, nausea, and vomiting, and also to maintain control of parkinsonian symptoms
    D. the combined use of levodopa with a decarboxylase inhibitor greatly reduces the incidence of nausea and vomiting
    E. the major dose-limiting side effect of levodopa therapy is the occurrence of adventitious involuntary movements, usually choreiform in pattern, in about 80% of patients

122. Concerning therapy with L-dopa,

    A. the appearance of dyskinetic movements in a patient while the dose of L-dopa is being increased indicates that optimum dosage has been attained
    B. toxic psychic effects of levodopa develop less often than with the centrally acting anticholinergic agents and, in general, are similar to those of amphetamines, usually requiring dosage adjustment

C. orthostatic hypotension is a commonly occurring side effect of L-dopa therapy and is occasionally severe enough to cause light-headedness, dizziness, or even syncope

D. cardiac arrhythmias may occasionally develop in patients receiving levodopa

E. all of the above

Questions 123 to 132

A 26-year-old male is referred to a cardiologist because of sporadic episodes of palpitations which have occurred paroxysmally for several years. Physical examination is completely within normal limits. An electrocardiogram is taken, and it shows a heart rate of 78. The P-R interval is 0.10 sec with a QRS interval of 0.12 sec. Slurring of the upstroke of the QRS complex is noted.

123. The most likely diagnosis is

A. idiopathic hypertrophic subaortic stenosis

B. Lown-Ganong-Levine syndrome

C. hyperthyroidism

D. Wolff-Parkinson-White syndrome

E. anxiety state

124. All of the following are true of this patient's condition *except*

A. the anomalous pathway may result not only in disorders of impulse conduction, but also in disorders of impulse formation such as first-degree, second-degree, and complete heart block, as well as bundle branch block

B. the tachyarrhythmias occurring in association with the preexcitation syndrome may be explained by the mechanism of reentrant excitation

C. electrically produced, premature atrial or ventricular systoles may terminate the tachyarrhythmia, possibly by blocking one of the reentrant paths

D. it would appear that the preexcitation syndrome is a congenital disorder, possibly hereditary

E. this syndrome is usually associated with cardiac disease

125. Recognition of this syndrome is important because

A. it is associated with paroxysmal tachyarrhythmias which, at times, do not respond to conventional therapy

B. the abnormal QRS complexes may mask underlying cardiac disease (acute myocardial infarction)

C. the anatomic and mechanistic explanations of the conduction abnormality and tachyarrhythmia provide clinical and experimental support for the mechanism of other tachyarrhythmias and serve to explain electrocardiographic variations of the short P-R interval with QRS prolongation

D. the syndrome may provide a clinical clue to underlying congenital heart disease, for example Ebstein's anomaly, with which it is frequently associated

E. all of the above

126. Electrocardiographic features of this syndrome include all the following *except*

A. the classic electrocardiographic features of the syndrome are a P-R interval less than 0.10 to 0.12 sec and a QRS complex that is prolonged greater than 0.11 sec in the presence of normal sinus rhythm

B. the prolonged QRS duration is due to the initial inscription of a delta wave; the remainder of the QRS complex is usually slender, representing normal ventricular activation

C. the delta wave indicates premature anomalous activation of the ventricles via bypass fibers

D. if the fibers bypassing the A-V node enter both ventricles posteriorly, the delta wave is upright in V-1 and V-6 (type A); if they enter the right ventricle, the delta wave is upright in V-6 and negative in V-1 (type B)

E. the P-J interval (interval from the onset of the P wave to the end of the QRS complex) is usually abnormal

127. Which of the following is *not* true of this syndrome?

    A. a third type of this syndrome may exist (type C) if the bypass fibers enter the left ventricle to produce an upright delta wave in V-1 and a negative delta wave in V-6

    B. secondary ST and T wave abnormalities do not occur

    C. variants of the classic features of this syndrome include a short P-R interval with a normal QRS complex

    D. in the classic syndrome and its variants, a variety of anatomic bridges have been demonstrated, which may provide partial or complete A-V nodal bypass from the atria to the bundle branch, or to the right and left ventricular myocardium

    E. in the preexcitation syndrome, ventricular fusion beats may be produced by a single impulse dividing in the A-V junction entering the ventricle in two anatomically separate areas

128. Paroxysmal tachyarrhythmias occur in approximately what percentage of patients with this syndrome?

    A. 1 to 5%
    B. 10 to 20%
    C. 30 to 45%
    D. 50 to 75%
    E. over 95%

129. Patients who have this condition exhibit all of the following *except*

    A. they are asymptomatic between paroxysms of tachycardia

    B. physical examination is normal

    C. because the aberrant pathway may bypass the normal A-V delay, a rapid ventricular rate is common during the supraventricular tachyarrhythmias

    D. ventricular tachycardia is common

    E. no exceptions

130. In this syndrome, aberrant ventricular conduction is present in about what percentage of the tachyarrhythmias?

    A. less than 1%

    B. 5%
    C. 15%
    D. 30%
    E. 60%

131. Patients with the preexcitation syndrome

    A. usually die before reaching adulthood

    B. usually enjoy a good prognosis

    C. usually present to a physician with refractory congestive heart failure

    D. invariably have abnormal electrocardiograms between attacks of tachycardia

    E. should be put on prophylactic antibiotics

132. In the treatment of the preexcitaion syndrome,

    A. therapy is directed toward the management or prevention of the tachyarrhythmias

    B. the usual approaches regarding the management of paroxysmal atrial tachycardia, atrial flutter and atrial fibrillation are employed

    C. digitalis may be ineffective in slowing the ventricular rate in the presence of atrial flutter or atrial fibrillation because the drug appears to preferentially slow conduction over the normal pathway, allowing conduction to persist over the anomalous pathway

    D. in patients refractory to digitalis, quinidine or procaineamide usually slows the ventricular rate by depressing impulse conduction over the anomalous pathway

    E. all of the above

Questions 133 to 151

A 30-year-old female sees her physician with multiple complaints. These include malaise, vague muscle cramps, and paresthesia. She has noted some dysphagia and twitching of her eyelids. She had recently seen a psychiatrist because she had become less alert mentally and felt much more anxious than usual.

On physical examination, spotty alopecia was

noted and her skin was coarse, scaly, and brownish in color. A thyroidectomy scar was present. Her nails were brittle and atrophied, with horizontal ridging. There was some wheezing present on auscultation of the chest. While taking her blood pressure, the nurse was distracted while the cuff was inflated and it remained inflated for several minutes. This was not only painful to the patient but resulted in a spasmodic twitching of the involved hand.

133. The patient's signs and symptoms were most likely due to

   A. hypothyroidism
   B. hypoparathyroidism
   C. anxiety neurosis
   D. diabetic neuropathy
   E. none of the above

134. The patient's spasmodic hand movement indicated a positive

   A. Trendelenberg sign
   B. Trousseau's sign
   C. Erb's sign
   D. Chvostek sign
   E. none of the above

135. During physical examination, the physician applied a sharp blow over the facial nerve just in front of the parotid gland; this resulted in an immediate twitch of the mouth, nose, and eye. He considered this a positive

   A. Erb's sign
   B. Trendelenberg sign
   C. Chvostek sign
   D. Trousseau's sign
   E. Myerson sign

136. The patient's illness

   A. need not be treated
   B. is probably familial
   C. occurs most frequently as a result of surgery on the thyroid gland
   D. will respond rapidly to phosphate administration
   E. all of the above

137. Which of the following is true of hypoparathyroidism?

   A. clinical hypoparathyroidism has been reported in a rare patient after I^{131} therapy of Graves' disease
   B. hypoparathyroidism is occasionally familial and may be associated with Addison's disease
   C. exfoliative dermatitis and monilial infection of the nails may occur
   D. lenticular cataracts may develop with time
   E. all of the above

138. In a patient with decreased renal function, hypocalcemia may be due to

   A. hyperproteinemia
   B. hypophosphatemia
   C. increased renal production of 1, 25-dihydroxycholecalciferol
   D. all of the above
   E. none of the above

139. In such a patient as described above,

   A. the administration of a diet limited in phosphate to 350 mg/day and supplemented with 60 ml aluminum hydroxide 4 times per day may correct the hyperphosphatemia and improve the hypocalcemia
   B. measurement of 1, 25-dihydroxycholecalciferol will be especially helpful when available
   C. treatment with vitamins may be necessary to normalize the serum calcium level and improve any associated osteomalacia
   D. all of the above
   E. none of the above

140. In the hospital workup of hypoparathyroidism and hypocalcemic states, which of the following series of tests would *least* likely be indicated?

   A. amylase, serum protein electrophoresis, stool fat
   B. creatinine, creatinine clearance, electrolytes, serum magnesium
   C. free thyroxine index and (if low) TSH level

D. total alkaline phosphatase and bone alkaline phosphatase
E. LE preparation, ANA and rheumatoid factor

141. X-rays that may be useful in the workup of hypoparathyroidism and hypocalcemic states may include

A. skull, chest, hands, and feet
B. small bowel for possible malabsorption pattern
C. long bones and pelvis for possible osteomalacia
D. all of the above
E. none of the above

142. In hypoparathyroidism, one might expect all of the following *except*

A. increased serum phosphate levels
B. normal serum alkaline phosphatase
C. decreased urine calcium
D. increased urine hydroxyproline
E. decreased levels of parathyroid hormone

143. Hypocalcemia may be associated with increased levels of parathyroid hormone and lack of end organ response. Which would be an *unexpected* finding in this condition?

A. increased serum phosphate
B. normal to increased alkaline phosphatase
C. urine hydroxyproline decreased or increased
D. decreased urine calcium
E. increased urine phosphate

144. Hypocalcemia may be associated with

A. laryngeal stridor
B. convulsions
C. pylorospasm
D. papilledema
E. all of the above

145. Overt tetany is the presenting complaint in approximately what percentage of cases of hypoparathyroidism?

A. 1%
B. 10%
C. 30%
D. 70%
E. over 95%

146. An electrocardiogram was ordered on the patient described in the case report. It most probably showed

A. atrial fibrillation
B. shortened PR interval
C. prolongation of the QT interval
D. all of the above
E. none of the above

147. Which of the following is true of hypoparathyroidism?

A. Erb's sign is positive when less than a 6 milliamp cathodal current induces a motor nerve response
B. in treated patients, the Sulkowitch test on the patient's urine should rarely be negative and provides an easy guide to therapy
C. over-treatment of the disorder is especially dangerous when normal or elevated serum calcium levels are present without an accompanying lowering of the serum phosphorus; under such conditions, nephrocalcinosis, kidney stones, uremia, and death may ensue
D. all of the above
E. none of the above

148. Which of the following would *not* be used in the treatment of acute hypocalcemia?

A. sodium bicarbonate
B. 10 ml of 10% calcium gluconate by slow intravenous injection
C. 50 to 150 units of parathyroid extract intramuscularly every 12 hr
D. A and B
E. B and C

149. In the control of chronic hypocalcemia secondary to hypoparathyroidism,

A. vitamin D is prescribed in doses from 50,000 to 200,000 units/day
B. calcium gluconate or calcium lactate in doses of 8 to 30 g/day is prescribed to raise the serum calcium level to within

physiologic range

C. occasionally hypomagnesemia may be found in some cases of tetany not responding to calcium treatment alone

D. phosphorus should be limited by dietary measures such as the elimination of dairy products or by the use of aluminum hydroxide gel or Benemid (probenecid)

E. all of the above

150. In a subject who has normal renal function, a normal serum magnesium level, and who has had an adequate diet including one quart of milk per day for three days, hypocalcemia and hyperphosphatemia most likely signify hypoparathyroidism; in such a patient

A. the serum level of parathyroid hormone is inappropriately low

B. the serum level of 25-hydroxycholecalciferol is normal

C. parathyroid extract increases the urinary excretion of phosphate and cyclic 3', 5'-AMP

D. all of the above

E. none of the above

151. Severe vitamin D deficiency

A. may be accompanied by hypocalcemia usually associated with hypophosphatemia

B. a low level of 25-hydroxycholecalciferol on admission with a rise after the administration of vitamin D_2 confirms the diagnosis

C. a failure of 25-hydroxycholecalciferol level to rise or a failure of the serum and urine calcium levels to rise after the administration of vitamin D_2 points to vitamin D resistance

D. all of the above

E. none of the above

Questions 152 to 163

A 49-year-old executive with a history of upper gastrointestinal surgery for peptic ulcer disease has noticed several disturbing signs and symptoms. These include fatigue, hunger, mild confusion, sweating, paresthesias, tremor, and tachycardia. These typically occur a few hours after a meal. His physician performed a five-hr glucose tolerance test which showed a peak glucose value of 250 mg% in one hr. The two-hr glucose is 40 mg% and the patient exhibited signs and symptoms similar to those described above.

152. This patient probably has

A. the dumping syndrome

B. insulinoma

C. a prediabetic state

D. alimentary hypoglycemia

E. fasting hypoglycemia

153. Concerning hypoglycemic symptoms, all of the following are true *except*

A. the symptoms of hypoglycemia may be related to the rate of fall in glucose, its nadir, or some combination of the two

B. a rapid fall in blood sugar stimulates catecholamine release with resulting epinephrine excess symptoms including sweating, palpitations, tremor, nervousness, acral and perioral numbness, faintness, weakness, and hunger

C. a slow decline in blood glucose levels produces primarily central nervous system effects which can mimic a wide variety of neurological and psychiatric abnormalities

D. the symptoms and signs of hypoglycemia are generally irreversible

E. in patients with cerebral vascular disease, hypoglycemic symptoms may occur at higher blood glucose levels and correlate with underperfused regions of the central nervous system

154. Fasting hypoglycemia would be most likely to be associated with

A. reactive hypoglycemia

B. maturity-onset diabetes mellitus

C. alimentary hypoglycemia

D. insulinoma

E. leucine sensitivity

155. Fasting hypoglycemia would be *least* likely to be associated with

    A. insulinoma
    B. oral hypoglycemic agents
    C. extrapancreatic tumors
    D. alimentary hypoglycemia
    E. alcohol ingestion

156. Hypoglycemia induced by food ingestion is associated with all the following *except*

    A. generally occurs within one to five hr after ingestion of a meal
    B. is characterized by symptoms related to catecholamine release
    C. significant central nervous system symptoms are common
    D. in the adult, seizures and coma are rare
    E. the symptoms usually subside within 30 min if no therapy is undertaken

157. In adults, hypoglycemia is usually related to intake of

    A. fructose
    B. glucose
    C. galactose
    D. leucine
    E. fatty acids

158. The procedure of choice to document postprandial hypoglycemia is a

    A. fasting blood sugar determination
    B. two-hr postprandial glucose
    C. five-hr glucose tolerance test
    D. upper gastrointestinal series
    E. serum insulin level

159. The most common of the postprandial hypoglycemias is

    A. alimentary hypoglycemia
    B. maturity-onset diabetes mellitus
    C. reactive (functional or idiopathic) hypoglycemia
    D. adrenal insufficiency
    E. alcohol ingestion

160. All of the following are true of reactive, functional hypoglycemia *except*

    A. the glucose tolerance test tends to be flat with a blunted early rise in serum glucose
    B. serum insulin level is inappropriate for the blood sugar level
    C. symptoms usually appear three to five hours after a meal, but occasionally occur during the first hour after glucose ingestion
    D. symptoms may be limited to mild anxiety and restlessness, but some patients describe more severe complaints associated with blatant epinephrine excess
    E. individuals who develop reactive, functional hypoglycemia tend to be asthenic, hyperkinetic, obsessive-compulsive persons who are tense and often emotionally labile

161. Concerning treatment of reactive, functional hypoglycemia, all of the following are true *except*

    A. therapy is directed toward attempts to maintain euglycemia through multiple small feedings high in protein and the avoidance of concentrated sweets
    B. if dietary measures are not totally successful, anticholinergic drugs such as tincture of belladonna or atropine sulfate may help to control symptoms by slowing gastric emptying and inhibiting vagal stimulation of insulin secretion
    C. diphenylhydantoin (Dilantin) has been used with apparent success in some patients
    D. psychotherapy is advisable for many patients since the symptoms of hypoglycemia often abate with improved psychiatric status
    E. without treatment, symptoms usually persist for many years

162. The syndrome of alimentary hypoglycemia would be *least* likely to be present in patients with

    A. thyrotoxicosis
    B. duodenal ulcer or a history of upper

gastrointestinal surgery
C. diabetes mellitus
D. rapid gastric emptying of unknown cause
E. A and D

163. In alimentary hypoglycemia,

A. hypoglycemia usually does not appear until several hours after eating
B. patients should be advised to eat more rapidly
C. patients should be advised to eat larger meals
D. patients should be advised to consume more carbohydrates
E. drugs that slow intestinal motility may be effectively employed

Answers and Commentary

1. **E.** The most likely diagnosis is lung abscess.
(8:1228–1229)

2. **D** Copious amounts of foul-smelling sputum are most consistent with an anaerobic infection.
(8:1228)

3. **E.** All statements are true of the pathogenesis of lung abscess.
(8:1228–1229)

4. **E.** A condition favoring aspiration and/or oral sepsis can be found in nearly 80% of patients with lung abscesses caused by anaerobic microorganisms. All other statements are true.
(8:1228–29)

5. **B.** Tubercle bacilli are more likely to reach the upper lobes by bloodstream dissemination than through the airways. All other statements are correct.
(8:1228–1229)

6. **E.** All statements are true of the treatment of lung abscesses.
(8:1229)

7. **A.** In the treatment of lung abscesses, the antibiotic regimen should be changed only when there is definite clinical or radiographic evidence of relapse, and not simply on the basis of changing flora in serial sputum cultures. All other statements are true.
(8:1229)

8. **C.** Incomplete resolution of a chronic lung abscess is not sufficient reason for resectional surgery, since delayed closure is common. All other statements are true of the role of surgery in patients with lung abscesses.
(8:1229)

9. **C.** For the patient described, proper dental care would be most appropriate in managing the patient after successful medical treatment of the lung abscess.
(8:1229)

10. **C.** The most likely diagnosis in this patient is acute tubular necrosis.
(8:1295–97)

11. **D.** Pregnancy appears in some way to predispose to ischemic renal insults; in a large proportion of most published series, acute renal failure followed placenta previa, septic abortion, postpartum hemorrhage, or eclampsia. All other statements are correct.
(8:1298)

12. **E.** All the listed factors are common causes of acute tubular necrosis.
(8:1293)

13. **A.** In most patients, casts appear to be a result of diminished urinary flow rather than its cause. All other statements are correct.
(8:1294)

14. **E.** Leukocytosis is the rule with or without infection in patients with acute tubular necrosis. All other statements are true of this disorder. (8:1296)

15. **D.** In acute tubular necrosis, oliguria usually lasts 10 to 14 days.
(8:1295)

16. **E.** All the statements are true of acute renal failure.
(8:1296)

17. **B.** Pericarditis may develop in patients with acute renal failure, but it does not have the grave prognosis attached to its appearance in chronic renal disease.
(8:1296)

18. **C.** Infection is the most frequent complication of acute tubular necrosis and the most common cause of death.
(8:1297)

19. **E.** In acute renal failure, neurologic manifestations are common, the two most important being coma and convulsions. Hyponatremia may be responsible for somnolence or seizures early in the course of the disease, and may be corrected by hypertonic saline solution, with proper regard for the complications of overhydration and heart failure. Hypocalcemia may also predispose to convulsions, as may too vigorous administration of alkali without accompanying calcium in the treatment of acidosis. Seizures may be focal in nature or generalized; some may have a vascular basis.
(8:1296)

20. **D.** All the statements are true. (8:1295)

21. **E.** All the findings listed may occur during the early diuretic phase of recovery from acute renal failure. (8:1297)

22. **D.** Hypertension is not a sequel in those who recover from acute tubular necrosis. All other statements are correct. (8:1297)

23. **E.** All statements are true of this patient's electrocardiogram. (8:1296)

24. **D.** In the treatment of hyperkalemia, calcium does not 'lower serum potassium levels but the deleterious action of potassium on the heart may be counteracted to some extent by infusions of calcium or by the administration of digitalis. (8:1298) 387)

25 **A.** Heart failure should be treated initially with digitalis in usual doses. All other statements are correct. (8:1298)

26. **D.** The most likely diagnosis is subacute thyroiditis. (2:2131)

27. **D.** Subacute thyroiditis (granulomatous thyroiditis, acute thyroiditis, De Quervain's thyroiditis) is an inflammatory condition of the thyroid causing painful enlargement, lasting over a period of weeks or months, with a prominent tendency to relapse. (2:2131)

28. **A.** The incidence of subacute thyroiditis is not known, but it appears to be about one-tenth as common as Graves' disease. (2:2131)

29. **D.** In patients with subacute thyroiditis, there is poor correlation between the histologic abnormalities, which may be extreme, and the clinical picture. (2:2131)

30. **B.** Fibrosis is prominent in patients with subacute thyroiditis. (2:2131)

31. **E.** All the statements are true of subacute thyroiditis. (2:2131)

32. **E.** All statements are true of the diagnosis of subacute thyroiditis. (2:2131)

33. **D.** In subacute thyroiditis, antibody titers against thyroid antigens may be transiently demonstrable, but they rarely reach the levels found in Hashimoto's thyroiditis, and the responses are not sustained. All other statements are characteristic of this disorder. (2:2131)

34. **E.** Radioactive iodine is the least useful of the treatments listed. (2:2131)

35. **B.** It is reported that up to 10% of patients with subacute thyroiditis develop permanent hypothyroidism. (2:2131)

36. **B.** The symptoms described would most likely be attributable to staphylococcal food poisoning. (2:65)

37. **E.** Foods may produce illness by any of the means listed. (2:64)

38. **B.** Staphylococcal food poisoning is the most common bacterial food poisoning in the United States. (2:64)

39. **A.** If food is held at ambient temperature in a warm climate after preparation, later reheating or even boiling will not prevent staphylococcal food poisoning which is caused by preformed, heat-stable toxin. (2:65)

40. **B.** In the toxin type of bacterial food poisoning such as that associated with staphylococci, the illness does not depend on the ingestion of living organisms. All other statements are true of this illness. (2:65)

41. **D.** In staphylococcal food poisoning, diarrhea is variable; it may be profuse, mild, or absent entirely. Although often violent, staphylococcal food poisoning is short-lived, usually subsiding in six or eight hr and rarely lasting as long as 24 hr. Enterotoxin is not produced at ordinary domestic refrigerator temperatures. Epidemiologic work on outbreaks of staphylococcal food poisoning involves standard methods of bacteriophage typing in identifying the source of the responsible strain. (2:65)

42. **E.** The patient is often recovering from staphylococcal food poisoning when first seen by a doctor but may require an intramuscular injection of an anti-nausea drug to control vomiting. Patients with evidence of serious depletion of extracellular fluid may require intravenous treatment using isotonic sodium chloride with added potassium. (2:65)

43. **B.** The most likely diagnosis is polyarteritis nodosa. (7:724–26)

44. **E.** In polyarteritis nodosa, virtually any organ may be involved, but most frequently affected are the kidneys and heart. (7:724–25)

45. **E.** All the changes listed may occur with this disease. (7:724)

46. **D.** The prognosis in patients with polyarteritis who have clinically evident multisystem disease is poor, with death the usual outcome after weeks or months of illness. (7:726)

47. **C.** The finding of a striking eosinophilia in a patient with this disorder would suggest involvement of the lungs. (7:726)

48. **C.** Relief from many of the symptoms and signs of illness may be observed promptly after initiating treatment with corticoids or corticotropin. This clinical improvement has been confirmed histologically. In serial biopsy specimens, one may see a resolution of the arterial inflammation within a few weeks. Large doses are often required to control the active manifestations of polyarteritis and the side reactions may be troublesome. However, adequate data are not available to determine whether or not life is prolonged by steroid therapy. (7:726–27)

49. **C.** The most probable cause of the patient's complaints and findings is acute, intermittent porphyria. (8:497)

50. **C.** The freshly voided urine of a patient with acute intermittent porphyria is frequently normal in color and on standing in the sunlight turns to a burgundy wine, or even black, color. This color change can be hastened by adding a small amount of acid to the urine and boiling for 30 min. The explanation for these color changes is that porphobilinogen (colorless) and not uroporphyrin (red) is excreted in the urine. Heating of porphobilinogen in an acid medium results in the nonenzymatic formation of uroporphyrin, together with a dark-brown or reddish-brown nonporphyrin pigment. (8:498)

51. **B.** The qualitative determination of porphobilinogen by the Watson-Schwartz modification of the Ehrlich reaction is a simple and valuable screening procedure. (8:498)

52. **D.** In patients with acute intermittent porphyria, the porphyrin content of the bone marrow is normal. All other statements are true. (8:497–8)

53. **C.** Acute, intermittent porphyria has a marked familial occurrence. It is probably transmitted as a mendelian dominant characteristic. All other statements are true. (8:497)

54. **E.** Acute, intermittent porphyria is characterized by all the clinical features listed. (8:497–8)

55. **D.** In acute intermittent porphyria, except for pain in the extremities, sensory changes are usually not prominent, and signs of upper motor neuron changes are usually absent. The neurologic manifestations may simulate a wide variety of conditions, including poliomyelitis, encephalitis, and arsenic or lead poisoning. The mortality rate is high. Abdominal pain, not neuromuscular and psychotic symptoms, is usually the presenting complaint. (8:497–8)

56. **E.** All the factors listed may precipitate acute intermittent porphyria. (8:494, 498–99)

57. **C.** The Watson-Schwartz test is quite specific for acute, intermittent porphyria. The test is negative in erythropoietic porphyria and in porphyria cutanea tarda symptomatica. It is positive in patients with porphyria cutanea tarda hereditaria during acute attacks but is negative in the interval between such episodes. (8:499)

58. **C.** The most effective treatment of the acute attack is to provide a liberal intake of glucose, either orally or intravenously. A low carbohydrate intake enhances ALA induction and a high intake suppresses the induction of this enzyme, the so-called "glucose effect." Rapid remissions may be induced by a high carbohydrate intake. (8:498)

59. **B.** In this patient the most likely diagnosis is carcinoid syndrome. (8:476)

60. **A.** Serotonin was the first agent to be discovered, and overproduction of this amine is the most consistent biochemical indicator of the carcinoid syndrome. Serotonin, however, is not the sole mediator of the clinical syndrome. All other statements are correct. (8:476)

61. **E.** Patients with this syndrome may have tumors which elaborate serotonin, histamine, adrenocorticotropic hormone (ACTH), bradykinin, or an additional unidentified substance which helps to produce flushing. (8:476)

62. **C.** Carcinoid tumors have an unusually slow rate of growth; most patients survive for five to ten years after the disease is recognized. (8:476)

63. **C.** A rise in blood pressure during flushing is rare, and carcinoid syndrome is not a cause of sustained hypertension. Malabsorption may occur in this syndrome, and the cardiac manifestations mentioned occur primarily in the right side of the heart. (8:476)

64. **A.** The diagnostic hallmark of this syndrome is overproduction of 5-hydroxyindoles with

increased urinary excretion of 5-hydroxyin-doleacetic acid. (8:478)

65. **D.** Tumors from all the locations listed may produce this syndrome before metastatic disease occurs. (8:476)

66. **E.** All the statements are true concerning the treatment of this disorder. (8.478–79)

67. **D.** The most likely diagnosis in this patient is heavy metal poisoning. (5:225–28)

68. **E.** Lead in the bootleg whiskey is the most probable cause of the patient's coma. (5:224)

69. **D.** The most serious toxic effect of lead poisoning results from its effect on the brain and peripheral nervous system. (5:225)

70. **A.** In acute lead poisoning, pathologic findings include inflammation of the gastrointestinal mucosa and renal tubular degeneration. All other statements are true of chronic lead poisoning. (5.225)

71. **A.** The most serious toxic effects result from effects of lead on the brain and peripheral nervous system. The lead in these tissues is only slowly removable by deleading agents. Since only uncombined lead is removed effectively by deleading agents, the increased excretion of lead brought about by such agents is only temporary. The deleading agent only becomes effective again when further lead has been released from combination. All other statements are correct. (5:225, 228–29)

72. **A.** In patients with lead intoxication, the urine coproporphyrin is 0.5 mg/liter or above. All other factors listed are correct. (5:227)

73. **E.** Lead poisoning may result in an increase in reticulocytes. All other factors are correct. (5:226)

74. **C.** Blood changes may include an increase in all forms of basophilic cells. All other changes listed are true. In addition, there may be an increase in reticulocytes and decreased platelets. (5:226)

75. **C.** The most likely diagnosis is hepatitis B. (*Public Health Reports*, III:149, 1974)

76. **E.** The treatment will not likely involve any of the modalities listed. (*Public Health Reports*, III:149, 1974)

77. **E.** Direct spread of hepatitis B infection by person-to-person contact has only recently been recognized. In the 1940s, experiments with volunteers failed to demonstrate transmission of hepatitis B virus by fecal-oral routes. Nonetheless, even at that time, it was suggested that nonparenteral spread could have occurred among close contacts of patients who contracted hepatitis B from immunization with icterogenic pooled yellow fever vaccine. In 1967, in experimental studies at Willowbrook State School, Krugman demonstrated serum-oral transmission of hepatitis B virus. Others have shown that this type of spread can also occasionally occur naturally under unique epidemiological circumstances. Skin rash and joint pains are more frequently associated with hepatitis B infection than with hepatitis A. Hepatitis B symptoms are usually more severe than those of hepatitis A and last longer. Chronic complications occur more frequently in hepatitis B; 5 to 10% of patients have such problems as fulminant hepatic necrosis, chronic active hepatitis, or cirrhosis. (*Public Health Reports*, III: 149, 1974)

78. **A.** For persons without serious underlying disease, the incidence of chronic antigenemia following acute hepatitis B infection has been shown to be less than 10%. (*Public Health Reports*, III:152, 1974)

79. **C.** In the United States and western Europe, 0.1 to 0.6% of asymptomatic adults are chronic carriers of hepatitis B antigen. (*Public Health Reports*, III:153, 1974)

80. **A.** Failure to detect hepatitis B antigen in a patient with acute hepatitis does not always exclude the diagnosis of hepatitis B. All other statements are correct. (*Public Health Reports*, III:153,156, 1974)

81. **E.** Immune serum globulin (ISG) is effective in preventing infection when it is administered prior to exposure to hepatitis A virus. All other statements are true. (*Public Health Reports*, III:154,160, 1974)

82. **E.** Transmission of hepatitis B by stool, urine, or saliva containing hepatitis B antigen has not yet been convincingly demonstrated, although antigen has been detected in urine, stool, and saliva from patients in the acute phase of hepatitis B infection. (*Public Health Reports*, III:156, 1974)

83. **B.** No increased prevalence of antigenemia has been observed in spouses of chronic hepatitis B antigen carriers, and women who acquire acute hepatitis B while pregnant can transmit the infection to their infant. (*Public Health Reports*, III:156,158, 1974)

84. **E.** ISG is of no value in the treatment of hepatitis A. All other statements are correct. The administration of ISG after exposure to hepatitis A acts to lessen the severity of clinical manifestations of disease rather than prevent infection.
(*Public Health Reports,* III:160, 1974)

85. **B.** The most likely diagnosis in the patient described would be mitral-valve prolapse syndrome. (*JAMA,* 236:867, 1976)

86. **B.** This disorder occurs more commonly in women than in men. (*JAMA,* 236:867, 1976)

87. **B.** An unexpected electrocardiographic finding in this patient would be a shortened QT interval; the interval in this disorder is often prolonged. (*JAMA,* 236:867, 1976)

88. **C.** There is a general lack of patient awareness of the recorded arrhythmias contrasted with a frequent lack of recorded arrhythmias during subjective experiences of palpitations.
(*JAMA,* 236:867, 1976)

89. **A.** There are some patients with typical clinical findings—i.e., typical history, midsystolic click, and late systolic murmur, arrhythmias, and a left ventricular angiogram suggesting mitral valve prolapse—in whom the echocardiogram is normal. Therefore, the echocardiogram cannot be used as the single hallmark for the diagnosis of this condition. In addition, there are no angiocardiographic criteria for the diagnosis of this condition that are acceptable to all angiographers; therefore, the angiogram is not a perfect tool for diagnosing this condition.
(*JAMA,* 236:867, 1976)

90. **E.** All statements are true.
(*JAMA,* 236:867, 1976)

91. **D.** The chronic fatigue found in this condition is relatively refractory to therapy and often worsens with propranolol hydrochloride. All other statements are true. (*JAMA,* 236:870, 1976)

92. **E.** All the disorders listed may be complications of the mitral-valve prolapse syndrome.
(*JAMA,* 236:870, 1976)

93. **D.** The most likely diagnosis is Parkinson's disease. (1:613)

94. **C.** Diagnosis of this disorder is best made by history and physical examination. (1:613)

95. **E.** Blacks are rarely affected by Parkinson's disease. All other statements are true of this disorder. (1:614)

96. **C.** This form of postencephalitic parkinsonism is felt to be caused by von Economo's encephalitis. (1:613)

97. **D.** The cause of classic Parkinson's disease is believed to be idiopathic. (1:613)

98. **E.** A parkinsonian syndrome is sometimes seen following manganese poisoning, and in lead, carbon monoxide, and carbon disulfide intoxication. (1:614)

99. **C.** Paralysis agitans has recently been attributed to emotional factors, but there is no good evidence that emotional strain is capable of producing a genuine disorder of this type. All other statements are correct. (1:614—616)

100. **B.** In cases of parkinsonism, there is a striking reduction in the dopamine content of the striatum. (1:616)

101. **A.** The disease process chiefly affects the substantia nigra and the pallidum, the striatum (caudate and putamen) generally being affected to a lesser degree. Lesions have also been found on occasion in the corpus subthalamicum, medulla, hypothalamus, central gray matter, around the aqueduct and the third ventricle, and the cerebral cortex. (1:615)

102. **C.** The neostriatal cells are actually in a state of equilibrium under ordinary circumstances, modulated by the inhibitory dopaminergic system on one hand and by facilitory cholinergic changes on the other. (1:616)

103. **B.** The relative specificity of derangement in the dopamine-influenced inhibition in parkinsonism in particular is underscored by the fact that in other diseases of the basal ganglia presenting with disorders of movement such as Huntington's chorea, the dopamine and homovanillic acid concentrations are normal. (1:617)

104. **D.** The clinical features of the parkinsonian state may be lessened by any of the methods listed. (1:617)

105. **E.** The manifestations of paralysis agitans are usually bilateral but it is not uncommon for them to be unilateral, either in the beginning of the illness or throughout its course. All other features listed are correct. In addition, fatigue is a frequent symptom. Other and less common complaints may bring the patient to the physician for relief. Among these are awareness of difficulty with speech or of change in facial appearance. Drag-

ging of the legs in walking or difficulty in lifting the legs to negotiate steps may also be early symptoms. (1:617)

106. **D.** As Parkinson's disease advances, the rigidity becomes greater and the tremor more severe until the patient is confined to a chair or bed. All other statements are true.

107. **E.** In the tremor of Parkinson's disease, flexion and extension movements are not uncommon. All other statements are true. (1:618)

108. **E.** Tremor of the legs is much less common than in the hands. It usually involves the calves but may spread to the thighs. All other statements are correct. (1:619)

109. **D.** All tremors of Parkinson's disease are increased by emotional stress, fatigue, and anxiety, and disappear during sleep. (1:619)

110. **E.** All statements are true. (1:619)

111. **B.** In patients with Parkinson's disease, the handwriting is tremulous and often micrographic. All other statements are correct. (1:620)

112. **D.** In Parkinson's disease, the glabellar reflex is negative. All other statements are correct. (1:620)

113. **D.** All statements are true of the oculogyric crises in Parkinson's disease. (1:620)

114. **D.** Tremor may be less prominent in the postencephalitic than in idiopathic paralysis agitans, and choreoathetosis is sometimes encountered. All other statements are correct. (1:621)

115. **E.** All of the statements are true. (1:621, 622)

116. **E.** Drug therapy is at times of great benefit in patients with Parkinson's disease. Many drugs have been advocated. No single drug treatment is effective, and the dosage and type must be worked out in every case individually. (1:622)

117. **E.** All the principles listed are important to remember when dealing with the drug treatment of Parkinson's disease. (1:622)

118. **A.** All the drugs listed are helpful in controlling the rigidity of Parkinson's disease; there is no known drug at present that is uniformly capable of controlling tremor or akinesia. (1:622)

119. **E.** Symmetrel, unlike the other drugs listed, is not a synthetic belladonna-like agent, nor does it possess significant anticholinergic properties. (1:623)

120. **E.** A patient being treated for Parkinson's disease with one of the synthetic belladonna-like agents may experience any of the side effects listed. (*Clin Symp*, 28:23, 1976)

121. **A.** L-Dopa is not effective in iatrogenic parkinsonism caused by phenothiazines and related medication. All other statements are true. (*Clin Symp*, 28:26, 1976)

122. **E.** All statements are true of therapy with L-dopa. (*Clin Symp*, 28:28, 1976)

123. **D.** The most likely diagnosis in this patient is Wolff-Parkinson-White syndrome. (3:363)

124. **E.** This syndrome is usually not associated with cardiac disease. All other statements are true. (3:363, 366)

125. **E.** All the statements are true. (3:363, 364)

126. **E.** The P-J interval is usually normal in patients with this syndrome, since the shortened P-R interval compensates for the QRS prolongation. All other statements are correct. (3:364)

127. **B.** ST and T wave abnormalities may occur in this syndrome. All other statements are correct. (3:364, 365)

128. **D.** Paroxysmal tachyarrhythmias occur in approximately 50 to 75% of patients with this syndrome. (3:366)

129. **D.** Ventricular tachycardia has been reported in patients with this condition, but such an arrhythmia may be misdiagnosed and probably represents a supraventricular tachycardia with aberrant conduction in almost all such cases. All other statements are correct. (3:366)

130. **D.** In this syndrome, aberrant ventricular conduction is present in about 30% of the arrhythmias. (3:366)

131. **B.** Patients with the preexcitation syndrome usually enjoy a good prognosis. All other statements are false. (3:366)

132. **E.** All statements are true of the treatment of the preexcitation syndrome. (3:366)

133. **B.** The most likely diagnosis is hypoparathyroidism. (4:421)

134. **B.** The patient's spasmatic hand movement indicated a positive Trousseau's sign. (4:421–22)

135. **C.** The reaction described would indicate a positive Chvostek sign. (4:421)

136. **C.** This illness occurs most frequently as a result of surgery on the thyroid gland, and a thyroidectomy scar suggests the acquired disease. (4:421)

137. **E.** All the statements are true of hypoparathyroidism. (4:421)

138. **E.** Patients with decreased renal function may have hypocalcemia due to hypoproteinemia, hyperphosphatemia, and decreased renal production of 1,25-dihydroxycholecalciferol. (4:425)

139. **D.** All statements are true of this patient. (4:425)

140. **E.** LE preparation, ANA and rheumatoid factor would be least indicated in the workup of a patient with hypoparathyroidism and hypocalcemia. (4:425)

141. **D.** All the X-rays listed may be helpful in the workup of hypoparathyroidism and hypocalcemic states. (4:425)

142. **D.** In hypoparathyroidism, one would not expect increased urine hydroxyproline. All other results listed are correct. (4:412)

143. **E.** Serum phosphate would be elevated with a decreased urine phosphate. (4:412)

144. **E.** Hypocalcemia may be associated with any of the disorders listed. (4:421)

145. **D.** Overt tetany is the presenting complaint in approximately 70% of cases of hypoparathyroidism. (4:421)

146. **C.** The electrocardiogram would probably show prolongation of the QT interval. (4:422)

147. **D.** All of the statements are true of hypoparathyroidism. (4:422, 426)

148. **A.** Sodium bicarbonate would not be used in the treatment of acute hypocalcemia. (4:424–25)

149. **E.** All statements are true of the control of chronic hypocalcemia secondary to hypoparathyroidism. (4:425–26)

150. **D.** All the statements listed are true. (4:425)

151. **D.** All statements are true of severe vitamin D deficiency. (4:425)

152. **D.** This patient probably has alimentary hypoglycemia. (6:817–18)

153. **D.** The symptoms and signs of hypoglycemia are generally reversible, but permanent brain damage can result from prolonged, severe hypoglycemia. (6:816)

154. **D.** Insulinoma would be most likely associated with fasting hypoglycemia. (6:817)

155. **D.** Alimentary hypoglycemia is classified under postprandial hypoglycemic states. The other conditions listed can induce a fasting hypoglycemia. (6:817)

156. **C.** In hypoglycemia induced by food ingestion, significant central nervous system symptoms are uncommon. (6:817)

157. **B.** In adults, hypoglycemia is usually related to the intake of glucose. (6:817)

158. **C.** The procedure of choice to document postprandial hypoglycemia is a five-hour glucose tolerance test. (6:817)

159. **C.** Reactive (functional or idiopathic) hypoglycemia is the most common of the postprandial hypoglycemias. (6:817)

160. **B.** In reactive, functional hypoglycemia, serum insulin levels are generally appropriate for the blood sugar levels. All other statements are correct. (6:817)

161. **E.** Even without treatment, symptoms of reactive, functional hypoglycemia are frequently self-limited to a period of 6 to 18 months. (6:818–819)

162. **C.** The syndrome of alimentary hypoglycemia would be least likely to occur in patients with diabetes mellitus. (6:818)

163. **E.** In alimentary hypoglycemia, a precipitous rise in blood glucose levels, resulting from the rapid entry of large amounts of glucose into the small intestine, provokes dramatic secretion of insulin and subsequent hypoglycemia as early as the first hour of a glucose tolerance test. Patients should be advised to eat slowly and to consume small meals which contain little concentrated sweets. (6:818)

Textbook References for Chapter 3

1. Alpers, B.J. and Mancall, E.L. (1971): *Clinical Neurology*, F.A. Davis Company, Philadelphia.

2. Beeson, P.B. and McDermott, W. (1979): *Cecil Textbook of Medicine*, Fifteenth Edition, W.B. Saunders Company, Philadelphia.

3. Conn, H.L. and Horwitz, O. (1971): *Cardiac and Vascular Disease*, Volume I, Lea & Febiger, Philadelphia.

4. Dillon, R.S. (1980): *Handbook of Endocrinology: Diagnosis and Management of Endocrine and Metabolic Disorders*, Lea & Febiger, Philadelphia.

5. Dreisbach, R.H. (1980): *Handbook of Poisoning*, Tenth Edition, Lange Medical Publications, Los Altos, California.

6. Harvey, A.M. (1980): *The Principles and Practice of Medicine*, Twentieth Edition, Appleton-Century-Crofts, New York.

7. McCarty, D.L., Editor (1979): *Arthritis and Allied Conditions*, Ninth Edition, Lea & Febiger, Philadelphia.

8. Isselbacher, K.J., Editor (1980): *Harrison's Principles of Internal Medicine*, Ninth Edition, McGraw-Hill Book Company, New York.

CHAPTER 4

Alterations in Normal Function

Directions: Indicate whether each of the following statements is true or false.

1. In severe accidental hypothermia, external rewarming is indicated.

2. Exertion causes a further fall in plasma glucose in patients with insulinomas or other types of fasting hypoglycemia, but causes a rise in plasma glucose in patients without fasting hypoglycemia such as functional hypoglycemia states.

3. A 10% increase in hematocrit for clinical purposes may generally be taken to indicate similar contraction of the extracellular fluid volume.

4. Hyponatremic patients with congestive heart failure who are rapidly diuresed usually show a depression in BUN levels.

5. Deviations from normal in plasma pH will alter the ratio of ionized calcium to total calcium, acidosis producing a decreased and alkalosis, an increased ratio.

6. Hypercalcemia occurring in neoplastic conditions may be related to immunoglobulin deficiency.

7. Oculocephalic reflexes (doll's eye movements) are present in the normal person.

8. All factors that affect protein binding influence the T_4 and T_3 tests in opposite directions.

9. Most patients with hypercalcemia and sarcoidosis have hypergammaglobulinemia.

10. The often dramatic effect of dexamethasone in relieving cerebral edema may be partly due to increased ion exchange accompanying a fall in intracellular $3',5'$-cyclic AMP.

11. Rectal temperature averages one-half to one degree lower than oral.

12. That water intoxication in association with neoplasm is due to an ADH abnormality is borne out by the finding of ADH-like materials in tumor extracts, especially the oat-cell variety of the lung.

13. Deficiency of blood supply to the sinus node has been demonstrated to occur in sinus bradycardia complicating myocardial infarction.

14. In systemic allergic vasculitis, only the larger vessels are usually involved.

15. Glucose tends to increase serum potassium levels.

16. Patients with emphysema usually have more difficulty breathing when recumbent.

Directions: For each of the incomplete statements below, ONE or MORE of the completions given is correct. In each case, select
  A. if 1, 2, and 3 are correct
  B. if 1 and 3 are correct
  C. if 2 and 4 are correct
  D. if only 4 is correct
  E. if all are correct

17. Nocturia may be seen in association with
  1. benign prostatic hypertrophy
  2. diabetes mellitus
  3. urinary tract infections
  4. reversed diurnal rhythm as occurs with renal and circulatory insufficiency

18. Major gastrointestinal pain mechanisms include
  1. capsular stretching, as in liver congestion due to heart failure
  2. irritation of the mucosa, as in acute gastritis
  3. severe smooth muscle spasm, as in acute enterocolitis
  4. peritoneal inflammation, as in acute appendicitis

19. The usual causes of hyponatremia in patients who are *not* edematous include
  1. volume (salt) depletion
  2. inappropriate ADH secretion
  3. adrenal insufficiency
  4. congestive heart failure

20. Patients secreting ADH because of hypovolemia require
  1. replacement of sodium deficits
  2. replacement of water deficits
  3. specific hormonal therapy
  4. correction of the underlying disease state

21. Postural syncope tends to occur under which of the following conditions?
  1. in otherwise normal persons who for some unknown reason have defective postural reflexes
  2. rarely, as a part of a syndrome named primary autonomic insufficiency, which includes chronic orthostatic hypotension, as well as symptoms of peripheral preganglionic autonomic and extrapyramidal disorder
  3. after physical deconditioning; e.g., after prolonged illness with recumbency, especially in elderly individuals with flabby muscles
  4. in diabetic and other neuropathies, tabes dorsalis, and diseases of the nervous system which cause muscular atrophy and paralysis of vasopressor reflexes

22. Aortic systolic ejection murmurs occur with
  1. valvular stenosis
  2. primary dilatation of the ascending aorta
  3. subvalvular stenosis
  4. decreased left ventricular stroke output

23. Exercise-induced bronchospasm may be prevented by
  1. beta-adrenergic agonist
  2. theophylline
  3. carbon dioxide breathing
  4. atropine

24. Diseases and conditions which are occasionally accompanied by seizures include
  1. polycythemia
  2. carbon monoxide poisoning
  3. Raynaud's disease
  4. Stokes-Adam's syndrome

Directions: For each of the following statements, fill in the correct word.

25. _____ is involuntary, repetitive, rapid movement of the eyeball.

26. Amyloid is structurally related to the _____ chains of immunoglobulins.

27. Cerebral _____ is a more or less diffuse disturbance to the brain following head injury characterized by edema and capillary hemorrhaging, which are most frequently present at the poles of the hemispheres.

28. The presence of nodules within the palm associated with firm fibrous bands which limit extension of the fingers suggests _____ contracture.

29. _____ is a polypeptide enzyme which cleaves kinin from its circulating liver-synthesized precursor—kininogen or prokinin.

30. Trotter has defined _____ as a condition of widespread paralysis of the functions of the brain which comes on as an immediate consequence of a blow on the head, has a strong tendency to spontaneous recovery, and is not necessarily associated with any gross organic change in the brain substance.

31. Homonymous _____ is the loss of vision in the nasal half of the visual field in one eye and the temporal half in the other.

32. Almost all focal cerebral lesions of sudden onset are in one way or another _____ in origin.

33. A failure to execute certain acts in the correct context while retaining the ability to carry out the individual movements upon which such acts depend is the main feature of _____ .

34. The beta-adrenergic theory offers the most plausible postulate to date with which to explain the varied etiologic relationship of bronchial hyperreactivity in _____ .

35. _____ is a state of increased amounts of body and facial hair, especially in the female.

36. Digitalization _____ the threshold for potassium toxicity.

37. A primary embolus in the lung is lysed by _____ released from the pulmonary arterial endothelium, but there is a continuous formation of secondary thrombus in response to the primary emboli.

38. For each 0.1 unit rise in the blood pH, the serum potassium level will _____ by 0.5 to 1.0 mEq/liter.

39. _____ is a sudden, brief loss of muscular power evoked by strong emotion, usually laughter.

40. Cells which have acquired excess intracellular sodium at the expense of the extracellular compartment may lie at the root of hyponatremia in various different conditions. This has been termed the _____ -cell syndrome.

Directions: Use the key below to answer the following questions. Select
  A. **if 1, 2, and 3 are correct**
  B. **if 1 and 3 are correct**
  C. **if 2 and 4 are correct**
  D. **if all statements are correct**
  E. **if none of the statements is correct**
  F. **if another combination is correct**

41. Lysosomes
  1. are cytoplasmic granules of polymorphonuclear leukocytes
  2. are separated from the rest of the cell by a lipoprotein membrane
  3. are functionally related to the inflammatory and microcirculatory responses, the

clotting system, complements, kinins, and fever generation
4. are stabilized by endotoxin

42. Autoimmune processes that may be forerunners of the neoplastic process include

1. hemolytic anemia
2. idiopathic thrombocytopenia purpura
3. Hashimoto's disease
4. rheumatoid arthritis
5. systemic lupus erythematosus

43. Physiological manifestations of chronic obstructive pulmonary disease include

1. decreased closing volume
2. increased frequency-dependent compliance
3. decreased airway resistance
4. increased maximum voluntary ventilation
5. increased first-second forced expiratory volume

44. Hypotheses for pathogenesis of asthma include

1. increased parasympathetic activity
2. beta-adrenergic blockade
3. beta-adrenergic amine deficiency
4. release of histamine and slow reacting substance of anaphylaxis from mast cells.

45. Low or normal digitalis blood levels may induce toxicity when associated with

1. hypokalemia
2. hypomagnesemia
3. pulmonary disease and hypoxia
4. excessive end-organ sensitivity, as in myocardial infarction
5. excessive end-organ sensitivity, as in hypothyroidism

Directions: If the following disorder is found in females more commonly than in males, select the letter A; if it is more common in males, select the letter B.

46. Habitual hyperthermia

Directions: For each of the following multiple-choice questions, select the ONE CORRECT answer.

47. When renal function is normal, the half-life of digoxin in serum or plasma is 1.6 days, whereas in a totally anuric patient, it is prolonged to about how many days?

A. 2.0
B. 2.5
C. 3.2
D. 4.4
E. 7.2

48. As revealed by radiolabeling, endotoxin localizes in the endothelium and walls of

A. arterioles
B. capillaries
C. venules
D. all of the above
E. none of the above

Directions: For each of the following multiple-choice questions, select the ONE INCORRECT answer.

49. Goodpasture's syndrome

A. is characterized by hematuria associated with hemoptysis
B. may follow a respiratory-tract infection
C. is described chiefly in young women
D. is characterized by typical, bilateral pulmonary lesions
E. characteristically, on immunofluorescent staining, IgG and complement are deposited along glomerular basement membrane in a continuous and linear fashion

50. Aleutian disease in mink is characterized by

A. Coombs'-positive hemolytic anemia
B. hypergammaglobulinemia
C. diffuse plasma-cell infiltrates
D. fibrinoid arteritis
E. changes in the tissues suggesting a conversion to multiple myeloma

51. Elevated creatine phosphokinase levels may be associated with

    A. intramuscular injections
    B. alcohol ingestion
    C. strenuous exercise
    D. hypothyroidism
    E. small muscle mass

52. Kinins

    A. are polypeptides, 9 to 11 amino acids in length
    B. produce hypertension and decreased blood vessel permeability
    C. influence smooth muscle contractility, produce leukotaxis, and cause pain
    D. or more specifically, the kinin cascade, is activated by endotoxin, antigen-antibody complexes, or cold, with the Hageman factor acting as an essential intermediate
    E. inactivated by kinases, result in a very short half-life

53. Hemodynamic alterations considered peculiar to septic shock include

    A. moderate hypertension
    B. oliguria
    C. dry, and/or warm skin
    D. abnormally high cardiac output
    E. appreciable decrease in general systemic vascular resistance

Directions: Use the key below to answer the following question.
   A. if both the statement and reason are true and are related as to cause and effect
   B. if both the statement and reason are true, but are not related as to cause and effect
   C. if the statement is true, but the reason is false
   D. if the statement is false, but the reason is true
   E. if both the statement and reason are false

54. There is increasing evidence that endotoxin tolerance is an immunologic phenomenon **because** it can be passively transferred with 19S immunoglobulins, and animals previously immunized manifest a good anamnestic response.

Directions: Use the key below to answer the following question.
   A. if A is more appropriate than B
   B. if B is more appropriate than A
   C. if A and B are equal or approximately equal

55. Raised circulating levels of immunoreactive parathyroid hormone-like substance have been described in

    A. hypernephroma
    B. breast cancer

Directions: For each of the incomplete statements below, ONE or MORE of the completions given is correct. In each case, select
   A. if 1, 2, and 3 are correct
   B. if 1 and 3 are correct
   C. if 2 and 4 are correct
   D. if only 4 is correct
   E. if all are correct

56. In the NZB mouse strain,

    1. there is a higher incidence of autoimmune hemolytic anemia with positive Coombs and LE tests
    2. there is a high incidence of membranous glomerulonephritis
    3. the lymphoid tissues show increasingly bizarre changes with the passage of time
    4. virus particles (mostly C-type) may be present in lymphoid tissues

57. Horner's syndrome

    1. is caused by sympathetic paralysis
    2. is characterized by ptosis of the upper lid
    3. is characterized by constriction of the pupil
    4. is characterized by increased sweating

58. Disorders which can cause a bounding pulse include

    1. fever
    2. anemia
    3. hepatic failure
    4. thyrotoxicosis

59. Falsely elevated temperature readings may result from

    1. inadequate shaking down of the thermometer
    2. previous ingestion of warm substances
    3. recent strenuous activity
    4. a very warm bath

60. A hydrocele

    1. is a fluid-containing cystic mass, usually arising as a result of incomplete obliteration of the processus vaginalis
    2. is common in infancy and is often bilateral
    3. may occur in the scrotum as a hydrocele of the testis
    4. may appear anywhere along the inguinal canal as a hydrocele of the cord

    Directions: For each of the following questions select
    A. **if the question is associated with A only**
    B. **if the question is associated with B only**
    C. **if the question is associated with both A and B**
    D. **if the question is associated with neither A nor B**

61. Intravenous administration of bradykinin produces marked

    A. systemic arteriolar contraction
    B. venoconstriction
    C. both
    D. neither

62. Cerebral concussion is associated with

    A. no loss of consciousness
    B. loss of memory regarding the accident
    C. both
    D. neither

63. In patients with diabetes mellitus, there is

    A. no evidence that immunologic competence is impaired
    B. a defect in chemotaxis of PMN leukocytes
    C. both
    D. neither

64. In gram-negative bacteremia,

    A. respiratory alkalosis may be an early manifestation
    B. metabolic acidosis is an infrequent accompaniment of the shock
    C. both
    D. neither

65. Studies on digoxin absorption in patients with malabsorption syndromes indicate that digoxin

    A. is poorly and erratically absorbed by patients with malabsorption on the basis of mucosal defects or hypermotility
    B. may be more normally absorbed by patients with pancreatic insufficiency
    C. both
    D. neither

66. The eosinopenic effect of epinephrine

    A. is purely a beta-adrenergic effect and can be completely reversed with propranolol
    B. glucocorticoids exert a permissive effect
    C. both
    D. neither

67. Carcinoma of the prostate

    A. occurs in approximately 20% of men over 60 years of age
    B. (the initial lesion) usually involves the posterior lobe and is readily palpable at rectal examination
    C. both
    D. neither

68. Nystagmoid movements of the eyes are

    A. irregular jerks observed in many normal individuals when the eyes are turned far to the side
    B. probably similar to the tremulousness of a muscle that is contracted maximally
    C. both
    D. neither

69. Serum levels that decrease with age include

    A. serum cholesterol
    B. serum triglyceride
    C. both
    D. neither

70. Largely blocked by atropine in normal subjects:

    A. hypocapnia-induced bronchospasm
    B. exercise-induced bronchospasm
    C. both
    D. neither

71. Normal subjects excrete more than 50% of a water load in three hours and the urine osmolality falls to less than 100 mOsm/kg coincidentally with a fall in plasma osmolality and disappearance of urinary ADH. In the presence of the inappropriate ADH syndrome,

    A. water excretion is unimpaired
    B. urinary ADH persists although initial plasma osmolality is low and falls further during water loading
    C. both
    D. neither

72. Pain may

    A. cause coronary artery dilatation
    B. stimulate excretion of catecholamines which can cause an increase in heart rate, cardiac output, and heart work
    C. both
    D. neither

73. Pseudohyponatremia

    A. is a misleading reduction in the serum sodium concentration that occurs when there is an osmotic material, usually glucose, in the extracellular fluid
    B. may occur in association with hyperlipidemia or hyperproteinemia in which there are large quantities of lipids or globulin in the plasma
    C. both
    D. neither

74. Normal subjects, given 8.5 liters of daily fluid during a 4-week period, have shown

    A. decreased serum osmolality
    B. a tendency to reduce urine osmolality
    C. both
    D. neither

75. Which of the following can result in hyponatremia and persistent antidiuresis and may also be mediated by a decrease in "effective" extracellular fluid volume and persistent volume receptor stimulation?

    A. cirrhosis with ascites
    B. advanced cardiac failure
    C. both
    D. neither

76. Hypercalcemia is a frequent finding in metastatic, osteolytic breast cancer occurring

    A. spontaneously
    B. after the administration of sex steroids
    C. both
    D. neither

77. Mutism refers to complete loss of speech in a conscious patient in the presence of

    A. aphasia
    B. anarthria
    C. both
    D. neither

78. In grand mal seizures,

    A. in some patients, particularly women, there is an apparent periodicity to the attacks which can be associated with menstrual periods
    B. approximately 50% of the patients experience some sort of aura
    C. both
    D. neither

Directions: Indicate whether each of the following statements is true or false.

79. Patients with congestive heart failure often have an elevation of body temperature between 0.5 and 1.5°F.

80. Since most blood tests of thyroid hormone primarily measure the bound fraction, medications which affect the thyroxine-binding relationships will alter the test results.

81. Extensive bleeding into the thyroid has been observed in thyrotoxic patients who have received radioactive iodine therapeutically while on anticoagulant therapy.

82. The same mechanism responsible for the giant "a" wave with right ventricular hypertrophy, namely very forceful atrial contraction, may result in a palpable presystolic component to the apex impulse with left ventricular hypertrophy.

83. In acidosis, blood is still able to unload oxygen to the tissues and circulation is therefore functional, while alkalosis inhibits this oxygen release and renders circulation less effective.

84. In myxedematous persons, hypertension occurs at a greater frequency than in nonmyxedematous persons.

Answers and Commentary

1. **False.** In accidental hypothermia, therapy should be instituted at once and consist of maintenance of the airway and intravenous administration of glucose, saline, or other agents to expand blood volume and to prevent infarctions which have been a hallmark in fatal cases. External rewarming is contraindicated in serious cases because, while it tends to dilate the constricted peripheral blood vessels, it diverts blood from the visceral organs; many patients who have been rewarmed externally have died. On the other hand, restoration of the core temperature by hemodialysis, during which the blood is warmed externally, or by peritoneal dialysis during which the dialysate is warmed to 98.6°F is helpful. Corticosteroids, vasopressors, and prophylactic antibiotics have not proved valuable. Large volumes of fluid may be needed. The prognosis in accidental hypothermia remains poor, primarily because many of these patients are old and have associated debilitating disease. One young patient was saved even after her temperature dropped to 69°F (20.6°C).

   (5:58)

2. **True.** Exertion causes a further fall in plasma glucose in patients with insulinomas or other types of fasting hypoglycemia, but causes a rise in plasma glucose in patients without fasting hypoglycemia as in functional hypoglycemic states. (*Mod Med*, 41:24, (1973)

3. **True.** A 10% increase in hematocrit, for clinical purposes, may generally be taken to indicate similar contraction of the extracellular fluid volume. In a man weighing 70 kg, this would reflect a deficit of approximately 1.4 liters (10% of the 14 liters). (*Ann Intern Med*, 82:64, 1975)

4. **False.** On occasion, strong diuretics may cause such a rapid diuresis that the edema stores cannot replace the vascular stores fast enough, and a prerenal azotemia may result. What is frequently overlooked, however, is that a patient with congestive heart failure may have started with a BUN that was actually higher than his report showed because the BUN was "diluted" in the same manner as the sodium. After diuresis, the dilutional state that was previously present may be eased with an apparent rise in BUN.

   (*Patient Care*, 9:22, 1975)

5. **False.** Deviations from normal in plasma pH will alter the ratio of ionized calcium to total calcium, acidosis producing an increased and alkalosis, a decreased ratio.

   [*Condenser* (Bio-Science Labs), 5:3, 1974]

6. **True.** Brugarolas and Takita of the Roswell Park Memorial Institute, working on the hypothesis that "hypercalcemia occurring in neoplastic conditions could be related to an immunoglobulin deficiency," administered 2 ml of human gammaglobulin to each of 16 patients with hypercalcemia resistant to conventional therapy. These patients all had advanced, progressive malignancies, including 12 with carcinoma of the lung, three with hypernephroma, two with carcinoma of the breast, and one with carcinoma of the nasopharynx. With just this one dose of gammaglobulin, nine of the 16 patients showed a progressive drop in serum calcium levels to within normal limits in 7 to 12 days. They then remained normocalcemic for one to four months, despite continued progression of their malignancies. After varying lengths of time, four patients relapsed into hypercalcemia, and again responded to a dose of gammaglobulin. By contrast, the

seven patients who did not respond promptly to gammaglobulin administration showed no improvement whatever.   (*Inf Dis*, 3:21, 1973)

7.   **False.**   Ocular movements are altered in a variety of ways. In light coma from metabolic abnormalities, the eyes may rove from side to side in random fashion like the slow eye movements of light sleep, with disappearance as brainstem function becomes depressed. Oculocephalic reflexes (doll's eye movements), elicited by briskly turning or tilting the head with eyes moving conjugately in the opposite direction, are exaggerated. They are not present in the normal person, and if they are elicitable, evidence is obtained of the integrity of the tegmental structures of the midbrain and pons which integrate ocular movements, and of the third, fourth, and sixth cranial nerves.   (5:119)

8.   **True.**   All factors which affect protein binding influence the T₄ and T₃ tests in opposite directions.   (*Am Fam Physician*, 3:73, 1971)

9.   **True.**   The majority of sarcoid patients with hypercalcemia have been found to have elevated gammaglobulin levels.   (*Mod Med*, 41:83, 1973)

10.   **False.**   The often dramatic effect of dexamethasone in relieving cerebral edema may be partly due to increased ion exchange accompanying a rise in intracellular 3', 5'-cyclic AMP.   (*Lancet*, 1:342, 1974)

11.   **False.**   Rectal temperature averages one-half to one degree higher than oral.   (2:35)

12.   **True.**   Tumor extracts have been found to contain neurophysin, a protein normally found only in the posterior pituitary.   (*Mod Med*, 41:39, 1973)

13.   **True.**   Deficiency of blood supply to the sinus node has been demonstrated to occur in sinus bradycardia complicating myocardial infarction.   (*Hosp Med*, 7:141, 1971)

14.   **False.**   In systemic allergic vasculitis, only the small vessels are usually involved.   (*N Engl J Med*, 291:195, 1974)

15.   **False.**   Glucose tends to lower serum potassium levels.   (*JAMA*, 231:631, 1975)

16.   **False.**   Patients with emphysema actually breathe much easier when recumbent. Difficulty in breathing, except in an upright position, is a hallmark of left heart failure and is rare in emphysema.   (*Res Int Consult*, 2:17, 1973)

17.   **E.**   Nocturia is usually a significant symptom seen in association with benign prostatic hypertrophy, diabetes mellitus, urinary tract infections, and reversed diurnal rhythm as occurs with renal and circulatory insufficiency.   (2:247)

18.   **E.**   Pain of gastrointestinal origin varies greatly, depending on its underlying cause. The causes listed are all major pain mechanisms. Direct splanchnic nerve stimulation, as in retroperitoneal extension of a neoplasm such as pancreatic carcinoma, can also cause GI pain.   (2:208)

19.   **A.**   Patients with hyponatremia may be separated into those with edema and those without. In the former, hyponatremia is usually related to the primary disorder as heart failure, cirrhosis, or the nephrotic syndrome. In the latter, the usual causes are volume (salt) depletion, inappropriate ADH secretion, and adrenal insufficiency. Hyperglycemia, hyperlipemia, and drug use are easily determined. The correct diagnosis in the vast majority of patients with hyponatremia can be easily and quickly reached and the condition treated appropriately.

(*JAMA*, 228:825, 1974)

20.   **E.**   Patients secreting ADH because of hypovolemia require replacement of the sodium and water deficits, specific hormonal therapy, and correction of the underlying disease state. Severe dilutional hyponatremia may necessitate intravenous hypertonic saline solution. This may temporarily elevate the serum sodium concentration. Water intake may have to be restricted to as little as 500 ml total, including that contained in food.   (*Mod Med*, 41:39, 1973)

21.   **E.**   All of the conditions listed may result in postural hypotension. It may also occur in persons with varicose veins because of pooling of blood in the abnormally enlarged venous channels, in patients in whom a sympathectomy has abolished vasopressor reflexes, and in patients receiving antihypertensive and certain sedative and antidepressive drugs.   (5:78)

22.   **A.**   Aortic systolic ejection murmurs occur with valvular and subvalvular stenosis, primary dilatation of the ascending aorta, and increased left ventricular stroke output. The latter may be due simply to hyperkinetic states or may be a compensatory increase in forward flow through the valve because of diastolic backflow with aortic regurgitation.   (2:185)

23. **A.** Exercise-induced bronchospasm may be prevented by beta-adrenergic agonists, theophylline, and carbon dioxide breathing.
(*Ann Intern Med*, 78:401, 1973)

24. **E.** The list of diseases and conditions which may be accompanied by seizures is extensive and includes developmental and congenital defects, cerebral aplasias, birth injuries, acute infectious diseases of childhood, meningitis, encephalitis, cerebral trauma, tumors, abscesses, granulomas, parasitic cysts, degenerative diseases of the nervous system, metabolic disturbances or intoxications such as uremia, water, and alcoholic intoxication, cerebral edema, polycythemia, asphyxia, carbon monoxide poisoning, protein shock, anaphylaxis, Raynaud's disease, Stokes-Adam's syndrome, carotid sinus sensitivity, tetany, insulin shock, hyperventilation, and the ingestion of convulsant drugs. (4:847)

25. **Nystagmus.** Nystagmus is involuntary, repetitive rapid movement of the eyeball. (2:341)

26. **Light.** Amyloid is structurally related to the light chains of immunoglobulins.
(*N Engl J Med*, 287:1138, 1972)

27. **Contusion.** Cerebral contusion is a more or less diffuse disturbance to the brain following head injury and characterized by edema and capillary hemorrhaging which are most frequently present at the poles of the hemispheres. (1:246–47)

28. **Dupuytren's.** The presence of nodules within the palm associated with firm fibrous bands which limit extension of the fingers suggests Dupuytren's contracture. (2:295)

29. **Kallikrein.** Kallikrein is a polypeptide enzyme which cleaves kinin from its circulating liver-synthesized precursor—kininogen or prokinin. (3:49)

30. **Concussion.** Trotter has defined concussion as a condition of widespread paralysis of the functions of the brain which comes on as an immediate consequence of a blow on the head, has a strong tendency to spontaneous recovery, and is not necessarily associated with any gross organic change in the brain substance. (1:246)

31. **Hemianopsia.** Homonymous hemianopsia is the loss of vision in the nasal half of the visual field in one eye and the temporal half in the other. (2:355)

32. **Vascular.** Almost all focal cerebral lesions of sudden onset are in one way or another vascular in origin. (1:278)

33. **Apraxia.** A failure to execute certain acts in the correct context while retaining the ability to carry out the individual movements upon which such acts depend is the main feature of apraxia. (5:87–88)

34. **Asthma.** The beta-adrenergic theory offers the most plausible postulate to date with which to explain the varied etiologic relationship of bronchial hyperreactivity in asthma.
(*Curr Med Digest*, 39:1117, 1972)

35. **Hirsutism.** Hirsutism is a state of increased amounts of body and facial hair, especially in the female. (2:39)

36. **Lowers.** Digitalization lowers the threshold for potassium toxicity. (*Postgrad Med*. 50:101, 1970)

37. **Fibrinolysins.** A primary embolus in the lung is lysed by fibrinolysins released from the pulmonary arterial endothelium, but there is a continuous formation of secondary thrombus in response to the primary emboli.
(*Chest*, 63:1006, 1973)

38. **Decrease.** For each 0.1 unit rise in the blood pH, the serum potassium level will decrease by 0.5 to 1.0 mEq/liter. (*JAMA*, 231:631, 1975)

39. **Cataplexy.** Cataplexy is a sudden, brief loss of muscular power evoked by strong emotion, usually laughter. Although a few of the reported cases are doubtless examples of hysteria, there is unquestionably a well-defined clinical entity which bears no relationship to neurosis or any other known psychiatric condition. (5:129)

40. **Sick.** Cells which have acquired excess intracellular sodium at the expense of the extracellular compartment may lie at the root of hyponatremia in various different conditions. This has been termed sick-cell syndrome.
(*Lancet*, 1:342, 1974)

41. **A.** Endotoxin labilizes lysosomes. All other statements are true of lysosomes. (3:49)

42. **D.** All the autoimmune processes listed may be forerunners of the neoplastic process.
(*Lancet*, 2:596, 1970)

43. **E.** Physiological manifestations of chronic obstructive pulmonary disease include increased closing volume, decreased frequency-dependent compliance, increased airway resistance, and decreased maximal voluntary ventilation. Other

findings may include decreased first-second forced expiratory volume, decreased maximal midexpiratory flow rate, increased residual volume, increased residual volume/total lung capacity ratio, hypoxemia, and hypercapnia-respiratory acidosis. (*Mod Med,* 41:32, 1973)

44. **D.** All the hypotheses listed have been offered to explain pathogenesis of asthma.
(*Ann Intern Med,* 78:401, 1973)

45. **D.** Low or normal digitalis blood levels may induce toxicity when associated with all conditions listed. (*N Engl J Med,* 285:1540, 1971)

46. **A.** A special problem termed habitual hyperthermia is encountered in young females. The patient may have temperatures of 99.0° to 100.5°F regularly or intermittently for years and also usually has a variety of complaints characteristic of psychoneurosis, such as fatigability, insomnia, bowel distress, vague aches, and headache. Prolonged careful study and observation fail to reveal evidence of organic disease.
(5:65–66)

47. **D.** When renal function is normal, the half-time of digoxin in serum or plasma is 1.6 days, whereas in a totally anuric patient it is prolonged to about 4.4 days. Five digoxin half-times thus may range from 8.0 to 22.0 days, indicating that the steady-state will not be closely approached for about 1 to 3 weeks if a loading dose of digoxin is omitted.
(*J Chron Dis,* 24: 1971)

48. **D.** As revealed by radiolabeling, endotoxin localizes in the endothelium and walls of arterioles, capillaries, and venules. (3:51)

49. **C.** Goodpasture's syndrome is described chiefly in young men. All other statements are true.
(*N Engl J Med,* 291:195, 1974)

50. **E.** Aleutian disease in mink is not characterized by changes in the tissues, suggesting a conversion to multiple myeloma. All other statements are true. Additionally, Bence Jones protein may appear in the urine and the condition has been transferred by cell-free extracts from infected tissues. (*Lancet,* 2:596, 1970)

51. **E.** Elevated creatine phosphokinase levels may be associated with large muscle mass. All other conditions listed may be associated with elevated creatine phosphokinase levels, as will skeletal muscle diseases and cerebrovascular disease.
(*JAMA,* 228:1395, 1974)

52. **B.** Kinins produce hypotension and increased blood vessel permeability. All other statements are true. (3:49)

53. **A.** Several investigations have emphasized the hemodynamic alterations considered peculiar to septic shock: moderate hypotension, oliguria, dry and even warm skin, abnormally high cardiac output, appreciable decrease in general systemic vascular resistance, decrease in oxygen transport, increase in lactate production, and progressive acidosis. (3:98)

54. **A.** There is increasing evidence that endotoxin tolerance is an immunologic phenomenon because it can be passively transferred with 19S immunoglobulins, and animals previously immunized manifest a good anamnestic response. (3:44)

55. **A.** In hypernephroma, unlike breast cancer, raised circulating levels of immunoreactive parathyroid hormone-like substance have been described. (*Lancet,* 1:1082, 1973)

56. **E.** All of the conditions listed may be found in the NZB mouse strain. About one-third of the animals eventually die of malignant lymphoma, with or without leukemia. (*Lancet,* 2:596, 1970)

57. **A.** Horner's syndrome causes decreased sweating and involves only one side of the head and face. All other statements are true. (2:341)

58. **E.** Bounding pulse is characterized by a wide pulse pressure with a normal or slightly lower diastolic pressure. Fever, anemia, hepatic failure, thyrotoxicosis, and complete heart block are all capable of producing a bounding pulse. (2:172)

59. **E.** Falsely elevated temperature readings may occur as a result of any of the listed items. (2:35)

60. **E.** All statements are true of hydroceles. (2:255)

61. **B.** Intravenous administration of bradykinin produces marked systemic arteriolar dilation, venoconstriction, and hypotension. (3:49)

62. **B.** Cerebral concussion is associated with loss of consciousness and memory regarding the accident. The patient may appear to be well when seen initially, but observation is important, since there is the possibility of delayed intracranial hemorrhage. (2:311)

63. **B.** In patients with diabetes mellitus there is considerable evidence that immunologic competence is impaired and that a defect in chemotaxis of PMN leukocytes exists.
(*N Engl J Med,* 284:621, 1973)

64. **A.** Respiratory alkalosis may be an early manifestation of gram-negative bacteremia; metabolic acidosis is a frequent accompaniment of

the shock which occurs in approximately 40% of these patients. (3:22)

65. **C.** Both statements are true of digoxin absorption in patients with malabsorption syndromes.
(*N Engl J Med,* 285:257, 1971)

66. **C.** Both statements are true of the eosinopenic effect of epinephrine. (*J Allergy,* 49:142, 1972)

67. **C.** Carcinoma of the prostate occurs in approximately 20% of men over 60 years of age. The initial lesion usually involves the posterior lobe and is readily palpable at rectal examination. The early lesion feels like a small nodule on the posterior surface of the gland. Similar nodules can also be caused by calculi, chronic infection, or benign adenoma. More advanced malignant lesions usually are stony hard, irregular, and painless on palpation. (2:251)

68. **C.** A few irregular jerks are observed in many normal individuals when the eyes are turned far to the side. These so-called "nystagmoid movements" are probably similar to the tremulousness of a muscle that is contracted maximally. (5:107)

69. **D.** Both serum cholesterol and serum triglyceride levels increase with age.
(*JAMA,* 233:275, 1975)

70. **A.** Hypocapnia-induced bronchospasm is largely blocked by atropine in normal subjects.
(*Ann Intern Med,* 78:401, 1973)

71. **B.** Normal subjects excrete more than 50% of a water load in three hours and the urine osmolality falls to less than 100 mOsm/kg coincidentally with a fall in plasma osmolality and disappearance of urinary ADH. In the presence of the inappropriate ADH syndrome, water excretion is impaired and urinary ADH persists although initial plasma osmolality is low and falls further during water loading. (*Postgrad Med,* 52:232, 1972)

72. **B.** Pain can cause coronary artery spasm and stimulate excretion of catecholamines which can cause an increase in heart rate, cardiac output, and heart work. (*Postgrad Med,* 50:143, 1970)

73. **C.** Pseudohyponatremia, a misleading reduction in serum sodium concentration, is seen basically in two different circumstances. The first occurs when there is osmotic material—almost always glucose but occasionally mannitol—in the extracellular fluid. The osmotic material attracts water from the cells, reducing the sodium concentration in the extracellular fluid. This type of pseudohyponatremia may occur in hyperglycemia with mannitol administration, as

well as during marked alcohol intoxication. The second type of pseudohyponatremia may occur in association with hyperlipidemia and hyperproteinemia. In hyperlipidemia there is a measurement problem, not a physiologic disturbance. The sodium concentration in plasma is altered if there is a large quantity of lipids in the plasma; the concentration appears to be reduced. However, if you measure the sodium concentration in plasma water, you find the concentration normal. In hyperproteinemia, you will find a misleading reduction in the serum sodium only if the patient has extraordinary hyperglobulinemia such as that seen in multiple myeloma; enormously high concentrations of globulin—greater than 10 g/100 ml—are needed to produce pseudohyponatremia. Partial explanation is that proteins, like lipids, take up space in the plasma.
(*Patient Care,* 9:22, 1975)

74. **D.** Normal subjects, given as much as 8.5 liters of daily fluid during a 4-week period, showed no change in serum osmolality, nor did they show a tendency to reduce urine osmolality.
(*Ann Intern Med,* 83:676, 1975)

75. **C.** The hyponatremia and persistent antidiuresis of cirrhosis with ascites and advanced cardiac failure may be mediated by a decrease in "effective" extracellular fluid volume and persistent volume receptor stimulation. The osmoreceptors also are implicated in these conditions as well as in some of the inappropriate ADH disorders. A reset of osmoreceptor sensitivity often occurs and the osmoreceptor will respond to any further fall in plasma osmolality by appropriate suppression of ADH release aimed at preserving the existing steady state. (*Mod Med,* 41:37, 1973)

76. **C.** Hypercalcemia may occur spontaneously in metastatic, osteolytic breast cancer. It may also occur immediately upon the administration of sex steroids. For this reason, sex steroid therapy must be discontinued at the first symptom or sign of hypercalcemia—thirst, nausea, drowsiness, vague malaise, or elevated serum levels of calcium.
(*JAMA,* 223:913, 1973)

77. **D.** Mutism is the term applied to complete loss of speech in a conscious patient in the absence of both aphasia and anarthria. It is usually a symptom of a psychological disorder, either a psychosis or hysteria. (1:118)

78. **C.** Both statements are true of grand mal seizures. (4:852)

79. **True.** Patients with congestive heart failure often have an elevation of body temperature between 0.5 and 1.5°F. Perhaps this elevation is caused by impairment of heat dissipation as a result of diminished cardiac output, decline in cutaneous blood flow (with increasing insulation of the central temperature core), the insulating effect of edema, and the increased heat production incident to the muscular activity of dyspnea. On the other hand, patients with congestive heart failure are likely to have other causes of fever such as venous thrombosis, pulmonary embolism and infarction, myocardial infarction, rheumatic fever, and urinary tract infection. However, since slight fever is so regularly present even in the absence of such complications, the circulatory disturbance may be responsible. (5:55)

80. **True.** Since most blood tests of thyroid hormone primarily measure the bound fraction, medications which affect the thyroxine-binding relationships will alter the test results. (*AFP*, 3:73, 1971)

81. **True.** Extensive bleeding into the thyroid has been observed in thyrotoxic patients who have received radioactive iodine therapeutically while on anticoagulant therapy. (*JAMA*, 228:757, 1974)

82. **True.** Left ventricular hypertrophy produces a sustained, systolic apex impulse which may be displaced laterally and downward. The same mechanism responsible for the giant "a" wave with right ventricular hypertrophy, namely, very forceful atrial contractions, may result in a palpable presystolic component to the apex impulse with left ventricular hypertrophy. (2:176)

83. **True.** In acidosis, blood is still able to unload oxygen to the tissues and circulation is therefore functional, whereas alkalosis inhibits this oxygen release and renders circulation less effective. (*Emerg Med*, 5:182, 1973)

84. **True.** In myxedematous persons, blood pressure is usually normal; however, hypertension occurs at a greater frequency than in nonmyxedematous persons. (2:48)

Textbook References for Chapter 4

1. Bannister, R. (1978): *Brain's Clinical Neurology*, Fifth Edition, Oxford University Press, New York.

2. Judge, R.D., and Zuidema, G.D., Editors. (1974): *Methods of Clinical Examination: A Physiologic Approach*, Third Edition, Little, Brown and Company, Boston.

3. Lauler, D.P., Editor-in-Chief. (1971): *Gram Negative Sepsis*, MedCom., Clifton, N.J.

4. Merritt, H.H. (1979): *A Textbook of Neurology*, Sixth Edition, Lea & Febiger, Philadelphia.

5. Isselbacher, K.J., Editor. (1980): *Harrison's Principles of Internal Medicine*, Ninth Edition, McGraw-Hill-Company, New York.

CHAPTER 5

Cardiology

Directions: Indicate whether each of the following statements is true or false.

1. Pericarditis is not a contraindication to systemic anticoagulation.

2. In uncomplicated myocardial infarction, evidence suggests the presence of transient left ventricular failure with pulmonary vascular congestion and transudation of fluid into the interstitial space, leading to premature airway closure.

3. VMA values may be lowered by monoamine oxidase inhibitors and clofibrate and may be slightly lowered by methyldopa, although the last agent usually would not lower it sufficiently to obscure the presence of pheochromocytoma.

4. Mitral regurgitation occurs in a minority of patients with idiopathic hypertrophic subaortic stenosis.

5. The combined action of digitalis and propranolol appears to be less effective than either agent alone in controlling rapid ventricular rates in the presence of supraventricular arrhythmias.

6. Propranolol, which decreases the force of cardiac contraction, is contraindicated with acute dissection of the aorta.

7. Although digoxin in the serum comprises only 1% or less of the total body digoxin in a digitalized subject, there is evidence of a relatively constant relation between serum and tissue levels.

8. S-T segment depression, as well as elevations which are usually seen in patients with infarction and observed in a few patients during anginal attacks, appear related to alterations in cellular ionic balance.

9. Pulsus paradoxus is an important sign of cardiac tamponade.

10. Several studies have shown that patients with angina pectoris have a death rate of 3 to 5% per year.

11. A normal resting electrocardiogram excludes severely obstructive coronary artery disease.

Directions: Use the key below to answer the following questions. For the following numbered words or phrases, select
 A. if the mean pressure is 8 mm Hg
 B. if the mean pressure is 3 mm Hg
 C. if the pressure is 25/3 mm Hg
 D. if the pressure is 25/15 mm Hg
 E. if the pressure is 115/7 mm Hg
 F. if the mean pressure is 9 mm Hg
 G. if the mean pressure is 7 mm Hg
 H. if the pressure is 115/80 mm Hg
 I. if the pressure is 120/75 mm Hg

12. brachial artery

13. right atrium

14. right ventricle

15. pulmonary veins

16. aorta

17. brachial vein

18. left atrium

19. left ventricle

20. pulmonary artery

Directions: Each of the questions or incomplete statements below is followed by five suggested answers or completions. Select the one BEST answer in each case.

21. The Framingham study reported that what percentage of patients with congestive heart failure survived five years?

 A. 10%
 B. 25%
 C. 50%
 D. 75%
 E. 90%

22. Analysis of cardioversion energies for ventricular tachycardia has demonstrated that what percentage of episodes are reversed with energies of 10 W sec or less?

 A. 0%
 B. 3%
 C. 19%
 D. 57%
 E. 93%

23. About what percentage of pheochromocytomas occur in the adrenal gland?

 A. 10%
 B. 20%
 C. 40%
 D. 60%
 E. 80%

24. About what percentage of patients with high blood pressure have the essential form?

 A. 5%
 B. 10%
 C. 20%
 D. 40%
 E. 80%

25. In coronary artery-vein-aorta bypass, occlusion rate in the first year is

 A. less than 5%
 B. 10 to 15%
 C. 20 to 25%
 D. 50%
 E. 75%

26. The Framingham study reported that high blood pressure preceded the development of congestive heart failure in what percentage of cases?

A. 10%
B. 25%
C. 50%
D. 75%
E. 90%

27. Marfan's syndrome is most frequently associated with what type of dissecting aneurysm of the aorta?

A. Type 1
B. Type 2
C. Type 3
D. Type 4
E. Type 5

28. When a patient's endogenous creatinine clearance is 100 ml/min, approximately what percentage of the digoxin present in the body is lost each day?

A. 10%
B. 22%
C. 34%
D. 46%
E. 85%

Directions: For each of the following statements, fill in the correct word answer.

29. _____ is the most potent risk factor for coronary heart disease.

30. The most common cause of mitral regurgitation is _____ valvulitis.

31. A syndrome has been described consisting of protein-loss enteropathy, anergy, lymphocytopenia, and severe _____ regurgitation.

32. Asymmetrical left ventricular hypertrophy with disproportionate septal thickness is characteristic of _____ cardiomyopathy and has not been reported in any other condition.

33. In high doses, digitalis _____ junctional or ventricular pacemakers.

34. The use of coumarin drugs in patients with _____ complicating acute myocardial infarction increases the possibility of hemopericardium.

35. _____ is the predominant organism in endocarditis occurring in narcotic addicts.

36. Complete atrioventricular block is the commonest arrhythmia that leads to fainting; syncopal episodes associated with this arrhythmia are known as the _____-Adams-Morgagni syndrome.

37. Left atrial _____ must be considered in any case of obstruction of the mitral valve, especially if the features of the lesion are not entirely typical.

38. A postinfarction syndrome, _____ syndrome, has been described, occurring one week or more after acute infarction and characterized by pericarditis with pleuritis and pleural effusions.

Directions: Use the key below to answer the following questions. Select
  A. **if the statement is characteristic of systemic circulation**
  B. **if the statement is characteristic of pulmonary circulation**

39. High-resistance, high-pressure circuit requiring relatively high stroke work.

40. Distensible, low-pressure, low-resistance system.

Directions: Select the ONE INCORRECT answer to the following questions.

41. Type IV hyperlipoproteinemia may be mimicked by

    A. obstructive jaundice
    B. dysproteinemia as in multiple myeloma, macroglobulinemia, and systemic lupus erythematosus (SLE)
    C. poorly controlled diabetes mellitus
    D. hyperthyroidism
    E. nephrotic syndrome

42. Common features of idiopathic hypertrophic subaortic stenosis include

    A. mitral regurgitation
    B. left ventricular heave
    C. prominent fourth heart sound
    D. aortic pulse slow in upstroke
    E. left ventricular hypertrophy and strain
    F. left atrial enlargement

43. In adult patients with significant valvular aortic stenosis in whom the severity of obstruction has been documented by hemodynamic measurement and in whom the natural history was not interrupted by operation,

    A. the overall prognosis was poor
    B. the percentage of mortality was over 50% at five years and 90% at ten years
    C. the age of onset was related to the duration of survival
    D. there was no clear relation between the type of symptoms and the duration of survival
    E. hemodynamic parameters could not be correlated with symptoms or survival

44. Patients with cerebrovascular accidents, particularly with subarachnoid hemorrhage, may develop

    A. electrocardiographic patterns resembling acute myocardial ischemia or nontransmural infarction
    B. shortening of Q-T interval
    C. wide, large inverted T waves in the left precordial leads
    D. increased amplitude of U waves
    E. ventricular arrhythmias
    F. shortened P-R intervals

45. In the sick sinus syndrome pacemaker insertion may be indicated

    A. in most patients
    B. when syncope occurs
    C. when digitalis is required
    D. when cardiac output is significantly decreased

46. Apical fourth heart sound gallop

    A. is regularly audible with severe aortic stenosis or severe systemic hypertension
    B. is common with aortic insufficiency of severe degrees, especially when accompanied by an Austin Flint's murmur
    C. is increased on inspiration and is loudest along the left sternal edge and occasionally over the right jugular vein; is often heard when the right ventricle is hypertrophied or dilated (as in acute pulmonary embolism, pulmonary hypertension of any cause, including left heart failure, or pulmonary valvular stenosis)
    D. presumably originating in the left heart, is very common in hyperdynamic states
    E. is very common in severe mitral stenosis

Directions: For each question select
    A. if the question is associated with A only
    B. if the question is associated with B only
    C. if the question is associated with A and B
    D. if the question is associated with neither A nor B

47. Lidocaine is contraindicated in

    A. paroxysmal supraventricular tachy-
       cardia
    B. Wolff-Parkinson-White syndrome
    C. both
    D. neither

48. Wolff-Parkinson-White syndrome is
    characterized by

    A. a long P-R interval
    B. delta waves
    C. both
    D. neither

49. Diazoxide is

    A. a nondiuretic thiazide
    B. a non-thiazide diuretic

50. A hypertensive patient with minimal abnor-
    malities in urinary constituents but with
    polyuria and nocturia suggests presence of

    A. hyperkalemia
    B. hypocalcemia
    C. both
    D. neither

51. Which of the following do(es) not cross the
    placental barrier?

    A. coumarin derivatives
    B. heparin
    C. both
    D. neither

52. The first heart sound is accentuated with

    A. hyperkinetic disorders
    B. mitral stenosis
    C. both
    D. neither

53. Which of the following is/are related experi-
    mentally to an increase in sodium content in
    the arterial wall?

    A. decreased peripheral resistance
    B. decreased vascular tone
    C. both
    D. neither

54. Emboli from thrombosed veins in the ex-
    tremities can reach the left side of the cir-
    culation through an atrial septal defect or
    patent foramen ovale; this occurrence is

    A. termed paradoxical embolism
    B. usually not preceded by recurrent
       pulmonary embolism
    C. both
    D. neither

55. Slow ventricular tachycardia

    A. may occur transiently in acute myocardial
       infarction
    B. may not require specific treatment
    C. both
    D. neither

56. Temporary ventricular pacing may be indi-
    cated for

    A. second and third degree A-V block dur-
       ing myocardial infarction
    B. "overdrive" suppression of ventricular
       tachycardia with A-V block
    C. both
    D. neither

57. Tangier disease involves

    A. partial absence of alpha-lipoprotein
    B. deposition of cholesterol esters in the
       reticuloendothelial system of blood
       vessels, liver, and spleen
    C. both
    D. neither

58. Hypertension associated with contraceptive therapy is probably based on increased

    A. renin secretion
    B. hepatic angiotensinogen production
    C. both
    D. neither

59. An indicator of pacemaker battery decay, as measured by a rate meter, is

    A. a decrease in rate
    B. an increase in rate
    C. both
    D. neither

Directions: For each of the incomplete statements below, ONE or MORE of the completions given is correct. In each case, select
    A. **if 1, 2, and 3 are correct**
    B. **if 1 and 3 are correct**
    C. **if 2 and 4 are correct**
    D. **if only 4 is correct**
    E. **if all are correct**

60. Edrophonium (Tensilon), in doses ranging from 5 to 20 mg,

    1. has been shown to convert supraventricular tachycardia to normal sinus rhythm in 75% of cases
    2. has its effects dissipated in three to five min
    3. has a vagotonic effect
    4. significantly depresses myocardial function

61. Oral diuretics

    1. enhance the effect of other antihypertensive agents
    2. counteract the sodium retention that may follow the use of other agents
    3. lower pressure both in the supine and standing position
    4. have an antihypertensive effect that is not maintained during long-term administration

62. Echocardiography may identify

    1. idiopathic hypertrophic subaortic stenosis
    2. prolapse of the mitral leaflets in regurgitation
    3. mitral stenosis including valve thickness and calcification
    4. atrial myxoma and left atrial enlargement

63. Multifocal atrial ("chaotic") tachycardia

    1. has at least two different atrial foci discharging at an irregular rate, usually over 100/min
    2. is seen in older patients, often diabetic, postoperative, or with chronic obstructive lung disease
    3. has a P-R interval that usually does not vary from beat to beat
    4. has a relatively high mortality rate

64. The important factors limiting the success of any coronary bypass graft include the

    1. size of the anastomosed vessels
    2. magnitude of perfusion through the shunt
    3. gradient across the proximal obstruction
    4. extent of collaterals

65. Uremic pericarditis occurs with increased frequency in

    1. younger patients
    2. older patients
    3. women
    4. men

66. A-V nodal block

    1. presents in some cases of Wenckebach periods
    2. has a wide QRS morphology
    3. has an escape focus in complete block with a rate of 50 or faster and a form identical to that found with conducted beats
    4. usually requires permanent pacemaking

67. In congestive cardiomyopathy,

    1. the condition may be primary or secondary
    2. there is low-voltage QRS
    3. atrial fibrillation is common
    4. antemortem thrombi are rare

68. Lutembacher's syndrome is characterized by

    1. atrial septal defect
    2. ventricular septal defect
    3. mitral stenosis
    4. mitral regurgitation

69. Diphenylhydantoin (Dilantin)

    1. is contraindicated in treating digitalis toxicity
    2. checks premature beats by suppressing ventricular irritability
    3. exerts considerable effect on the sino-atrial node
    4. increases conduction through the atrio-ventricular node relieving any block that may have been caused by digitalis

70 Idiopathic hypertrophic subaortic stenosis involves

    1. massive asymmetrical hypertrophy of the septum and outflow tract of the left ventricle
    2. diffuse hypertrophy of the ventricular wall
    3. a systolic murmur, typically midsystolic crescendo-decrescendo, heard best at the apex or lower left sternal border
    4. obstruction of the left ventricular outflow in all cases

71. Factors which are important in the genesis of arrhythmias during a myocardial infarction include

    1. pain
    2. anxiety

    3. straining
    4. hypoxia

72. Regarding patients with anatomically isolated aortic valve stenosis,

    1. half have congenitally bicuspid or unicuspid valves
    2. most have a history of rheumatic fever
    3. anticipated survival after the onset of angina or syncope is three to four years
    4. most are female

73. Demand pacemakers

    1. are "R wave inhibited"
    2. avoid competition with spontaneous ventricular depolarization
    3. are valuable in treating patients with intermittent heart block since the generator is inhibited at rates of 70 beats/min or above
    4. require vagal stimulation or special "overdrive" units used to verify the function of the pacemaker when the patient's own rhythm predominates

74. Causes of isolated aortic regurgitation include

    1. leaflet deformity
    2. ankylosing spondylitis
    3. rheumatic or bacterial endocarditis
    4. Ehlers-Danlos syndrome

75. Congenital causes of obstruction of left ventricular inflow include

    1. congenital mitral stenosis
    2. "parachute" mitral valves
    3. supravalvular stenosing ring
    4. congenital pulmonary vein stenosis

76. The potentially audible component of the atrial systolic wave, normally inaudible, may become audible under certain circum-

stances when it is usually called a fourth heart sound gallop (S₄). This may occur with

1. prolonged A-V conduction time with first-degree A-V block
2. decreased compliance of the left ventricle, as in aortic stenosis, systemic hypertension, or aortic insufficiency
3. acute myocardial infarction and angina pectoris because of decreased compliance of the left ventricle
4. right ventricular dilatation or hypertrophy

77. Congenital mitral regurgitation occurs with

1. Marfan's syndrome
2. endocardial fibroelastosis
3. endocardial cushion defect
4. anomalous origin of the left coronary artery from the pulmonary artery

78. Intra-aortic balloon counterpulsation (IABC)

1. has been used successfully to improve myocardial performance in patients with cardiogenic shock
2. is based on the principle of diastolic augmentation with a resultant increase in coronary blood flow and the reduction of afterload with a resultant decrease in myocardial oxygen requirements
3. has been used principally in acute myocardial infarction and shock, both as primary treatment and to stabilize such patients to permit coronary arteriography in preparation for emergency coronary artery bypass
4. has been successfully used for circulatory support following cardiopulmonary bypass

Directions: Use the key below to answer the following questions. Select
  A. **if the numbered item is characteristic of valvular aortic stenosis**
  B. **if the numbered item is characteristic of idiopathic hypertrophic subaortic stenosis (asymmetric septal hypertrophy)**

79. Delayed carotid pulse

80. Systolic murmur located in second right intercostal space, neck, and apex

81. Murmur is increased as an effect of Valsalva maneuver

82. Soft aortic closure sound

83. Systolic ejection clicks are rare

84. Diastolic murmur of aortic regurgitation is common

85. Electrocardiogram shows marked left ventricular hypertrophy, deep Q waves (septal in origin), and left atrial enlargement

86. Chest roentgenogram shows cardiomegaly (left ventricular) and left atrial enlargement

87. Post-stenotic dilatation of the aorta is present

88. Calcium is present in the aortic valve

Directions: Use the key below to answer the following questions. Select
  A. **if A is greater or more appropriate than B**
  B. **if B is greater or more appropriate than A**
  C. **if A and B are equal or approximately equal**

89. Blood pressure is better correlated with

  A. body fat
  B. body weight

90. Wide pulse pressure

  A. aortic stenosis
  B. aortic regurgitation

91. Obesity

  A. hypertension
  B. increased serum cholesterol

92. Ball variance

  A. aortic position
  B. mitral position

Answers and Commentary

1. **False.** Pericarditis is a contraindication to systemic anticoagulation. Regional heparinization may be necessary during dialysis of patients with uremic pericarditis. (1.13)

2. **True.** In uncomplicated myocardial infarction, evidence suggests the presence of transient left ventricular failure with pulmonary vascular congestion and transudation of fluid into the interstitial space, leading to premature airway closure. (*N Engl J Med*, 290:761, 1974)

3. **True.** VMA values may be lowered by monoamine oxidase inhibitors and clofibrate and may be slightly lowered by methyldopa, although the last agent usually would not lower it sufficiently to obscure the presence of pheochromocytoma. (*N Engl J Med*, 288:1010, 1973)

4. **False.** Mitral regurgitation occurs in at least one-half of the patients with idiopathic hypertrophic subaortic stenosis. (1:3)

5. **False.** The combined action of digitalis and propranolol appears to be more effective than either agent alone in controlling rapid ventricular rates in the presence of supraventricular arrhythmias. (*Am Fam Physician*, 9:178, 1974)

6. **False.** Propranolol, which decreases the force of cardiac contraction, is useful with acute dissection of the aorta. (1:12)

7. **True.** Although digoxin in the serum comprises only 1% or less of the total body digoxin in a digitalized subject, there is evidence of a relatively constant relation between serum and tissue levels. (*N Engl J Med*, 285:258, 1971)

8. **True.** There is strong experimental evidence that S-T depressions, as well as the elevations which are usually seen in patients with infarction and observed in a few patients during anginal attacks, are related to alterations in cellular ionic balance. (4:29)

9. **True.** Pulsus paradoxus is an important sign of cardiac tamponade. It is found with tense pericardial effusions and with chronic constrictive pericarditis. The term refers to a weakening of the pulse during normal inspiration. Lowering of the diaphragm tenses the indistensible pericardium, compressing the heart, and reducing diastolic filling. The resultant fall in stroke output narrows the pulse pressure. The systolic pressure may fall by 10 mm or more with inspiration. The estimation of blood pressure is more reliable than palpation for distinguishing pulsus paradoxus. As the pressure is reduced, the first Korotkoff's sounds appear only during expiration (upper systolic level). Further reduction produces a point at which all beats are heard (lower systolic level). A difference of greater than 10 mm is evidence of cardiac tamponade. (3:172-73)

10. **True.** Several studies have shown that patients with angina pectoris have a death rate of 3 to 5% per year. (1:2)

11. **False.** A normal resting electrocardiogram by no means excludes severely obstructive coronary artery disease, and a frankly abnormal electrocardiogram, characterized by generalized T wave inversion, may occur in patients with a normal heart. (*Am J Cardiol*, 30:298, 1972)

12. **I.** (3:152)

13. **B.** (3:152)

14. **C.** (3:152)

15. **F.** (3:152)

16. **H.** (3:152)

17. **A.** (3:152)

18. **G.** (3:152)

19. **E.** (3:152)

20. **D.** (3:152)

21. **B.** The Framingham study reported that 25% of patients with congestive heart failure survived five years. (1:1)

22. **E.** Analysis of cardioversion energies for ventricular tachycardia has demonstrated that 93% of episodes are reversed with energies of 10 W sec or less. (*N Engl J Med*, 283:1192, 1970)

23. **C.** About 40% of pheochromocytomas occur in the adrenal gland. (*N Engl J Med*, 288:1010, 1973)

24. **E.** About 80% of patients with high blood pressure have the essential form. (1:14)

25. **B.** In coronary artery-vein-aorta bypass, occlusion rate in the first year is 10 to 15%. (1:2)

26. **D.** The Framingham study reported that high blood pressure preceded the development of congestive heart failure in 75% of cases with both systolic and diastolic pressure proving of equal risk. (1:1)

27. **B.** Marfan's syndrome is most frequently associated with Type 2 dissecting aneurysm of the aorta. (*JAMA*, 217:1533, 1971)

28. **C.** The percentage of digoxin lost from the body each day is highly dependent upon renal function. When a patient's endogenous creatinine clearance is 100 ml/min, approximately 34% of the digoxin present in the body is lost each day. When a patient is anuric, only 14% of body digoxin is lost each day. (*J Chron Dis*, 24:411, 1971)

29. **Hypertension.** It is agreed that hypertension is the most potent risk factor for coronary heart disease. (*N Engl J Med*, 291:178, 1974)

30. **Rheumatic.** The most common cause of mitral regurgitation is rheumatic valvulitis. (1:3)

31. **Tricuspid.** A syndrome has been described consisting of protein-loss enteropathy, anergy, lymphocytopenia, and severe tricuspid regurgitation. (1:4)

32. **Hypertrophic.** Asymmetrical left ventricular hypertrophy with disproportionate septal thickness is characteristic of hypertrophic cardiomyopathy and has not been reported in any other condition. (*N Engl J Med*, 289:118, 1973)

33. **Accelerates.** In high doses, digitalis accelerates junctional or ventricular pacemakers. (1:8)

34. **Pericarditis.** The use of coumarin drugs in patients with pericarditis complicating acute myocardial infarction increases the possibility of hemopericardium. (*JAMA*, 228:757, 1974)

35. **Staphylococcus.** Staphylococcus is the predominant organism in endocarditis occurring in narcotic addicts. (1:11)

36. **Stokes.** Complete atrioventricular block is the commonest arrhythmia that leads to fainting; syncopal episodes associated with this arrhythmia are known as the Stokes-Adams-Morgagni syndrome. (4:79)

37. **Myxoma.** Left atrial myxoma must be considered in any case of obstruction of the mitral valve, especially if the features of the lesion are not entirely typical. (1:3)

38. **Dressler's.** A postinfarction syndrome, Dressler's syndrome, has been described, occurring one week or more after acute infarction and characterized by pericarditis with pleuritis and pleural effusions. This condition is similar to the postpericardiectomy syndrome observed after cardiac surgery. It responds dramatically to moderate doses of corticosteroids. (2:1237)

39. **A.** (3:152–53)

40. **B.** (3:152, 53)

41. **D.** Type IV hyperlipoproteinemia may be mimicked by obstructive jaundice, dysproteinemia as in multiple myeloma, macroglobulinemia, and systemic lupus erythematosus, poorly controlled diabetes mellitus, nephrotic syndrome, and hypothyroidism. (1:6)

42. **D.** Idiopathic hypertrophic subaortic stenosis is characterized by an aortic pulse which is rapid in upstroke with peak pressure occurring early in systole. All other statements are true. (1:5)

43. **C.** In adult patients with significant valvular aortic stenosis in whom the severity of obstruction has been documented by hemodynamic measurement and in whom the natural history was not interrupted by operation, the age at the onset of symptoms was not related to duration of survival; there was no clear relation between the type of symptoms and survival. All other statements are true of this study. Additionally, patients with a combination of symptoms (angina pectoris, syncope, and congestive heart failure) tended to have the worse prognosis.
(*Br Heart J*, 35:41, 1973)

44. **B.** Patients with cerebrovascular accidents, particularly with subarachnoid hemorrhage, may develop all the changes listed except there is prolongation of the Q-T interval. (1:14)

45. **A.** In the sick sinus syndrome pacemaker insertion may be indicated in all instances listed but most patients do not require specific treatment.
(1:7)

46. **E.** The fourth heart sound gallop is very rare in severe mitral stenosis, and may be either right- or left-sided in ventricular hypertrophy as is found in cardiomyopathy. (*JAMA*, 224:1133, 1973)

47. **D.** Lidocaine may be useful in both paroxysmal supraventricular tachycardia and Wolff-Parkinson-White syndrome.
(*Am Fam Physician*, 7:152, 1973)

48. **B.** In the Wolff-Parkinson-White syndrome a short P-R interval and delta waves are characteristic. (1:8)

49. **A.** Diazoxide, which appears to be highly effective in the emergency reduction of high blood pressure, is a nondiuretic thiazide. (1:15)

50. **D.** A hypertensive patient with minimal abnormalities in urinary constituents but with polyuria and nocturia suggests hypokalemia (hyperaldosteronism) or hypercalcemia (hyperparathyroidism). (4:1169)

51. **B.** Since heparin does not cross the placental barrier, it is recommended in pregnancy when an anticoagulant is indicated. Coumarin derivatives do cross the placental barrier. (1:12)

52. **C.** The first heart sound is accentuated with hyperkinetic disorders and mitral stenosis. (3:179)

53. **D.** Elevated peripheral resistance and vascular tone are related experimentally to an increase in sodium content in the arterial wall. (1:14)

54. **A.** The occurrence described may be termed paradoxical embolism, and is usually preceded by recurrent pulmonary embolism.
(*N Engl J Med*, 282:968, 1970)

55. **C.** Both statements are true of slow ventricular tachycardia. (1:8)

56. **C.** Both statements are true of temporary ventricular pacing. (*Am Fam Physician*, 3:84, 1971)

57. **B.** In Tangier disease, there is total absence of alpha-lipoprotein. The deposition of cholesterol esters in the reticuloendothelial system of blood vessels, liver, and spleen can occur. (1:6)

58. **C.** Both statements are true of hypertension associated with contraceptive therapy. (1:12)

59. **C.** The most accurate indication of battery decay in a pacemaker is an increase or decrease in the rate, as measured by a rate meter. (1:12)

60. **A.** A significant advantage with edrophonium is that it apparently does not depress myocardial function. All other statements are true.
(*Arch Intern Med*, 130:221, 1972)

61. **A.** Oral diuretics have an antihypertensive effect that is maintained during long-term administration. All other statements are true. (1:15)

62. **E.** Echocardiography may be useful in identifying all the conditions listed, as well as pericardial effusion and tricuspid stenosis. (1:13)

63. **C.** Multifocal atrial ("chaotic") tachycardia shows at least three different atrial foci discharging at an irregular rate, usually over 100/min. The P-R interval usually varies from beat to beat. Digitalis does not produce this disorder. (1:8)

64. **E.** All the factors listed limit the success of any coronary bypass graft. Runoff or degree of obstruction by atherosclerosis of the distal vessels can also be a limiting factor.
(*JAMA*, 223:767, 1973)

65. **B.** Uremic pericarditis occurs with increased frequency in younger females. (1:13)

66. **B.** A-V nodal block is present in some cases of Wenckebach periods, is usually reversible, has an escape focus in complete block with a rate of 50 or faster and a form identical to that found with

conducted beats, has a narrow QRS morphology, and permanent pacemaking is not usually required. (1:7)

67. **A.** In congestive cardiomyopathy, antimortem thrombi are common, the coronary arteries are usually normal, and long-term anticoagulation therapy is recommended. All other statements are true. (1:4)

68. **B.** Lutembacher's syndrome is characterized by atrial septal defect and mitral stenosis. (1:9)

69. **C.** Diphenylhydantoin (Dilantin) may be useful in treating digitalis toxicity. This drug exerts little effect on the sinoatrial node. All other statements are true. (*Res Int Consult*, 2:20, 1973)

70. **A.** In idiopathic hypertrophic subaortic stenosis, obstruction of the left ventricular outflow is not invariable and murmurs increase with upright position and decrease with squatting. (1:5)

71. **E.** All the factors listed are important in the genesis of arrhythmias during a myocardial infarction. Other factors include acidosis, hyperkalemia, pulmonary embolism, shock, and congestive heart failure. (*Hosp Med*, 7:141, 1971)

72. **B.** Patients with anatomically isolated aortic valve stenosis usually do not have a history of rheumatic fever, are usually male, and angina may occur with normal coronary arteries. (1:4)

73. **E.** All statements are true of demand pacemakers. (*Am Fam Physician*, 3:84, 1971)

74. **E.** All factors listed cause isolated aortic regurgitation. Syphilis and Marfan's syndrome can also cause this disorder. (1:4)

75. **E.** All factors listed are congenital causes of obstruction of left ventricular inflow. Another congenital cause is cor triatriatum. (1:3)

76. **E.** The potentially audible component of the atrial systolic wave, normally inaudible, may be-

come audible under certain circumstances when it is usually called a fourth heart sound gallop (S₄). This may occur with all the circumstances listed, in hyperdynamic states such as hyperthyroidism, severe anemia, and severe liver disease, and in ventricular hypertrophy, as in obstructive or nonobstructive cardiomyopathy. (*JAMA*, 224:1133, 1973)

77. **E.** All disorders may be associated with congenital mitral regurgitation. (1:3)

78. **E.** All statements are true of intra-aortic balloon counterpulsation. (*JAMA*, 224:1133, 1973)

79. **A.** (2:1192)

80. **A.** (2:1192)

81. **B.** (2:1192)

82. **A.** (2:1192)

83. **B.** (2:1192)

84. **A.** (2:1192)

85. **B.** (2:1192)

86. **B.** (2:1192)

87. **A.** (2:1192)

88. **A.** (2:1192)

89. **B.** Blood pressure is better correlated with body weight than with body fat. (*N Engl J Med*, 291:178, 1974)

90. **B.** Wide pulse pressure is associated with aortic regurgitation. (1:4)

91. **A.** There is a significant association between obesity and hypertension, and a less significant association between obesity and increased serum cholesterol. (*JAMA*, 221:378, 1972)

92. **A.** Ball variance is more common in the aortic position than the mitral position. (1:14)

Textbook References for Chapter 5

1. American College of Physicians. (1974): *Medical Knowledge Self-Assessment, Program III: Recent Developments in Internal Medicine*, R.G. Petersdorf, General Editor, American College of Physicians, Philadelphia.

2. Beeson, P.B. and McDermott, W. (1979): *Cecil Textbook of Medicine*, Fifteenth Edition, W.B. Saunders Company, Philadelphia.

3. Judge, R.D. and Zuidema, G.D. (1974): *Methods of Clinical Examination: A Physiologic Approach*, Third Edition, Little, Brown and Company, Boston.

4. Isselbacher, K.J., Editor. (1980): *Harrison's Principles of Internal Medicine*, Ninth Edition, McGraw-Hill Company, New York.

CHAPTER 6

Dermatology

1. Regarding hordeolum (sty),

   A. it is a staphylococcal infection of the eyelid glands, characterized by a localized, red, swollen, and tender area

   B. it is essentially an abscess, since there is pus formation within the lumen of the affected gland

   C. when infection is in the meibomian gland, the lesion is relatively large and is known as an internal hordeolum

   D. when smaller and more superficial, external hordeolum is an infection of the glands of Zeis or Moll, which are adjacent to the hair follicles

   E. pain is uncommon

   F. treatment may consist of hot compresses, antibiotics and possible drainage

2. Blepharitis

   A. is an acute or chronic inflammation of the eyelid margins

   B. is uncommon

   C. frequently occurs in patients with seborrhea of the scalp, ears, chest, or brow

   D. causes the eyelids to be red and swollen and have scales at the base of the lashes

   E. scales may form crusts which occa-

sionally cause the lids to stick together in the morning

   F. is associated with ocular discomfort and burning, and chronic conjunctivitis

   G. requires treatment for the lids consisting of removing the scale on the lashes twice daily and applying steroid-sulfur drops to the lid margin

   H. is chronic and treatment is not curative

3. Regarding urticaria pigmentosa,

   A. it appears in adulthood

   B. rubbing the lesions results in urtication of the involved area and surrounding tissues; i.e., a dermagraphia is found

   C. histologically, the lesions appear to be tumors of mast cells

   D. tumors may involve the bones, lymph nodes, liver, thymus, and gastrointestinal tract, and bleeding may result

   E. there is no known effective treatment

4. Mycosis fungoides

   A. may affect the lymph nodes, bones, and gastrointestinal tract

   B. may start as a nonspecific eruption possibly proceeding to an erythroderma with widespread redness, scaling, and thickening of the skin

   C. develops characteristic nodules which may become very large

D. is uncommonly associated with ulceration

E. has a poor prognosis

F. is characterized by comparatively radiosensitive lesions

5. Regarding rosacea,

A. it is usually malignant

B. it is more common in patients with polycythemia vera

C. it occurs mainly in the butterfly area of the face

D. vessel dilation may become chronic and telangiectasia develops

E. papules and pustules may be noted

F. the nose may be involved in an overgrowth of fibrous tissue producing scarring and lobulation (rhinophyma)

6. Regarding Raynaud's disease,

A. it is a benign, symmetrical disorder of unknown cause

B. onset is usually in the late teens or early twenties

C. males are more commonly afflicted

D. cold and emotional stimuli are the factors which trigger the response in the digits

E. the fingers become white, then blue, and finally red (triphasic color response)

7. Urticaria

A. is estimated to affect 10 to 20% of the population

B. attack which persists for more than eight weeks is considered chronic

C. has its greatest incidence between the third and fourth decades

D. affects only the superficial layers of the skin and mucous membranes in contrast to angioneurotic edema which is a well outlined edematous process involving blood vessels in the deeper

subcutaneous tissues of the skin and submucosa

E. only occurs on an immunological basis

Directions: For each of the following statements, fill in the correct word.

8. If a patient has a generalized eruption that involves the palms and the soles, the eruption is probably either _____ syphilis or a dermatitis medicamentosa.

9. A color change in the skin without elevation or depression is a _____ .

10. Each scalp hair grows about 0.3 to 0.4 mm/day during the growing or anagen phase, before entering resting periods (_____ phase), which occur every few months to a few years.

11. The commonest cause of trophic lesions in the skin in the upper limb is _____ .

12. The _____ is the smallest in a sequence of masses which elevate the skin.

13. Urticaria is more commonly found in _____ sex.

Directions: For each of the following multiple-choice questions, select the ONE CORRECT answer.

14. In most instances, the cause of erythema nodosum is

A. allergy

B. infection

C. unknown

D. birth control pills

15. The commonest site of the lesion of herpes zoster is the

    A.   dorsal root ganglia and the corresponding sensory ganglia of the cranial nerves

    B.   posterior horn of the grey matter

    C.   dorsal root

    D.   anterior root

    E.   peripheral nerves

Directions: Indicate whether each of the following statements is true or false.

16. Seborrheic dermatitis may be associated with central nervous system derangements.

17. Herpes zoster commonly develops after exposure to chickenpox.

18. The treatment of sunburn is straightforward—simple calamine lotion for mild cases, a corticosteroid cream for the more severely affected.

19. The Sturge-Weber syndrome is a capillary-venous malformation in one hemisphere associated with a facial nevus.

20. Spontaneous ecchymoses may occur beneath the conjunctivas in otherwise healthy patients, and usually have no significance unless signs of a bleeding tendency are present elsewhere.

21. Herpes simplex may cause an acute necrotizing encephalitis without concurrent skin lesions.

Directions: For questions 25 and 26, select ALL INCORRECT answers.

22. Regarding chalazion,

    A.   it is characterized by painless, localized, moderate swelling in the eyelid without signs of active inflammation

    B.   lipogranulomas which occur occasionally become secondarily infected

    C.   when the lid is everted, the conjunctiva over the chalazion appears reddened and elevated

    D.   if sufficiently large, the lesion may press on the eyelid and cause astigmatism, for which surgery may be required

    E.   it usually subsides spontaneously

    F.   if it recurs at the same site, a biopsy should be done to rule out sebaceous gland carcinoma

    G.   treatment with hot pack and antibiotic ointment is effective

23. Kaposi's sarcoma

    A.   is characterized by neoplasms similar to those seen on the skin which may develop in the gastrointestinal tract involving any area from the mouth to the anus

    B.   may affect the bones, liver, spleen, lymph nodes, and most other constituents of the body

    C.   lesions consist of red to purple to brown nodules that are especially common on the legs

    D.   is more common in women

    E.   lesions are usually smooth although they may be ulcerated or verrucous

    F.   occurs frequently in those of Jewish or Italian origin

    G.   is probably a low grade lymphoma

    H.   lesions are not radiosensitive

    I.   has a reasonably good prognosis

Directions: Use the key below to answer the following questions. Select

    A.   **if 1, 2, and 3 are correct**

    B.   **if 1 and 3 are correct**

    C.   **if 2 and 4 are correct**

    D.   **if all statements are correct**

    E.   **if none of the statements is correct**

    F.   **if another combination is correct**

24. Fowler's solution

    1.   was formerly used as a tonic for anemia and certain skin diseases

2. caused epitheliomas, especially on the palms and soles
3. caused systemic cancer involving especially the pelvis
4. is the drug of choice for Bowen's disease

25. Sarcoidosis

   1. may involve the eyes, lymph nodes, bones and almost any other structure of the body
   2. cutaneous manifestations consist of small superficial firm papules found most frequently on the face, neck, and upper trunk
   3. lesions may coalesce or the individual lesion may grow, become depressed in the center, and form an annular plaque
   4. treatment (systemic corticosteroid therapy) usually controls the systemic but not the cutaneous involvement

26. Regarding porphyria cutanea tarda,

   1. the patient, usually a middle aged man, develops bullae and ecthymatous lesions on the back of his hands
   2. lesions are apt to appear after exposure to sunshine or comparatively trivial trauma
   3. it is common in alcoholics
   4. response to therapy is reasonably good
   5. chloroquine may be very effective, but this is a comparatively dangerous treatment
   6. venesection is often effective

27. The majority of cases of erythema nodosum have been found to be secondary to

   1. tuberculosis
   2. sarcoidosis
   3. coccidioidomycosis
   4. streptococcal infections
   5. ulcerative colitis

28. Hereditary angioneurotic edema

   1. is characterized by nonpitting, nonpruritic edema
   2. is frequently precipitated by trauma
   3. is caused by absence of the alpha-2 globulin which inhibits the enzymatic activity of the first component of complement
   4. diagnosis is made by measuring levels of C4 and is confirmed by direct estimation of the amount of C1 inhibitor present

Directions: For each question select
A. if the question is associated with A only
B. if the question is associated with B only
C. if the question is associated with both A and B
D. if the question is associated with neither A nor B

29. Nevus flammeus is characterized by

   A. port-wine marks, especially in the distribution of the trigeminal nerve, which may be associated with angiomas of the choroid or pia mater
   B. lesions which rarely subside spontaneously in contradistinction to cavernous hemagiomas and "strawberry marks"
   C. both
   D. neither

30. Ichthyosis

   A. usually appears early and persists throughout the patient's life
   B. in some patients, develops during or after middle life and in these patients one should suspect a derangement of the liver on the basis of a malignancy, especially a lymphoma
   C. both
   D. neither

31. Regarding vasculitis,

   A. the prognosis for pure cutaneous vasculitis is generally poor
   B. necrotizing vasculitis is characterized pathologically by varying degrees of fibrinoid degeneration of the vessel wall accompanied by an inflammatory infiltrate primarily of neutrophils
   C. both
   D. neither

32. Scars or leg ulcers may be clues to the presence of

    A. hereditary spherocytosis
    B. sickle-cell anemia
    C. both
    D. neither

33. In erythema nodosum, lesions tend to

    A. occur in crops and are often accompanied by malaise and fever
    B. heal in the same manner as does a bruise, with hemorrhage and pigmentation
    C. both
    D. neither

34. Exfoliative erythroderma is a characteristic skin disease of

    A. lymphatic leukemia
    B. Hodgkin's disease
    C. both
    D. neither

35. Central cyanosis may be secondary to

    A. decreased arterial oxygen saturation
    B. hemoglobin abnormalities
    C. both
    D. neither

36. Erythroplasia of Queyrat

    A. is an uncommon precancerous dermatosis of the genital mucosa which occurs predominantly in circumcised men
    B. has been successfully treated with topically applied fluorouracil

37. Which of the following have been reported to relieve postherpetic pain?

    A. fluphenazine
    B. amitriptyline
    C. both
    D. neither

38. Topical steroids have been found to

    A. cause glaucoma
    B. aggravate glaucoma

C. both
D. neither

Directions: For each of the incomplete statements below, ONE or MORE of the completions given is correct. In each case, select
  A. if 1, 2, and 3 are correct
  B. if 1 and 3 are correct
  C. if 2 and 4 are correct
  D. if only 4 is correct
  E. if all statements are correct

39. Melanoma metastasizes commonly to the

    1. lymph nodes
    2. liver
    3. lungs
    4. bones

40. Malignant atrophic papulosis

    1. is Degos' disease
    2. involves endovasculitis of the cutaneous and gastrointestinal vessels
    3. produces pathognomonic skin lesions and strikingly similar lesions with focal infarction, perforation, and usually death from peritonitis
    4. involves the central nervous system, eye, kidney, and heart

41. Adenoma sebaceum

    1. lesions start in the nasolabial fold and spread to the cheeks, chin, nose, and even upper portions of the chest
    2. may be associated with tuberous sclerosis, which is characterized by certain potato-like tumors of the brain and is marked clinically by epilepsy and mental deficiencies
    3. is considered epiloia when all three conditions (skin lesions, brain tumors, and mental deterioration) are present
    4. is an acquired disorder

42. Peripheral cyanosis may occur secondary to

    1. reduced cardiac output
    2. cold exposure

3. redistribution of blood flow from extremities
4. venous or arterial obstruction

43. In Cushing's syndrome, the skin is thin and there are purplish striae located on the

   1. anterior and posterior axillary folds
   2. breasts
   3. abdomen
   4. lateral aspects of the buttocks and thighs

44. Peripheral cyanosis (acrocyanosis) is limited to the

   1. hands and feet
   2. tip of the nose
   3. earlobes
   4. lips

45. Paget's disease of the nipple

   1. is characterized by an excoriation or dry scaling lesion of the nipple
   2. may extend to involve the entire areola
   3. may only be diagnosed by biopsy
   4. does not bleed easily on contact

46. Conjunctivitis

   1. diagnosis is suggested by a short duration of symptoms, absence of pain, an inflamed appearance of the conjunctiva, and a history of exudate or sticky lids, especially in the morning
   2. is usually self-limited and responds quickly to antibiotics
   3. as a viral form is treated with a topical antibiotic to prevent secondary bacterial invasion
   4. if bacterial, is often treated by a sulfa preparation in drop form because of low cost and low antigenicity

Answers and Commentary

1. **E.** Pain is the primary symptom in patients with hordeolums, and the intensity of discomfort is usually in direct proportion to the amount of lid swelling. All other statements are true.
(*Am Fam Physician*, 3:104, 1971)

2. **B.** Blepharitis is a common disorder. All other statements are correct.
(*Am Fam Physician*, 3:104, 1971)

3. **A.** Urticaria pigmentosa is a comparatively unusual condition, appearing early in life in most instances. Additionally, the lesions of uticaria pigmentosa are comparatively radiosensitive. All other statements are true.
(*Hosp Med*, 7:9, 1971)

4. **D.** Ulceration is common in patients with mycosis fungoides. All other statements are correct.
(*Hosp Med*, 7:9, 1971)

5. **A.** Rosacea is usually a benign condition of the skin. All other statements are true of this disorder.
(*Hosp Med*, 7:9, 1971)

6. **C.** Raynaud's disease is a benign, symmetrical disorder of unknown cause which usually has its onset in the late teens or early twenties. Females are more commonly afflicted and cold or emotional stimu i are the factors which trigger the response in the digits. The fingers become white, then blue, and finally red (triphasic color response). Pain and paresthesias are common during the ischemic phase. Ulcerations are rarely observed.
(4:1184–85)

7. **E.** Most frequently, the basis of urticarial reaction is immunologic with antigen-antibody combining to release mediators such as histamine from the tissue mast cells and circulating basophils. Causes can be either immunologic or non-immunologic. All other statements are correct.
(*Lahey Clinic Found Bull*, 22:153, 1973)

8. **Secondary.** If a patient has a generalized eruption that involves the palms and the soles, the eruption is probably either secondary syphilis or a dermatitis medicamentosa. (*Hosp Med*, 7:9, 1971)

9. **Macule.** A color change in the skin without elevation or depression is a macule. (3:53)

10. **Telogen.** Each scalp hair grows about 0.3 to 0.4 mm/day during the growing or anagen phase, before entering resting periods (telogen phase), which occur every few months to a few years. Hair growth is not synchronous, and there is a variation by age and general health. (3:56)

11. **Syringomyelia.** The commonest cause of trophic lesions in the skin in the upper limb is syringomyelia. (1:323)

12. **Papule.** The papule is the smallest in a sequence of masses which elevate the skin; a nodule is larger; a tumor, the largest. (3:53)

13. **Female.** Urticaria is more commonly found in the female sex. (*Lahey Clinic Found Bull*, 22:153, 1973)

14. **C.** In most cases, the cause of erythema nodosum is unknown. (*Hosp Med*, 7:9, 1971)

15. **A.** The dorsal root ganglia and the corresponding sensory ganglia of the cranial nerves are the commonest sites of the lesion of herpes zoster, but the posterior horn of the gray matter of the spinal cord, the dorsal root, and, less often, the anterior root or the peripheral nerves may also be involved. (1:347)

16. **True.** Seborrheic dermatitis may be associated with central nervous system derangements.
(*Hosp Med,* 7:9, 1971)

17. **False.** It has long been recognized that chickenpox may develop after exposure to a patient with herpes zoster, although this is less likely than development of chickenpox after exposure to chickenpox. In contrast, zoster rarely develops after exposure to chickenpox or other cases of zoster. These observations are supported by the epidemiologic findings that chickenpox is a seasonal disease occurring mainly in the winter and spring, and occurring in epidemic proportions every two to four years. In contrast, zoster is not a seasonal disease, and there is no increase in incidence during the years of chickenpox epidemics. There is, in fact, some evidence that the incidence of zoster decreases slightly during years when there are large numbers of cases of chickenpox.
(2:825)

18. **True.** The treatment of sunburn is straightforward—simple calamine lotion for mild cases, and a corticosteroid cream for the more severely affected. (*Lancet,* 2:31, 1973)

19. **True.** The Sturge-Weber syndrome is capillary-venous malformation in one hemisphere associated with a facial nevus. (1:201)

20. **True.** Almost all diseases affecting the conjunctivas produce injection of the vessels together with discharge. In conjunctivitis of infectious origin, the injection usually increases in the fornices, and secretions are present. More severe involvement produces small hemorrhages beneath the conjunctivas. Spontaneous ecchymoses may occur beneath the conjunctivas in otherwise healthy patients, and usually have no significance unless signs of a bleeding tendency are present elsewhere. (3:75)

21. **True.** Herpes simplex is a rare cause of aseptic meningitis in adults and infants, causing acute encephalitis with disseminated visceral necrosis. More important, herpes simplex also causes an acute necrotizing encephalitis without concurrent skin lesions. (1:404)

22. **E,G.** Chalazion seldom subsides spontaneously. Treatment with hot packs and antibiotic ointment is of little value. All other statements are correct.
(*Am Fam Physician,* 3:104, 1971)

23. **D,H.** In Kaposi's sarcoma, the lesions are radiosensitive, responding best to ionizing radiation or certain chemotherapeutic approaches. This condition is more common in men than in women. All other statements are correct.
(*Hosp Med,* 7:9, 1971)

24. **A.** Fowler's solution is not the drug of choice for Bowen's disease. All other statements are correct.
(*Hosp Med,* 7:9, 1971)

25. **A.** In sarcoidosis, systemic corticosteroid therapy usually controls the cutaneous and systemic involvement. (*Hosp Med,* 7:9, 1971)

26. **D.** All statements are true of porphyria cutanea tarda. (*Hosp Med,* 7:9, 1971)

27. **E.** Erythema nodosum should be suspected when tender erythematous nodules appear in or under the skin and are associated with fever and joint pains. The articular manifestations often precede the appearance of the nodules. These lesions can be associated with a wide variety of diseases, some of which include tuberculosis, sarcoidosis, coccidioidomycosis, streptococcal infections, and ulcerative colitis. However, in the majority of cases, no underlying disease is found.
(4:244)

28. **D.** All statements are true of hereditary angioneurotic edema.
(*Lahey Clinic Found Bull,* 22:153, 1973)

29. **C.** Both statements are true of nevus flammeus.
(*Hosp Med,* 7:9, 1971)

30. **C.** Ichthyosis appears early and persists throughout the patient's life. In some individuals, ichthyosis develops during or after middle age. In these patients, one should suspect a derangement of the liver on the basis of a malignancy, especially a lymphoma. (*Hosp Med,* 7:9, 1971)

31. **B.** The prognosis for pure cutaneous vasculitis is generally good. The other statement is true regarding vasculitis. (*Mod Med,* 40:70, 1972)

32. **C.** Scars or leg ulcers may be clues to the presence of hereditary spherocytosis or sickle-cell anemia. (*Res Staff Phys*, 19:24, 1973)

33. **C.** Both statements are true of the lesions in patients with erythema nodosum. (*Hosp Med*, 7:9, 1971)

34. **C.** Exfoliative erythroderma is a characteristic skin disease of both lymphatic leukemia and Hodgkin's disease. (*Hosp Med*, 7:9, 1971)

35. **C.** Central cyanosis may be secondary to decreased arterial oxygen saturation such as found with decreased atmospheric pressure, impaired pulmonary function, or anatomic shunts. It may also be due to hemoglobin abnormalities, such as methemoglobinemia, sulfhemoglobinemia, and carboxyhemoglobinemia. The latter, however, is not true cyanosis. (4:166)

36. **B.** Erythroplasia of Queyrat occurs predominantly in uncircumcised men. The other statement is true. (*JAMA*, 232:934, 1975)

37. **C.** Both fluphenazine and amitriptyline have been reported to relieve postherpetic pain. (2:609)

38. **C.** Topical steroids have been found to both cause and aggravate glaucoma. (*Am Fam Physician*, 3:104, 1971)

39. **E.** Melanoma metastasizes most commonly to the lymph nodes, liver, lungs, and bones. (*Hosp Med*, 7:9, 1971)

40. **E.** All the statements are true of malignant atrophic papulosis. (*Mod Med*, 40:70, 1972)

41. **A.** Adenoma sebaceum is a genetic disorder which develops between the fourth and ninth years of life. (*Hosp Med*, 7:9, 1971)

42. **E.** Peripheral cyanosis may occur secondary to all the conditions listed. (4:167)

43. **E.** In Cushing's syndrome, purplish striae may be located on all the areas listed. (3:49)

44. **E.** Peripheral cyanosis (sometimes called acrocyanosis) is limited to the hands, feet, tip of the nose, earlobes, and lips. (3:166, 168)

45. **A.** In Paget's disease of the nipple, the nipple tends to bleed easily on contact and is always associated with an underlying carcinoma although the underlying carcinoma may not always be palpable. (3:268)

46. **E.** All the statements are true of conjunctivitis. This disorder may be associated with keratitis, iritis, and acute glaucoma. (*Am Fam Physician*, 3:104, 1971)

Textbook References for Chapter 6

1. Bannister, R. (1978): *Brain's Clinical Neurology*, Fifth Edition, Oxford University Press, New York.

2. Beeson, P.B. and McDermott, W. (1979): *Cecil Textbook of Medicine*, Fifteenth Edition, W.B. Saunders Company, Philadelphia, London, Toronto.

3. Judge, R.D. and Zuidema, G.D. (1974): *Methods of Clinical Examination: A Physiologic Approach*, Third Edition, Little, Brown and Company, Boston.

4. Isselbacher, K.J., Editor. (1980): *Harrison's Principles of Internal Medicine*, Ninth Edition, McGraw-Hill Company, New York.

CHAPTER 7

Electrocardiography

Directions: Indicate whether each of the following statements is true or false.

1. The U wave precedes the T wave.

2. By Einthoven's convention, the negative pole of the galvanometer is attached to the right arm and the positive pole of the galvanometer is attached to the left arm to record Lead I.

3. The magnitude of deflection on the augmented unipolar extremity leads is more than the magnitude of deflection on the bipolar extremity leads.

4. The vector method of electrocardiography aids in the recognition of arrhythmias.

5. The recognition of right ventricular hypertrophy from the direction of the QRS vector is less reliable than is the recognition of left ventricular hypertrophy from the direction of the mean QRS vector.

6. When stress tests fail to produce ST segment depression in a patient with known ischemic heart disease, the presence of ventricular aneurysm should be seriously considered.

7. Ventricular hypertrophy alone will not prolong the QRS duration beyond 0.12 sec.

8. Electrocardiographic localization of a myocardial infarct always coincides with pathologic localization.

9. Changes toward normal in serial electrocardiograms always indicate improvement.

10. Right bundle branch block may occur in young subjects with no history or evidence of heart disease and may represent a congenital defect of the conduction system.

11. QRS abnormalities frequently occur in uncomplicated pericarditis.

12. In pericarditis, the epicardial injury and ischemia are usually localized.

13. Epinephrine can convert a fine ventricular fibrillation to a coarser fibrillation which may be more amenable to defibrillation.

14. Ventricular tachycardia is defined as two or more consecutive premature ventricular beats that usually occur at a rate of 150 to 250/min.

15. The P wave usually decreases in amplitude with an increase in heart rate.

16. The entire P wave will be large, peaked, and positive in Lead V-1 when there is a pure left atrial abnormality.

17. When the P waves are identified in paroxysmal atrial tachycardia, they are usually of the same configuration as the normal sinus P waves of the same patient.

18. Aberrant conduction rarely occurs in the presence of atrial fibrillation.

19. Edrophonium (Tensilon), 10 mg intravenously, will not be as effective as carotid sinus pressure in terms of parasympathetic effect for differentiating various forms of tachycardia.

20. It is uncommon for atrial fibrillation to fail to respond to carotid sinus pressure.

21. In atrial or ventricular bigeminy, the premature beats are not triggered by nor are they dependent upon the normal beat.

Directions: For each of the incomplete statements below, ONE or MORE of the completions given is correct. In each case, select
- **A. if 1, 2, and 3 are correct**
- **B. if 1 and 3 are correct**
- **C. if 2 and 4 are correct**
- **D. if only 4 is correct**
- **E. if all statements are correct**

22. When there is sufficient right ventricular hypertrophy,
    1. the mean spatial QRS vector is directed to the right and anteriorly because the right ventricle lies to the right and is anterior to the left ventricle
    2. the R wave is largest in V-1 and becomes progressively smaller in an orderly sequence until it is smallest in V-6
    3. the S wave is smallest in V-1 but becomes progressively deeper until it is largest in V-6
    4. there is no "reversal of the R/S ratio"

23. Low amplitude of QRS complexes may be found in
    1. myxedema
    2. obesity
    3. pericardial effusion
    4. emphysema

24. Regarding digitalis,
    1. it lengthens electrical systole
    2. premature ventricular contractions, frequently occurring as bigeminy, are the most common cardiac arrhythmia associated with digitalis toxicity
    3. it alters the QRS complexes
    4. the P-R interval is frequently prolonged because of a delay of impulse conduction at the A-V node

25. P waves may be altered by
    1. tachycardia
    2. autonomic nervous system stimulation
    3. unimportant conduction defects
    4. atrial myocardial infarction

26. Electrocardiographic characteristics of a wandering pacemaker within the sinus node include
    1. rate changes as seen in ordinary sinus arrhythmia plus P wave variations and minor P-R interval changes with rate
    2. a tendency for taller P waves and larger P-R intervals with a faster rate
    3. a phasic or nonphasic respiratory cycle
    4. of itself, indication of disease

27. Rapid sinus tachycardia in adults
    1. does not usually exceed 150 to 160 beats/min
    2. occurs occasionally with rates as fast as 170 to 180/min

3. in a few individuals may reach or exceed 200/min during extreme exercise

4. responds to carotid sinus pressure by slowing followed by a gradual return to the original rate in a few seconds to a minute

28. Regarding ventricular parasystole,

1. a sinus node pacemaker drives the heart, while a second automatic pacemaker in the ventricles (which is protected from, and thus not discharged by, the descending sinus impulse because of a form of block) is intermittently discharging the ventricles

2. when the ventricular pacemaker is faster than the sinus pacemaker, it usurps the primary function of the heart and a ventricular tachycardia occurs

3. the electrocardiographic features are ventricular ectopic beats not coupled to the preceding sinus beats by fixed intervals and showing no fixed pattern of variability

4. it is the least common form of parasystole

Directions: For each of the following statements, fill in the correct word(s).

29. When a primary pacemaker of the heart is present at a nodal or ventricular level (as in nodal or ventricular tachycardia), block in the reverse direction, or _____ block from ventricle or A-V node to atria across the A-V junction, may occur.

30. When two pacemakers discharge at such time that each is able to depolarize part of the ventricular musculature before they physiologically interfere with each other, a ventricular _____ beat occurs. Electrocardiographically, its QRS-T complex is intermediate in contour between the configuration of the QRS complexes of each of the pacemakers.

31. A _____ beat results from simultaneous activation of the ventricles by both sinus and ectopic impulses.

32. If an inverted P wave precedes the QRS complex by .12 sec or more, it may be a premature atrial beat from a focus _____ in the atrium.

33. If the vector representing subendocardial injury develops and persists for hours or days in a patient with a clinical picture of myocardial infarction, one should suspect _____ infarction.

34. Perhaps the most common electrocardiographic finding observed after pulmonary embolism is nonspecific _____ _____ .

35. If inspection of the three bipolar extremity leads reveals that the resultant QRS complex is conspicuously larger on one lead than on the other two leads, then the mean QRS vector will be relatively _____ to that lead.

36. Lead I plus Lead III equals Lead _____ , and aVR plus aVF plus aVL equals _____ .

37. All electrocardiograms are standardized so that 1 mv of electrical force will move the recording stylus or string _____ mm.

38. The two physiologic properties of the heart of primary importance in rhythm disturbances are _____ and _____ .

39. Electrocardiographic changes of _____ consist of T wave flattening, ST-segment depression, and the appearance of a prominent U wave that gives the impression of a prolonged Q-T interval.

Directions: For each of the following multiple-choice questions, select the ONE CORRECT answer.

40. Which of the following is either uninfluenced by carotid sinus pressure or will abruptly revert to a normal sinus rhythm?

A. paroxysmal atrial tachycardia
B. atrial fibrillation

C.   atrial flutter
D.   sinus tachycardia
E.   all of the above

41.   The incidence of sinus bradycardia in myocardial infarction is approximately

A.   5%
B.   20%
C.   50%
D.   70%
E.   90%

42.   The frequency with which nonspecific T wave abnormalities occur in a population of individuals without evidence of clinical cardiac disease varies between

A.   1 and 4%
B.   5 and 9%
C.   10 and 18%
D.   25 and 30%
E.   40 and 60%

Directions: For each of the following multiple-choice questions, select the ONE INCORRECT answer.

43.   Regarding A-V dissociation,

A.   the common denominator is a nodal rate faster than the sinus rate
B.   two different pacemakers drive the heart—a sinus pacemaker controls the atria and an A-V nodal pacemaker controls the ventricles
C.   it is always associated with heart block
D.   A-V conduction is usually potentially normal
E.   the rhythm is basically regular, but the regularity is interrupted by capture beats

44.   Regarding the spatial QRS-T angle,

A.   it represents the relationship between the forces of depolarization and the forces of repolarization
B.   it varies with age
C.   in the average adult, it is frequently wider than 60 degrees

D.   when angles of 100–180° are found, this identifies an abnormal T vector for that particular QRS vector.

45.   Paroxysmal atrial tachycardia

A.   denotes an abnormal rhythm in which a rapid ectopic focus in the atrium has become the pacemaker of the heart
B.   heart rate is in the range of 140 and 240 (usually 170 to 220 beats/min)
C.   is frequent in normal younger people, more common in the male and in patients with Wolff-Parkinson-White syndrome
D.   almost always has 1:1 conduction of the ectopic atrial impulses, producing a ventricular rate equal to the ectopic atrial rate
E.   when accompanied by heart block (such as 2:1, 3:1, or higher, or variable block), the implication is that there is a relative or absolute abnormality of conduction which may be caused by digitalis or by disease of the A-V conduction system

46.   Accelerated idioventricular rhythm

A.   rates range from 60 to 100 beats/min
B.   is often seen with slow ventricular tachycardia
C.   often appears with an inferior myocardial infarction and sinus arrhythmia, especially when the ectopic rhythm exceeds the sinus rate during the slow phase of the sinus arrhythmia
D.   usually begins as a premature beat near the normally conducted sinus beat rather than as a late ventricular ectopic beat
E.   disappears as the rate of the sinus rhythm exceeds the rate of the ectopic rhythm, and if both occur at the same time, fusion complexes result

47.   Regarding atrial premature beats,

A.   they are uncommon
B.   they occur both with and without iden-

tifiable heart disease

C. frequent (often multifocal) premature atrial contractions often precede the onset of atrial tachycardia or atrial flutter or fibrillation

D. occasional unifocal atrial premature systoles are seen in the absence of heart disease, sometimes being precipitated by excesses of caffeine, tobacco, or alcohol, or by fatigue

E. they are recognized electrocardiographically as an early P wave, frequently different in configuration from the normal P wave

48. Regarding premature nodal beats,

A. complexes often have an identical configuration to those of the normal sinus beats

B. instead of following a pause or occurring in association with sinus bradycardia or sinus arrest, nodal extrasystoles may occur at any heart rate and occur early (i.e., a short interval preceding the nodal beat)

C. when an inverted P wave in inferior leads, occurring less than .12 sec before the premature QRS, is associated with the premature beat of normal configurations, it is usually positive evidence of nodal premature systole

D. in general, an inverted P wave preceding the QRS indicates an extrasystolic focus high in the node; an inverted P wave following the QRS indicates an extrasystolic focus low in the node, and a P wave concealed in the QRS indicates midnodal focus

E. when a normal anterograde P wave (with a normal or long P-R interval) is seen to precede an early beat, the early beat is more likely a premature nodal systole than a premature atrial systole

49. After digitalis medication,

A. the Q-T interval, normally over .34 sec at heart rates of 75 to 95, is frequently reduced to as low as .28 sec at these heart rates

B. the T waves may become smaller

C. at times, the entire recovery phase proceeds from endocardium to epicardium and no T waves may be found

D. the ST and T change may closely resemble the subendocardial injury of coronary insufficiency

E. persons with heart disease rarely show electrocardiographic effects in response to doses of digitalis which have no effect on the electrocardiogram of normal subject

50. Activation of the nodal escape mechanism may occur

A. in well-trained athletes whose physiologic bradycardia may become slow enough that nodal escape beats occur

B. with sinus bradycardia in the course of acute inferior myocardial infarction

C. with diminished vagal tone due to pharmacologic agents

D. with any degenerative or inflammatory lesion which may interfere with sinus node or atrial pacemaker function

51. In third degree (complete) A-V block,

A. both the atria and the ventricles have their own pacemaker

B. P waves and QRS complexes are independent of each other and occur at different rates

C. most cases are associated with an idioventricular pacemaker and the ventricular rate is usually in the range of 30 to 40 beats/min

D. there may be a nodal pacemaker with a rate of 40 to 60 beats/min

E. the atrial rate is usually subnormal

Directions: Use the key below to answer the following questions. Select

A. if the statement defines A-V dissociation
B. if the statement defines interference
C. if the statement defines coupling interval
D. if the statement defines parasystole
E. if the statement defines block

52. the interval between a sinus beat and a premature beat, or between any two beats occurring in pairs

53. independent activity of the atria and ventricles

54. two impulses traveling toward each other from different directions and preventing each other's passage

55. a pathologic state in the conducting system causing the propagation of an impulse to be slowed or stopped

56. a rhythm in which the heart is being paced by two independent pacemakers

Directions: For each of the following questions select
A. **if the question is associated with A only**
B. **if the question is associated with B only**
C. **if the question is associated with both A and B**
D. **if the question is associated with neither A nor B**

57. In left ventricular hypertrophy,
    A. the mean QRS vector is often directed farther to the left and more posteriorly than normal
    B. a narrow Q wave often appears in Lead I
    C. both
    D. neither

58. QS complexes
    A. are not recorded in V-1 in normal subjects
    B. may be recorded in V-1, V-2, and V-3 in cases of left ventricular hypertrophy
    C. both
    D. neither

59. When the left ventricular apex is the site of an infarction, little QRS abnormality other than reduced magnitude results because
    A. the myocardium generating a large portion of the normal initial forces is still intact
    B. there is little ventricular muscle diametrically opposite to the cardiac apex
    C. both
    D. neither

60. Left bundle branch block
    A. frequently occurs as the result of congenital heart disease
    B. may be associated with many types of myocarditis
    C. both
    D. neither

61. In the normal subject, the wave of depolarization producing the
    A. QRS complex proceeds from the epicardium to the endocardium
    B. T wave proceeds from the endocardium to the epicardium
    C. both
    D. neither

62. In patients in normal sinus rhythm, the electrocardiogram gives considerable information indicating when
    A. digitalis is needed
    B. the optimal digitalis effect has been reached
    C. both
    D. neither

63. The normal P wave is usually
    A. less than 2.5 mm in height
    B. less than .11 sec in duration
    C. both
    D. neither

64. The P wave
    A. axis is usually between +30° and +60°
    B. may have a smooth contour or be slightly notched
    C. both
    D. neither

65. Abnormal variations of sinus node impulse formation include

    A. sinus arrhythmia
    B. wandering pacemaker
    C. both
    D. neither

66. A-V dissociation may occur by

    A. an abnormal slowing of the sinus node to a rate below the intrinsic A-V nodal rate
    B. an increase of the intrinsic A-V nodal rate above the sinus node pacemaker rate
    C. both
    D. neither

67. Capture beat

    A. is an early beat preceded by a P wave which occurs beyond the refractory period of the preceding QRS complex
    B. has a normal P-R interval unless the P wave occurs in the relative refractory period of the preceding beat or else if first degree heart block coexists with the A-V dissociation
    C. both
    D. neither

68. Heart block

    A. may or may not coexist with "A-V dissociation"

    B. is an essential feature of "A-V dissociation"
    C. both
    D. neither

Directions: Use the key below to answer the following questions. Select
   A. **if the statement defines an ectopic beat**
   B. **if the statement defines an interpolated beat**
   C. **if the statement defines a fusion beat**
   D. **if the statement defines a reciprocal beat**
   E. **if the statement defines an escape beat**

69. a beat caused by an impulse originating in an area other than the sinus node

70. a beat originating in one of the lower pacemaker centers of the heart with a slower intrinsic rate, due to failure of the faster sinus node pacemaker to discharge

71. a complex intermediate in configuration between complexes of two different origins, due to simultaneous discharge of parts of the myocardium by each of the two sites of impulse formation

72. a complex triggered by an impulse which has left and then reentered its area of origin

73. an extra beat occurring between two sinus beats without affecting the sinus cycle or ventricular cycle

Answers and Commentary

1. **False.** The U wave follows the T wave and is sometimes of clinical significance. For example, it may aid in the diagnosis of hypokalemia. (1:4)

2. **True.** By Einthoven's convention, the negative pole of the galvanometer is attached to the right arm and the positive pole of the galvanometer is attached to the left arm to record Lead I; the negative pole of the galvanometer is attached to the right arm and the positive pole of the galvanometer is attached to the left leg to record Lead II, and the negative pole is attached to the left arm and the positive pole to the left leg to record Lead III. This must be memorized since it is a purely arbitrary arrangement. (1:14, 15)

3. **False.** The magnitude of deflection on the augmented unipolar extremity leads is less than the magnitude of deflection on the bipolar extremity leads. (1:17)

4. **False.** The portion of the electrocardiogram produced by the ventricular musculature, including the QRS complex, the T wave, and ST segment displacement, can be represented by spacial vectors and utilized to study the electrocardiogram. The vector method of electrocardiography does not aid in the recognition of arrhythmias. (1:43)

5. **False.** The recognition of hypertrophy of the right ventricle from the direction of the mean spatial QRS vector is much more reliable than is the recognition of left ventricular hypertrophy from the direction of the mean spatial QRS vector. (1:70)

6. **True.** When stress tests fail to produce ST segment depression in a patient with known ischemic heart disease, the presence of ventricular aneurysm should be seriously considered.
(*J Electrocardiol*, 5:317, 1972)

7. **True.** The QRS duration, though often normal, may be prolonged to .11 or even .12 sec in left ventricular hypertrophy. Most electrocardiographers state that ventricular hypertrophy alone will not prolong the QRS duration beyond .12 sec. (1:84)

8. **False.** At times, the electrocardiographic localization of a myocardial infarct will not coincide with pathologic localization. One difficulty arises from the fact that the vectors resulting from a myocardial infarction in a vertical heart may project on the routine leads in a different manner to the vectors of a similarly located infarction in a horizontal heart. Another reason for the lack of perfect parallelism in electrocardiographic and pathologic localization is the fact that the electrocardiogram reflects electrical death while the pathologist studies the morphologic evidence of necrosis. (1:99)

9. **False.** Two abnormal .04 vectors, resulting from two separate myocardial infarcts, may produce a perfectly normally directed .04 vector since the recorded vector is the vector sum of the two abnormal vectors. Similarly, two abnormal ST vectors may produce normally directed ST or T vectors. The fact that two abnormal vectors can at times produce a normal vector should cause one

to be cautious in assuming that changes toward the normal in serial electrocardiographic tracings always indicate improvement. (1:119)

10. **True.** Right bundle branch block may occur in young subjects with no history or evidence of heart disease and may represent a congenital defect of the conduction system. The etiology of right bundle branch block must be determined clinically. (1:158)

11. **False.** The electrocardiographic findings commonly found in pericarditis are due to associated epicardial myocardial damage. Under such circumstances, epicardial injury and ischemia develop and alter the ST-T portion of the electrocardiogram. Unlike myocardial infarction, QRS abnormalities never occur in uncomplicated pericarditis. (1:198)

12. **False.** In pericarditis, the epicardial injury and ischemia are generalized, involving all ventricular surfaces, and therefore the mean ST vector is directed toward the centroid of the area of epicardial ischemia. As a consequence, the mean ST vector is commonly relatively parallel with the mean QRS vector and the mean T vector directed opposite to the mean QRS vector. Often, the T vector change does not appear until the ST vector has largely vanished, which usually occurs in one to two weeks. (1:198)

13. **True.** Epinephrine can convert a fine ventricular fibrillation to a coarser fibrillation which may be more amenable to defibrillation.
(*Postgrad Med*, 48:168, 1970)

14. **False.** Ventricular tachycardia is defined as three or more consecutive premature ventricular beats that usually occur at a rate of 150 to 250 per minute. (*Postgrad Med*, 48:168, 1970)

15. **False.** The P wave may increase in amplitude with an increase in heart rate. (1:209)

16. **False.** The entire P wave will be large, peaked, and positive in Lead V-1 when there is a pure right atrial abnormality. (1:212)

17. **False.** Occasionally, a low, atrial ectopic focus may produce a slow, paroxysmal atrial tachycardia with a rate in the range of approximately 120/min in which the P waves are readily identifiable. When the P waves are identified in paroxysmal atrial tachycardia, they are usually of a different configuration from the normal sinus P waves of the same patient. (1:236)

18. **False.** Aberrant conduction often occurs in the presence of atrial fibrillation. (1:271)

19. **False.** Carotid massage should not be performed in patients with diseased carotid arteries or with known cerebrovascular disease and should be used only under extremely strong indications in patients with recent myocardial infarction. An alternative to the use of carotid sinus pressure is the use of the drug edrophonium (Tensilon), 10 mg intravenously. This will often be as effective as carotid pressure in terms of parasympathetic effect. (1:274)

20. **False.** Atrial fibrillation responds to carotid sinus pressure with an increased degree of block, and the slowing may make obscure fibrillatory waves demonstrable. In addition, the ventricular response will have the typical irregular response of atrial fibrillation unless complete block with nodal rhythm is temporarily induced, resulting in a regular response. It is not uncommon, however, for atrial fibrillation to fail to respond to carotid sinus pressure. (1:276–77)

21. **False.** In atrial or ventricular bigeminy, the premature beats are triggered by and dependent upon the normal beat. This type of premature beat only occurs after the beat to which it is coupled and does not occur during a pause. (1:288)

22. **A.** When there is sufficient right ventricular hypertrophy, the mean spatial QRS vector is directed to the right and anteriorly because the right ventricle lies to the right and is anterior to the left ventricle. The amount the mean QRS vector rotates to the right and anteriorly varies greatly from subject to subject. When the mean spatial QRS vector is rotated to the right and anteriorly, the precordial electrode deflections are greatly different from the normal. The R wave is largest in V-1 and becomes progressively smaller in an orderly sequence until it is smallest in V-6, while the S wave is smallest in V-1 but becomes progressively deeper until it is largest in V-6. This is the reverse of what is seen when the mean spatial R/S is normally directed and has been called "reversal of the R/S ratio"; the reversal of the R/S ratio is a result of the abnormal QRS loop. In space, the initial instantaneous forces of the QRS loop are directed to the left and anteriorly, the succeeding forces are directed more anteriorly and to the right, and the terminal forces are directed to the right and more posteriorly. In addition, the mean spatial T vector associated with right ventricular hypertrophy is usually directed to the left and is usually flush with the frontal plane or directed a variable number of degrees posteriorly. The spatial QRS-T angle is frequently 150 to 180 degrees. (1:69–71)

23. **E.** Low amplitude of the QRS complexes may be found in all the disorders listed.
(*Res Staff Phys*, 20:96, 1974)

24. **C.** There are several electrocardiographic effects of digitalis medication. It produces cardiac arrhythmias, prolongs conduction time, shortens electrical systole, and alters the manner of repolarization so that marked ST and T changes occur. Although premature ventricular contractions, frequently occurring as bigeminy, are the most common cardiac arrhythmia resulting from digitalis medication, virtually any cardiac rhythm can be produced. The P-R interval is frequently prolonged because of a delay of impulse conduction at the A-V node. Occasionally the P-R interval may gradually increase during several successive heart cycles until the auricular impulse fails to be conducted through the A-V node. Under such circumstances a P wave may not be followed by a QRS complex. This type of conduction defect is called the Wenckebach phenomenon. The QRS complexes are not altered by digitalis. (1:187)

25. **E.** Many benign conditions, such as tachycardia, autonomic nervous system stimulation, and unimportant conduction defects may alter the P waves. Atrial myocardial infarction may produce abnormal P waves. The P waves may also become abnormal in patients with valvular and myocardial disease. (1:212–213)

26. **A.** A wandering pacemaker within the sinus node is characterized electrocardiographically by rate changes as seen in ordinary sinus arrhythmia plus P wave variations and minor P-R interval changes with rate. The P waves tend to be taller and P-R intervals longer with a faster rate. It also may be phasic (i.e., related to the respiratory cycle) or nonphasic. A wandering pacemaker within the S-A node does not, in itself, indicate disease. (1:231)

27. **E.** All statements are true of rapid sinus tachycardia in adults. (1:233)

28. **A.** In ventricular parasystole, a sinus node pacemaker drives the heart, while a second automatic pacemaker in the ventricles (which is protected from, and thus not discharged by, the descending sinus impulse because of a form of block) intermittently discharges the ventricles. The ventricular pacemaker is slower than the sinus pacemaker. When the ventricular pacemaker is faster, it usurps the primary function of the heart and a ventricular tachycardia results. The electrocardiographic features of ventricular parasystole are ventricular ectopic beats not coupled to the preceding sinus beats by fixed intervals (i.e., the interval between the onset of the preceding sinus QRS and the onset of the parasystolic QRS is not constant) and showing no fixed pattern of variability. It is the most common form of parasystole,

but parasystole may occur between the sinus pacemaker and an ectopic atrial focus or the sinus pacemaker and an ectopic A-V nodal focus or, very rarely, between any other two automatic centers, one being the primary pacemaker and the other the parasystolic pacemaker. (1:291)

29. **Retrograde.** When a primary pacemaker of the heart is present at a nodal or ventricular level (as in nodal or ventricular tachycardia), block in the reverse direction, or retrograde block from ventricle or A-V node to atria across the A-V junction, may occur. (1:286–87)

30. **Fusion.** When two pacemakers discharge at such time that each is able to depolarize part of the ventricular musculature before they physiologically interfere with each other, a ventricular fusion beat occurs. Electrocardiographically, the fusion QRS-T complex is intermediate in contour between the configuration of the QRS complexes of each of the pacemakers. (1:295)

31. **Fusion.** A fusion beat results from simultaneous activation of the ventricles by both sinus and ectopic impulses. (*Postgrad Med,* 48:168, 1970)

32. **Low.** In general, an inverted P wave preceding the QRS indicates an extrasystolic focus high in the node, an inverted P wave following the QRS indicates an extrasystolic focus low in the node, and a P wave concealed in the QRS indicates mid-nodal focus. Conversely, if the inverted P wave precedes the QRS complex by .12 sec or more, it may be a premature atrial beat from a focus low in the atrium. (1:250)

33. **Subendocardial.** If the vector representing subendocardial injury develops and persists for hours or days in a patient with a clinical picture of myocardial infarction, one should suspect subendocardial infarction. (1:116)

34. **Sinus tachycardia.** Perhaps the most common electrocardiographic finding observed after pulmonary embolism is nonspecific sinus tachycardia. It is not uncommon for various abnormal cardiac rhythms to be precipitated by pulmonary embolism, particularly auricular fibrillation or auricular tachycardia. (1:202)

35. **Parallel.** If inspection of the three bipolar extremity leads reveals that the resultant QRS complex is conspicuously larger on one lead than on the other two leads, then the mean QRS vector will be relatively parallel to that lead. (1:24)

36. **II, zero.** By using the six extremity lead axes, one can learn the direction of a vector with an accuracy of about ±5 degrees. The vector positions

iying between those shown above can be determined by interpolation and constant recall that Lead I plus III equals Lead II and that aVR plus aVL plus aVF equals zero.   (1:25)

37. **10.** All electrocardiograms are standardized so that 1 mv of electrical force will move the recording stylus or string 10 mm.   (1:5)

38. **Automaticity, conductivity.** The two physiologic properties of the heart of primary importance in rhythm disturbances are automaticity and conductivity. Automaticity is the physiological term denoting the process of impulse formation. Conductivity is the term denoting the ability to transmit the formed impulse throughout the heart.   (1:217)

39. **Hypokalemia.** Electrocardiographic changes of hypokalemia consist of T wave flattening, ST segment depression, and the appearance of a prominent U wave that gives the impression of a prolonged QT interval.   (*JAMA*, 231:631, 1975)

40. **A.** Paroxysmal atrial tachycardia is either uninfluenced by carotid sinus pressure or will abruptly revert to a normal sinus rhythm. Atrial flutter and fibrillation exhibit a decrease in ventricular response, often rendering flutter or fibrillary waves obvious during the slower rate. This is a temporary response; the rate rapidly returns to its prior level.   (1:244)

41. **B.** The incidence of sinus bradycardia in myocardial infarction is approximately 20%.
(*Hosp Med*, 7:141, 1971)

42. **A.** The frequency with which nonspecific T wave abnormalities occur in a population of individuals without evidence of clinical cardiac disease varies between 1 and 4%.
(*Arch Intern Med*, 130:895, 1972)

43. **C.** A-V dissociation usually occurs by one or by a combination of two mechanisms, either by an abnormal slowing of the sinus node to a rate below the intrinsic A-V nodal rate or by an increase of the intrinsic A-V nodal rate above the sinus node pacemaker rate. In both instances, the common denominator is a nodal rate faster than the sinus rate. Two different pacemakers thus drive the heart—a sinus pacemaker controls the atria and an A-V nodal pacemaker controls the ventricles. While the nodal pacemaker is the faster, the rates of the two pacemakers are usually fairly close. The rhythm in A-V dissociation is basically regular, but the regularity is interrupted by capture beats.   (1:253, 256–57)

44. **C.** The spatial QRS-T angle represents the relationship between the forces of depolarization and forces of repolarization and varies with age. The QRS-T angle is a very useful tool. For example, in the average adult, the spatial QRS-T angle is seldom wider than 60 degrees. When angles of 100 or 180° are found, this identifies an abnormal T vector for that particular QRS vector.   (1:44)

45. **C.** Paroxysmal atrial tachycardia denotes an abnormal rhythm in which a rapid ectopic focus in the atrium has become the pacemaker of the heart. The heart rate is in the range of 140 to 240 (usually 170 to 220 beats/min). It is frequent in normal younger people, more commonly in the female and in patients with Wolff-Parkinson-White syndrome. There is almost always 1:1 conduction of the ectopic atrial impulses, producing a ventricular rate equal to the ectopic atrial rate. When an ectopic atrial tachycardia is accompanied by heart block (such as 2:1, 3:1, or higher or variable block), the implication is that there is a relative or absolute abnormality of conduction which may be caused by digitalis or by disease of the A-V conduction system.   (1:233, 236)

46. **D.** Accelerated idioventricular rhythm usually begins as a late ventricular rhythm beat rather than a premature beat near the preceding normally conducted sinus beat as is often seen with the conventional type of ventricular tachycardia. All other statements are true.
(*Postgrad Med*, 48:168, 1970)

47. **A.** Atrial premature beats are common and occur both with and without identifiable heart disease. Frequent (often multifocal) premature atrial contractions often precede the onset of atrial tachycardia or atrial flutter or fibrillation. On the other hand, occasional unifocal atrial premature systoles are often seen in the absence of heart disease, sometimes being precipitated by excesses of caffeine, tobacco, or alcohol, or by fatigue. Electrocardiographically, the premature atrial contraction is recognized as an early P wave, frequently different in configuration from the normal P wave. Conduction of the premature impulse, with a resulting QRS complex, may or may not occur. The premature P-QRS is followed by a pause, either compensatory or noncompensatory. The P-R interval of the premature complex may be prolonged because of residual refractoriness in parts of the A-V conduction system at the time of the early beat.   (1:244–45)

48. **E.** All of the statements are true of premature nodal beats, except that when a normal antegrade P wave (with a normal or long P-R interval) is seen to precede an early beat, the early beat is a premature atrial systole rather than a premature nodal systole.   (1:250)

49. **E.** After digitalis medication, persons with heart disease often show electrocardiographic effects in response to doses of digitalis which have no effect on the electrocardiogram of normal subjects. All other statements are true of digitalis medication. (1:189)

50. **C.** Excessive vagal tone due to pharmacologic agents may induce nodal escape. All other factors listed may activate the nodal escape mechanism. (1:248)

51. **E.** In third degree (complete) A-V block, the atrial rate is usually normal or may be increased, but it is not subnormal. All other statements are true of complete A-V block. (1:281–82)

52. **C.** (1:304)

53. **A.** (1:304)

54. **B.** (1:305)

55. **E.** (1:304)

56. **D.** (1:305)

57. **C.** In left ventricular hypertrophy, the mean QRS vector is often directed farther to the left and more posteriorly than normal. Usually the early forces of the QRS loop project a negative quantity on Lead I, producing a narrow Q wave in this lead. (1:83)

58. **B.** QS complexes may be recorded in V-1 in normal subjects and QS complexes may be recorded in V-1, V-2, and V-3 in cases of left ventricular hypertrophy. (1:97)

59. **C.** When the left ventricular apex is the site of an infarction, little QRS abnormality, other than reduced magnitude, results. This is because the myocardium generating a large portion of the normal initial forces is still intact and because there is little ventricular muscle diametrically opposite to the cardiac apex. (1:98)

60. **B.** The most common cause of left bundle branch block is coronary atherosclerosis with or without the clinical symptoms of coronary disease. This type of bundle block rarely occurs as a result of congenital heart disease, but may be associated with many types of myocarditis. The exact etiology and significance of left bundle branch block must be determined clinically. (1:164–65)

61. **D.** In the normal subject, the wave of depolarization producing the QRS complex proceeds from endocardium to epicardium and the wave of repolarization producing the T wave proceeds from epicardium to endocardium. (1:188)

62. **D.** In patients in normal sinus rhythm, the electrocardiogram gives no information relative to when digitalis is needed nor when the optimum effect has been reached. (1:189)

63. **C.** The normal P wave is usually less than 2.5 mm in height and less than .11 sec in duration. (1:209)

64. **C.** The P wave may have a smooth contour or be slightly notched. Its axis is usually located to the left of Lead axis AVF and below Lead axis I (most frequently between +30 and +60 degrees). (1:209)

65. **D.** Not all variations of sinus node impulse formation are abnormal. Two common mechanisms which fall into the category of normal variants are sinus arrhythmia and wandering pacemaker. (1:231)

66. **C.** A-V dissociation usually occurs by one or by a combination, of two mechanisms—either by an abnormal slowing of the sinus node to a rate below the intrinsic A-V nodal rate, or by an increase of the intrinsic A-V nodal rate above the sinus node pacemaker rate. (1:253)

67. **C.** A capture beat is recognized as an early beat preceded by a P wave which occurs beyond the refractory period of the preceding QRS complex. The P-R interval of a capture beat is normal unless the P wave occurs in the relative refractory period of the preceding beat or if first-degree heart block coexists with the A-V dissociation. (1:258)

68. **A.** Heart block may or may not coexist with "A-V dissociation," but heart block is not an essential feature of it. (1:258)

69. **A.** (1:304)

70. **E.** (1:304)

71. **C.** (1:304)

72. **D.** (1:305)

73. **B.** (1:305)

Textbook Reference for Chapter 7

1. Hurst, J.W. and Myerburg, R. (1973): *Introduction to Electrocardiography*, Second Edition, McGraw-Hill Book Company, New York.

CHAPTER 8

Endocrinology

Directions: For each of the following multiple-choice questions, select the ONE CORRECT answer.

1. The commonest form of hypercortisolism (Cushing's syndrome) is

   A. adrenal adenoma
   B. bilateral adrenocortical hyperfunction from excess ACTH
   C. adrenal carcinoma
   D. due to exogenous steroids
   E. none of the above

2. Elevated thyroxine-binding globulin and serum total thyroxine result from

   A. estrogens
   B. phenytoin (Dilantin)
   C. salicylates
   D. all of the above
   E. none of the above

3. About what percentage of the pancreas must be removed at operation for clinical diabetes to occur?

   A. 5 to 10%
   B. 15 to 25%
   C. 30 to 50%
   D. 60 to 85%
   E. 90 to 95%

4. According to Conn, abnormal glucose tolerance occurs in about what percentage of patients with primary aldosteronism?

   A. 5%
   B. 10%
   C. 25%
   D. 50%
   E. 90%

5. In general, what percentage of mortality exists in diabetic ketoacidosis?

   A. 1%
   B. 2%
   C. 5%
   D. 10%
   E. 25%

6. All the following are equivalent in terms of glucocorticoid activity *except*

   A. 25 mg of cortisone
   B. 20 mg of hydrocortisone
   C. 5 mg of prednisone or prednisolone
   D. 4 mg of methylprednisolone
   E. 75.0 mg of dexamethasone

7. Hypothyroidism has been reported to occur in what percentage of patients who have had subacute thyroiditis?

   A. 1%
   B. 5%
   C. 10%
   D. 25%
   E. 50%

8. In the Mayo Clinic Study, malignant islet cell tumors were found in what percentage of a large series of patients with insulinomas?

   A. less than 1%
   B. 3%
   C. 11%
   D. 32%
   E. 84%

9. Approximately what percentage of patients with Cushing's syndrome resulting from benign adrenal adenomas have bilateral tumors?

   A. 1%
   B. 2 to 4%
   C. 5 to 10%
   D. 20 to 25%
   E. 50 to 75%

10. Of the following clinical manifestations in Cushing's syndrome, the one reported to occur most frequently is

    A. central obesity
    B. hypertension
    C. oligomenorrhea
    D. osteoporosis
    E. impaired glucose tolerance

Directions: For each of the following multiple-choice questions, select the ONE INCORRECT answer.

11. Subtotal thyroidectomy is preferable to radioactive iodine in patients with Graves' disease

    A. who have unusually small goiters
    B. who have significant incidental nodules in the gland
    C. who have low uptake of RAI by the thyroid
    D. in children
    E. in pregnant women

12. Secondary hyperlipoproteinemias are seen in

    A. hyperthyroidism
    B. dysproteinemias
    C. corticosteroid therapy
    D. obesity
    E. poorly controlled diabetes mellitus

13. The diagnosis of pseudohyperparathyroidism or ectopic hyperparathyroidism is more likely than primary hyperparathyroidism under which of the following circumstances? When

    A. serum calcium exceeds 14 mg/100 ml
    B. serum alkaline phosphatase activity is increased
    C. radiographic evidence of osteitis fibrosa is absent
    D. there is a long-standing history of recurrent renal lithiasis
    E. there is a significant degree of anemia

14. Long-acting thyroid stimulator (LATS) is

    A. an IgM
    B. produced by lymphocytes
    C. found in some patients with Graves' disease
    D. passed through the placenta evoking transient hyperthyroidism in the baby

15. Alternate day steroid regimen

    A. consists of giving a single, large dose of prednisone in the morning every other day and none for the following 48 hours
    B. permits the peripheral tissues and the hypothalamic-pituitary-adrenal axis to recover before the next exposure to high levels of circulating glucocorticoids so that adverse metabolic effects and prolonged hypothalamic-pituitary-adrenal inhibition are less likely to occur
    C. is relatively free of serious side effects even when the prednisone dosage is as high as 120 mg every other morning
    D. evokes suppression of delayed-type hypersensitivity responses
    E. allows the response of the hypothalamic-pituitary-adrenal axis to insulin hypoglycemia, metyrapone, or stress to remain intact and the stigmata of Cushing's syndrome are avoided

16. In hypothyroidism,

    A. there is progressive infiltration of the skin by mucoprotein and mucopolysaccharides, giving a puffy appearance
    B. muscle fibers become frayed, and the cells may become necrotic
    C. there is a generalized decreased rate of nucleic acid and protein synthesis, and almost all enzyme systems are reported to be underactive
    D. the skin is thickened and dry, and sweating rarely occurs
    E. there is generalized thickening and puffiness of the face and extremities, and pitting is characteristic

17. In islet cell hyperinsulinism,

    A. classical hyperinsulinism is a relatively uncommon disease of the islets of Langerhans, characterized by hypersecretion of insulin and sometimes proinsulin
    B. neuropsychiatric symptoms and obesity predominate
    C. delay in diagnosis can be particularly dangerous in children, since severe brain damage or death may result
    D. the glucose tolerance test is usually of considerable help in establishing a diagnosis
    E. weight gain (possibly due to overeating to prevent symptoms) may be seen in many adults unless metastatic carcinoma is present

    Directions: For each of the incomplete statements below, ONE or MORE of the completions given is correct. In each case, select
    A. **if 1, 2, and 3 are correct**
    B. **if 1 and 3 are correct**
    C. **if 2 and 4 are correct**
    D. **if only 4 is correct**
    E. **if all are correct**

18. The combined effect of decreased production of thyroidal, adrenal, gonadal hormones, and melanocyte-stimulating hormone (MSH) results in skin which is

    1. pallid
    2. hairless
    3. smooth
    4. dry

19. The symptoms of pheochromocytoma related to excess beta (epinephrine) stimulation include

    1. facial flushing
    2. fever
    3. sweating
    4. occasional hypotension

20. Growth hormone levels have been shown to increase following

    1. rest
    2. prolonged fast
    3. hyperglycemia
    4. arginine infusion

21. Primary aldosteronism may be

    1. due to macronodular or micronodular hyperplasia of the adrenal cortex
    2. due to adrenocortical adenoma
    3. due to adrenocortical hyperplasia with suppressible hyperaldosteronism
    4. glucocorticoid-suppressible

22. In steroid withdrawal syndrome,

    1. weakness, lethargy, nausea, vomiting, arthralgias, myalgias, headaches, fever, anorexia, weight loss, and postural hypotension may occur
    2. a fine desquamation of the superficial layers of the skin may occur
    3. the symptoms can be rapidly suppressed by readministration of a glucocorticoid
    4. the syndrome is due to adrenocortical insufficiency

23. Patients who have become euthyroid and are taking

    1. T_3, may have a low serum total T_4 and free T_4
    2. T_4, may have a slightly elevated total T_4
    3. desiccated thyroid, may have a decreased total T_4
    4. an appropriate mixture of T_3 and T_4, will have a normal total T_4

24. Serum thyroid-stimulating hormone (TSH)

    1. measurement is the most sensitive way to distinguish primary from secondary hypothyroidism
    2. is increased in primary hypothyroidism
    3. is decreased or absent in secondary hypothyroidism
    4. will not be significantly elevated in primary hypothyroidism before the serum thyroxine value falls below normal

25. Which of the following is (are) antidiuretic in diabetes insipidus?

    1. clofibrate (Atromid-S)
    2. chlorpropamide (Diabinase)
    3. thiazides
    4. carbamazepine (Tegretol)

26. The principal actions of parathyroid hormone include

    1. inhibition of phosphate reabsorption resulting in increased urinary excretion of phosphate
    2. resorption of calcium and phosphate from bone
    3. enhancement of calcium resorption from the glomerular filtrate
    4. promotion of calcium absorption from the gastrointestinal tract

27. Nonparathyroid malignancy syndromes which have been associated with secretion of parathyroid hormone-like substances include

    1. hypernephroma
    2. bronchogenic carcinoma
    3. hepatoma
    4. cancer of the ovary, stomach, and pancreas

28. Hypoaldosteronism is associated with

    1. hypokalemia
    2. normal cortisol production
    3. hypernatremia
    4. reduced renin production or release

29. In adrenal medullary hyperfunction (pheochromocytoma), as a result of increased circulating epinephrine and norepinephrine, there may be

    1. tachycardia or bradycardia
    2. sweating
    3. blanching of the skin
    4. tremor of the hands

30. Calcitonin

    1. is a hypocalcemia-inducing polypeptide produced by C cells of the thyroid, thymus, and parathyroids
    2. has pharmacologic effects which include decreased bone resorption, hypophosphatemia, and natriuresis
    3. is used in hypercalcemia secondary to malignancy, hyperparathyroidism, and vitamin D intoxication
    4. has been used most importantly in the treatment of Paget's disease of the bone

31. Menstrual irregularities may be associated with which of the following endocrine disturbances?

    1. primary ovarian failure
    2. secondary ovarian failure
    3. hypothyroidism
    4. adrenogenital syndrome

32. Multiple endocrine adenomatosis may include

    1. pituitary tumor
    2. insulin-secreting islet cell adenomas of the pancreas
    3. gastrin-producing adenomas
    4. chief cell hyperplasia of the parathyroid

33. Which of the following appear(s) to have a prolonged depressive effect on the pituitary gland and should not be used in alternate day regimens?

    1. triamcinolone (Aristocort)
    2. dexamethasone (Decadron)
    3. paramethasone (Haldrone)
    4. betamethasone (Celestone)

34. Schmidt's syndrome is characterized by

    1. hyperthyroidism

2. thyroid insufficiency
3. Cushing's disease
4. adrenal insufficiency

35. Which of the following are helpful in the diagnosis of diabetes insipidus?

    1. persistent urinary hypo-osmolality in the presence of water restriction
    2. impaired antidiuretic response to intravenous hypertonic saline or nicotine administration
    3. correction of the antidiuretic response by administered ADH
    4. radioimmunoassay techniques for the determination of circulating vasopressin

36. In acromegaly,

    1. the disease is usually first manifested by changes in facial features and overgrowth of the head, hands, and feet which may necessitate an increase in hat, glove, or shoe size
    2. headache or visual disturbances from local effects of the expanding pituitary tumor may be the first indications of the disorder
    3. the hands and feet are broad and greatly enlarged, the ends of the digits are square, and prognathism may be so marked as to interfere with mastication
    4. arthritic manifestations are not unusual, and widespread osteoarthritic-like changes in the bones and joints are often demonstrable

Directions: Use the key below to answer the following questions. Select
    A. if the statement is characteristic of idiopathic myxedema
    B. if the statement is characteristic of secondary hypothyroidism resulting from pituitary failure

37. Thyroid is replaced by scar tissue containing a few scattered thyroid cells and many lymphocytes

38. Thyroid is small and inactive with flattened, cuboidal epithelium and acini filled with colloid

Directions: Indicate whether each of the following statements is true or false.

39. Although circulating antibodies to insulin are present within a few months after starting insulin treatment, the insulin-binding capacity of the serum remains low in most diabetic subjects.

40. The clinical syndrome of pseudohyperparathyroidism can be caused by humoral mechanisms other than excessive parathyroid hormone production.

41. Ketoacidosis may be artifactually underestimated in the presence of lactic acidosis; an unexpectedly weakly reacting serum nitroprusside test in the presence of severe metabolic acidosis should arouse suspicion of lactic acidosis.

42. The infertility of primary ovarian polycystic disease is best treated with wedge resection of the ovaries.

43. T_3 uptake varies in a direct manner to the thyroxine-binding globulin.

44. In diabetics, absolute glucagon levels are abnormal.

45. Decreased intracranial pressure accompanies the treatment of ketoacidosis.

46. Hypomagnesemia impairs the response of bone cells to parathyroid hormone and may induce hypocalcemia resistant to endogenous or administered parathyroid hormone or vitamin D.

47. Sarcoidosis with hypercalcemia is usually accompanied by increased serum concentrations of parathyroid hormone-like substances.

48. Widespread defects in tactile and special sensory perception are present only late after the onset of juvenile diabetes.

49. Patients with insulinoma never show high glucose values during a glucose tolerance test.

50. To establish the diagnosis of malignancy in a pheochromocytoma, clear-cut distant metastases must be demonstrated.

51. There is a decreased incidence of diabetes in patients with cirrhosis of the liver.

52. If there is myxedematous involvement of the pituitary gland, sex hair is usually increased.

53. Increased bone resorption is primarily responsible for hypercalcemia in hyperparathyroidism.

54. Pulse pressure is frequently widened in thyrotoxicosis due to an elevation of systolic pressure as a result of increased stroke volume of the heart.

55. Gross obesity in Cushing's syndrome is common.

56. Orally administered corticosteroids are nearly completely metabolized and excreted within 12 hours.

57. The true extent of ketoacidosis occurring in patients with lactic acidosis can be demonstrated only by assay of the individual ketones.

58. Adults with insulinomas frequently exhibit symptoms typical of the "insulin reaction" in the diabetic who requires insulin.

59. In contrast to the improvement in carbohydrate metabolism with the development of adrenal insufficiency in a diabetic, the development of diabetes in a patient with previously well-controlled Addison's disease is characterized by an apparent exacerbation of adrenal insufficiency.

60. When a patient with Cushing's syndrome exhibits marked evidence of androgen excess, the cause is likely to be adrenocortical carcinoma.

Directions: For each of the following questions select
A. if the question is associated with A only
B. if the question is associated with B only
C. if the question is associated with both A and B
D. if the question is associated with neither A nor B

61. In the syndrome of inappropriate secretion of antidiuretic hormone, life-threatening cerebral dysfunction may necessitate rapid elevation of the serum sodium concentration. In this situation,

    A. treatment with fluid restriction may be too slow
    B. infusions of hypertonic saline are excreted because these patients already have volume expansion
    C. both
    D. neither

62. The clinical syndrome of a nonparathyroid tumor associated with hypercalcemia and hypophosphatemia has been referred to as

    A. pseudohyperparathyroidism
    B. ectopic hyperparathyroidism
    C. both
    D. neither

63. Most obese patients, with or without diabetes, have excessive levels of plasma insulin in

    A. the fasting state
    B. response to a glucose load
    C. both
    D. neither

64. Inappropriate ADH syndrome

    A. is associated with impaired ability to excrete sodium
    B. may result from the production of ADH by carcinoma, particularly of the lung
    C. both
    D. neither

65. The secretion of insulin is
    A. inhibited by beta-adrenergic stimulation
    B. enhanced by alpha-adrenergic stimulation
    C. both
    D. neither

66. Hyperkalemia secondary to adrenal insufficiency should be treated by
    A. rapid volume expansion with saline
    B. appropriate steroid therapy
    C. both
    D. neither

67. Theoretic objections to the routine use of bicarbonate in diabetic ketoacidosis include
    A. a rapid elevation in arterial pH may be accompanied by an exaggerated fall in central nervous system pH and attendant worsening of central nervous system functioning
    B. the shift to the left in the oxygen dissociation curve brought about by alkalinization may limit tissue oxygen delivery since red-cell 2-3-diphosphoglycerate concentration is reduced in diabetic ketoacidosis and is not immediately restored by insulin treatment
    C. both
    D. neither

68. Congenital neurocutaneous syndromes often associated with a pheochromocytoma include
    A. neurofibromatosis
    B. von Hippel-Lindau syndrome
    C. both
    D. neither

69. Chemotherapy of Cushing's disease with adrenocorticocytolytic agents usually restores normal
    A. circadian production of cortisol
    B. suppressibility with dexamethasone
    C. both
    D. neither

Directions: For each of the following statements, fill in the correct answer.

70. _____ hyperparathyroidism develops as a result of hyperplasia compensatory to any state which produces hypocalcemia; e.g., chronic renal failure.

71. "Normocalcemic hyperparathyroidism" may result from a disproportionate increase in the _____ fraction of calcium.

72. In a hypertensive patient hyperglycemia, increased hematocrit, and/or orthostatic hypotension suggest _____ .

73. In rare instances mild diabetes comes from an alpha-cell pancreatic tumor (_____) that presumably alters glucose tolerance by oversupplying the hyperglycemic hormone glucagon.

74. It has been noted that a rapid blood sugar decline can result in the movement into the brain of markedly _____ fluid, causing increased intracranial pressure, neurologic disturbances, coma, and death.

75. In the absence of edema and hypertension, hyperaldosteronism with hypokalemia is characteristic of _____ syndrome (hyperplasia of the juxtaglomerular complex).

76. In hyperparathyroidism, calcium deposits may be detected in the cornea as a faint white band, principally at the 3 and 9 o'clock positions and separated from the limbus by a narrow uninvolved area (_____ keratopathy).

77. Thyrotropin-releasing hormone (TRH) produces an increase in _____ as well as thyroid-stimulating hormone (TSH).

78. Idiopathic empty- _____ syndrome occurs when an arachnoid pouch filled with cerebrospinal fluid extends below the

diaphragm of the sella through the foramen of the pituitary stalk.

79. Congenital or acquired _____ diabetes insipidus produces a syndrome identical to neurohypophysial diabetes insipidus, but does not respond to ADH since the lesion is in the target organ, the kidney.

80. When the activities of the thyroid, adrenals, gonads, growth hormone, and melanocyte-stimulating hormone (MSH) are reduced the patient is said to have _____ .

81. The estimation of fasting plasma levels of _____ may be helpful in the diagnosis of islet cell tumors, particularly when one cannot demonstrate absolute increases in plasma levels of total immunoreactive insulin.

82. The two most important factors influencing angiographic detection of islet cell tumors are _____ and vascularity.

Directions: Use the key below to answer the following questions.
   A. if A is greater than or more appropriate than B
   B. if B is greater than or more appropriate than A
   C. if A and B are equal or approximately equal

83. The primary factor in the pathogenesis of the hyponatremia in the syndrome of inappropriate secretion of ADH is

   A. water retention
   B. cation loss

84. Greater incidence exists of

   A. Cushing's syndrome
   B. Cushing's disease

85. Decrease in body hair growth in Addison's disease is most significant in

   A. males
   B. females

86. If a patient has a serum calcium level above 14 mg/100 ml, a high serum alkaline phosphatase in the absence of radiographic evidence of subperiosteal bone resorption or bone cysts, a hematocrit below 38%, and a serum chloride below 102 mEq/liter, the patient would be more likely to have

   A. pseudohyperparathyroidism
   B. primary hyperparathyroidism

87. The commonest form of undiagnosed diabetes occurs with

   A. abnormal fasting glucose
   B. undue hyperglycemia developing with a carbohydrate load

88. Storage of nutrients is favored by a

   A. high concentration of insulin relative to glucagon
   B. low concentration of insulin relative to glucagon

89. First to recover from prolonged hypothalamic-pituitary-adrenal suppression is/are the

   A. hypothalamus and pituitary
   B. adrenal cortex

Directions: For each of the following questions, select
   A. if the question is associated with A only
   B. if the question is associated with B only
   C. if the question is associated with both A and B
   D. if the question is associated with neither A nor B

90. Characteristics of chronic adrenal cortical insufficiency (Addison's disease) include

   A. orthostatic hypotension
   B. bradycardia
   C. both
   D. neither

91. Follicle-stimulating hormone (FSH)

   A. initiates ovulation and luteinization of

    the mature follicle in the female
B. in the male is testicular interstitial cell-stimulating hormone (ICSH)
C. both
D. neither

92. Hypothyroidism sometimes occurs as a part of the presentation of Graves' syndrome with coincident

A. exophthalmos
B. pretibial myxedema
C. both
D. neither

93. In patients with both diabetes mellitus and Addison's disease,

A. diabetes mellitus precedes adrenal insufficiency
B. there is increased insulin sensitivity, with lower insulin requirement and frequent hypoglycemic reactions
C. both
D. neither

94. Medullary carcinoma of the thyroid gland may

A. secrete calcitonin, ACTH, serotonin, histaminase, and prostaglandins
B. be associated with hyperparathyroidism, multiple pheochromocytomas, and ganglioneuromatosis of the mucous membranes
C. both
D. neither

95. In hyperinsulinism, there may be

A. prolonged hypoglycemia after tolbutamide administration
B. leucine sensitivity
C. both
D. neither

Answers and Commentary

1. **B.** The commonest form of hypercortisolism (Cushing's syndrome) is bilateral adrenocortical hyperfunction owing to excessive and unremitting secretion of pituitary ACTH. (1:23)

2. **A.** Estrogens and estrogen-containing oral contraceptives are the commonest causes of elevated thyroxine-binding globulin and TT₄; phenytoin and salicylates lower thyroxine-binding globulin. (1:21)

3. **E.** About 90 to 95% of the pancreas must be removed at operation for clinical diabetes to occur. (*JAMA*, 213:1676, 1970)

4. **D.** According to Conn, abnormal glucose tolerance occurs in about 50% of patients with primary aldosteronism. (*JAMA*, 213:1676, 1970)

5. **D.** 'In general, mortality of 10% exists in diabetic ketoacidosis. (*JAMA*, 223:1348, 1973)

6. **E.** All the doses listed are equivalent in terms of glucocorticoid activity except 75.0 mg of dexamethasone. The proper equivalent would be 0.75 mg dexamethasone. (*Ration Drug Ther*, 6:1, 1972)

7. **C.** Hypothyroidism is reported to occur in 10% of patients who have had subacute thyroiditis. (2:2132)

8. **C.** In the Mayo Clinic study, malignant islet cell tumors were found in 11% of a large series of patients with insulinomas. (*JAMA*, 230:1538, 1974)

9. **C.** Approximately 5 to 10% of patients with Cushing's syndrome resulting from benign adrenal adenomas have bilateral tumors. These patients require bilateral adrenalectomy followed by lifelong treatment, as for Addison's disease. (2:2156)

10. **E.** Impaired glucose tolerance in Cushing's syndrome is reported in 94% of cases. Central obesity is reported in 88% of cases; hypertension, 82%; oligomenorrhea, 72%; osteoporosis, 58%; purpura and striae, 42%; muscle atrophy, 36%; hirsutism, 30%; edema, 20%; hypokalemia (unprovoked), 18%; kidney stones, 12%; and psychotic mentation, 6%. (2:2153)

11. **A.** Subtotal thyroidectomy is preferable to radioactive iodine in patients with Graves' disease who have unusually large goiters, significant incidental nodules in the gland, low uptake of RAI by the thyroid, in children, and in pregnant women. (1:22)

12. **A.** Secondary hyperlipoproteinemias are seen in hypothyroidism, obstructive jaundice, nephrotic syndrome, dysproteinemias, corticosteroid therapy, obesity, and poorly controlled diabetes mellitus. (1:29)

13. **D.** Primary hyperparathyroidism is more likely than pseudohyperparathyroidism with a long history of recurrent renal lithiasis or with radiographic evidence of osteitis fibrosa. Pseudohyperparathyroidism is more likely when the other features described are present. (*Med Clin North Am*, 56:941, 1972)

14. **A.** Long-acting thyroid stimulator (LATS) is an immunoglobulin (IgG) produced by lymphocytes that is found in the serum of some patients with Graves' disease. The role of LATS in the pathogenesis of Graves' disease is not clear. Transplacental passage of LATS from a mother with Graves' disease will evoke transient hyperthyroidism in the baby. (1:21)

15. **D.** In an alternate day steroid regimen, normal delayed-type hypersensitivity responses are retained. All other statements are correct. (*Am Fam Physician*, 3:97, 1971)

16. **E.** Whatever the cause of thyroid hormone deprivation, the effects are similar. Although there is generalized thickening and puffiness of the face and extremities, pitting is not characteristic, but may occur in the presence of fluid retention or congestive heart failure. (2:2133)

17. **D.** The glucose tolerance test is of no help in establishing a diagnosis of islet cell hyperinsulinism. It is true that a high proportion of adult patients have signs of neuroglycopenia such as confusion, fainting, coma, visual disturbances, seizures, and nervousness. Most patients with this disorder demonstrate hypoglycemia, either following a brief fasting period (2 to 14 hours), or after 24 to 72 hours of fasting. During these periods of hypoglycemia, inappropriately high circulating insulin concentrations may appear, with glucose-insulin ratios of less than 2.0 mg of glucose per microunit of insulin. (*JAMA*, 230:1538, 1974)

18. **E.** Decreased melanocyte-stimulating hormone (MSH) production results in skin, areolar, and genital depigmentation. The combined effect of decreased production of thyroidal, adrenal, gonadal hormones, and MSH results in skin which is pallid, hairless, smooth and dry, and which may be called "alabaster" skin. (3:47)

19. **E.** Symptoms of pheochromocytoma related to excess beta (epinephrine) stimulation include facial flushing and sweating, fever, and occasional hypotension. (1:27)

20. **C.** Plasma growth hormone levels have been shown to increase following exercise, prolonged fast, and during hypoglycemia. Substances which may produce an increase in plasma growth hormone are arginine, vasopressin, pyrogens, and estrogens. (4:1670)

21. **E.** All the statements are true of primary aldosteronism. (1:24)

22. **A.** The steroid withdrawal syndrome is characterized by normal plasma cortisol levels.

The syndrome is not due to adrenocortical insufficiency. All other statements are true of this syndrome. (*Am Fam Physician*, 3:96, 1971)

23. **E.** All statements are true. (1:21)

24. **A.** In primary hypothyroidism, the serum thyroid-stimulating hormone (TSH) may be significantly elevated before the serum thyroxine value falls below normal limits. The serum TSH is low in almost all forms of hyperthyroidism. All other statements are true of TSH. (1:21)

25. **E.** All the drugs listed are antidiuretic in diabetes insipidus. (1:20)

26. **E.** All the actions listed are elicited by parathyroid hormone. (*Condenser*, Bio-Science Laboratories 5:2, 1974)

27. **E.** All the nonparathyroid malignancies listed have been associated with the secretion of parathyroid hormone-like substance. (*Med Clin North Am*, 56:941, 1972)

28. **C.** Hyperkalemia and hyponatremia with normal cortisol production are characteristic of hypoaldosteronism. The majority of these patients have hypoaldosteronism owing to reduced renin production or release rather than primary adrenal glomerulosa failure. (1:24)

29. **E.** Adrenal medullary hyperfunction (pheochromocytoma) is characterized by persistent or paroxysmal hypertension. As a result of increased circulating epinephrine or norepinephrine there may be tachycardia or bradycardia, sweating, blanching of the skin, tremor of the hands, and dilation of the pupils, along with an elevation of the blood pressure. (3:48)

30. **E.** All the statements are true of calcitonin. (1:22)

31. **E.** In addition to pregnancy and local disease of the uterus, menstrual irregularities are associated with four major endocrine disturbances: (1) primary ovarian failure, prior to natural menopause and characterized by hot flashes, gain in weight, increased emotional instability, and elevated urinary values of follicle-stimulating hormone, (2) secondary ovarian failure, associated with reduced or absent urinary gonadotropins and evidence of other target gland deficiencies, i.e., thyroid and adrenal, and (3) hypothyroidism, in which menorrhagia as well as oligomenorrhea frequently occurs, (4) adrenogenital syndrome in which oligomenorrhea or amenorrhea is seen in combination with increased muscular development, hirsutism, and other signs of masculinization. (4:1782–85)

32. **E.** All patients with chromophobe adenomas or acromegalic tumors of the pituitary should be screened for multiple endocrine adenomatosis (MEA) which, in addition to a pituitary tumor, may include one or more gastrin-producing adenomas of the pancreas or chief cell hyperplasia of the parathyroid glands, and, occasionally, functioning adenomas of the adrenal cortex and thyroid. (1:19)

33. **E.** All the drugs listed appear to have a prolonged depressive effect on the pituitary gland and should not be used in alternate day regimens.
(*Ration Drug Ther*, 6:1, 1972)

34. **C.** Schmidt's syndrome is characterized by thyroid and adrenal insufficiency.
(*Postgrad Med*, 55:62, 1974)

35. **E.** All the items listed are helpful in the diagnosis of diabetes insipidus. (1:20)

36. **E.** All statements listed are true of acromegaly. In addition, patients with acromegaly are particularly subject to psychologic disturbances and almost always exhibit considerable emotional instability. (4:1681–82)

37. **A.** (2:2132)

38. **B.** (2:2132)

39. **True.** Although circulating antibodies to insulin are present within a few months after starting insulin treatment, the insulin-binding capacity of the serum remains low in most diabetic subjects.
(*Diabetes*, 8:4, 1971)

40. **True.** The findings of Powell et al. suggest that in many patients with neoplasms and clinical and biochemical features typical of pseudohyperparathyroidism, some humoral substance other than parathyroid hormone must be responsible for hypercalcemia and other features of their disease. (*N Engl J Med*, 283:968, 1970)

41. **True.** Ketoacidosis may be artifactually underestimated in the presence of lactic acidosis; an unexpectedly weakly reacting serum nitroprusside test in the presence of severe metabolic acidosis should arouse suspicion of lactic acidosis.
(*N Engl J Med*, 283:968, 1970)

42. **True.** The ovulatory failure of the polycystic ovary syndrome responds to dexamethasone suppression when the circulating androgen is of adrenal origin. The infertility of primary ovarian polycystic disease is still best treated with wedge resection of the ovaries. (1:26)

43. **False.** Triiodothyronine (T_3) uptake varies in an inverse manner to the thyroxine-binding proteins because when there is an increase in thyroxine-binding proteins, more radioactive T_3 is bound to these proteins and less is available to bind to the erythrocytes or resin used in the measurement test. (1:21)

44. **False.** In diabetics, absolute glucagon levels are normal, but relative levels are high in the face of elevated glucose values. (1:29)

45. **False.** Increased intracranial pressure accompanies the treatment of ketoacidosis; this is usually well tolerated, but it occasionally results in cerebral edema. (1:29)

46. **True.** Hypomagnesemia impairs the response of bone cells to parathyroid hormone and may induce hypocalcemia resistant to endogenous or administered parathyroid hormone (and also vitamin D). (1:27)

47. **False.** Sarcoidosis with hypercalcemia is not accompanied by increased serum concentrations of parathyroid hormone-like substances unless there is coexistent hyperparathyroidism. (1:26)

48. **False.** Widespread defects in tactile and special sensory perception are present near the onset of juvenile diabetes. (*N Engl J Med*, 286:1233, 1972)

49. **False.** Patients with insulinoma often show high glucose values during a glucose tolerance test.
(*JAMA*, 213:1676, 1970)

50. **True.** To establish the diagnosis of malignancy in a pheochromocytoma clear-cut distant metastases must be demonstrated.
(*N Engl J Med*, 288:1010, 1973)

51. **False.** There is an increased incidence of diabetes in patients with cirrhosis of the liver.
(*JAMA*, 271:1517, 1971)

52. **False.** If there is myxedematous involvement of the pituitary gland, sex hair may be diminished.
(3:48)

53. **True.** Increased bone resorption is primarily responsible for hypercalcemia in hyperparathyroidism, though increased reabsorption of filtered calcium by the renal tubule and increased absorption of calcium from the intestine are additional factors.(*Med Clin North Am*, 56:941, 1972)

54. **True.** In thyrotoxicosis, the pulse rate is almost invariably elevated, and the pulse has a bounding quality. Pulse pressure is frequently widened due

to an elevation of systolic pressure as a result of the increased stroke volume of the heart. (3:47)

55. **False.** Gross obesity in Cushing's syndrome is rare; what is more common is loss of adipose tissue in the extremities with an increase in abdominal fat pad, striae, and "buffalo hump." (4:412)

56. **True.** Orally administered corticosteroids are nearly completely metabolized and excreted within 12 hours. (*Ration Drug Ther*, 6:1, 1972)

57. **True.** The true extent of ketoacidosis occurring in patients with lactic acidosis can be demonstrated only by assay of the individual ketones. (*N Engl J Med*, 283:968, 1970)

58. **False.** Adults with insulinomas rarely exhibit symptoms typical of the "insulin reaction" in the diabetic who requires insulin. Such symptoms usually suggest other diseases, i.e., stroke, seizure disorder, transient cerebral ischemia, or a psychiatric syndrome. (*JAMA*, 230:1538, 1974)

59. **True.** In contrast to the improvement in carbohydrate metabolism with the development of adrenal insufficiency in a diabetic, the development of diabetes in a patient with previously well-controlled Addison's disease is characterized by an apparent exacerbation of adrenal insufficiency. (*Postgrad Med*, 55:62, 1974)

60. **True.** When a patient with Cushing's syndrome exhibits marked evidence of androgen excess, the cause is likely to be adrenocortical carcinoma. In other varieties of Cushing's syndrome, virilism is usually mild or inapparent. (2:2157)

61. **C.** Both statements are true. Furosemide has been used as an alternative to hypertonic saline for the rapid correction of hyponatremia in the syndrome of inappropriate secretion of ADH. It was found that furosemide diuresis consistently diminished urine to plasma osmolality ratios, and a negative water balance could be achieved at all levels of urinary osmolality, provided the urinary electrolyte losses were replaced in a more concentrated solution. (*Ann Intern Med*, 78:870, 1973)

62. **C.** Both pseudohyperparathyroidism and ectopic hyperparathyroidism have been used as terms to describe the clinical syndrome of nonparathyroid tumor associated with hypercalcemia and hypophosphatemia. According to Lafferty, it is only a little less common than primary hyperparathyroidism. Moreover, differentiation of ectopic from primary hyperparathyroidism may be difficult. Patients with ectopic hyperparathyroidism may have all the biochemical characteristics of primary hyperparathyroidism including elevated concentrations of immunoreactive parathyroid hormone (iPTH), and the malignant tumor may not be clinically apparent when the patient is first seen. Although a variety of malignant tumors have produced ectopic hyperparathyroidism, hypernephromas and bronchogenic carcinomas accounted for 60% of the cases in Lafferty's series. (*Med Clin North Am*, 56:941, 1972)

63. **C.** Most obese patients, with or without diabetes, have excessive levels of plasma insulin in the fasting state and in response to a glucose load. (*JAMA*, 213:1676, 1976)

64. **B.** Inappropriate ADH syndrome is a term applied to the complex of persistent secretion of ADH in association with plasma hypotonicity, hypertonicity of urine, and unimpaired ability to excrete sodium. This syndrome may result from the production of ADH by carcinoma, particularly of the lung. (*Postgrad Med*, 52:232, 1972)

65. **D.** Beta-adrenergic stimulation enhances, whereas alpha-adrenergic stimulation inhibits the secretion of insulin. (*N Engl J Med*, 286:371, 1972)

66. **C.** Hyperkalemia secondary to adrenal insufficiency should be treated by rapid volume expansion with saline and appropriate steroid therapy. (*JAMA*, 231:631, 1975)

67. **C.** Theoretic objections to the routine use of bicarbonate in diabetic ketoacidosis include both objections listed. (*N Engl J Med*, 290:130, 1974)

68. **C.** Congenital neurocutaneous syndromes often associated with a pheochromocytoma include neurofibromatosis and Von Hippel-Lindau syndrome. (*N Engl J Med*, 288:1010, 1973)

69. **D.** Chemotherapy of Cushing's disease with adrenocorticocytolytic agents usually does not restore either the normal circadian production of cortisol or normal suppressibility with dexamethasone. (*N Engl J Med*, 285:289, 1971)

70. **Secondary.** Secondary hyperparathyroidism develops as a result of hyperplasia compensatory to any state which produces hypocalcemia; e.g., chronic renal failure. Progressive hyperparathyroidism is particularly apparent in many patients undergoing long-term hemodialysis therapy. (*Condenser*, Bio-Science Laboratories, 5:3, 1974)

71. **Ionized.** Reliable measurement of the ionized calcium concentration in the plasma by using ion-

specific electrodes can now be performed. It has been suggested that measurement of the ionized calcium fraction might aid in the diagnosis of hyperparathyroidism when serum calcium levels appear normal.

(*Med Clin North Am,* 56:941, 1972)

72. **Pheochromocytoma.** In a hypertensive patient, hyperglycemia (catecholamine inhibition of insulin release), increased hematocrit, and/or orthostatic hypotension (decreased plasma volume) suggest pheochromocytoma. (1:27)

73. **Glucagonoma.** In rare instances, mild diabetes comes from an alpha-cell pancreatic tumor (glucagonoma) that presumably alters glucose tolerance by oversupplying the hyperglycemic hormone glucagon. (*JAMA,* 213:1676, 1970)

74. **Hypotonic.** It has been noted that a rapid blood sugar decline can result in the movement into the brain of markedly hypotonic fluid, causing increased intracranial pressure, neurologic disturbances, coma and death.

(*Int Med News,* 4:4, 1971)

75. **Bartter's.** In the absence of edema and hypertension, hyperaldosteronism with hypokalemia is characteristic of Bartter's syndrome (hyperplasia of the juxtaglomerular complex). (1:24)

76. **Band.** Hyperparathyroidism is accompanied by physical signs that result from the accompanying hypercalcemia and bone disease. There may also be muscular weakness, mental confusion, obtundation, or coma due to the hypercalcemia. Calcium deposits may be detected in the cornea as a faint white band, principally at the 3 and 9 o'clock positions and separated from the limbus by a narrow uninvolved area (band keratopathy), and also detected as white flecks on the conjunctival surface of the tarsal plates of the eyelids and as calcifications of the eardrum. Demineralization of bone may result in fracture of the long bones or loss of height due to vertebral collapse. Bone cysts and tumors may be found as palpable enlargements, particularly at the ends of long bones, and in the jaw (epulides). (3:50)

77. **Prolactin.** Thyrotropin-releasing hormone (TRH) produces an increase in prolactin as well as thyroid-stimulating hormone (TSH). (4:1669)

78. **Sella.** Idiopathic empty-sella syndrome occurs when an arachnoid pouch filled with cerebrospinal fluid extends below the diaphragm of the sella through the foramen of the pituitary stalk. This pouch may become large enough to enlarge the sella and compress the pituitary gland. (1:20)

79. **Nephrogenic.** Congenital or acquired nephrogenic diabetes insipidus produces a syndrome identical to neurohypophysial diabetes insipidus but does not respond to ADH since the lesion is in the target organ, the kidney. (1:20)

80. **Panhypopituitarism.** Hypopituitarism in the adult frequently results in decreased activity of the thyroid, adrenals, and gonads. In addition, there may be diminished production of growth hormone and melanocyte-stimulating hormone (MSH). When the activities of all these hormones are reduced, the patient is said to have panhypopituitarism. (3:47)

81. **Proinsulin.** The estimation of fasting plasma levels of proinsulin may be helpful in the diagnosis of islet cell tumors, particularly when one cannot demonstrate absolute increases in plasma levels of total immunoreactive insulin.

(*Mod Med,* 41:24, 1973)

82. **Size.** The two most important factors influencing angiographic detection of islet cell tumors are size and vascularity. (*JAMA,* 230:1538, 1974)

83. **A.** Several investigations indicate that water retention rather than cation loss is the primary factor in the pathogenesis of the hyponatremia in the syndrome of inappropriate secretion of ADH; therefore, maneuvers that result primarily in a negative water balance rather than a positive sodium balance are the preferred modes of treatment. (*Ann Intern Med,* 78:870, 1973)

84. **B.** Cushing's syndrome resulting from adrenal tumor occurs in approximately 1 of every 10,000 hospital admissions. Cushing's disease occurs in approximately 1 of every 4000 admissions. The incidence of the ectopic ACTH syndrome is difficult to estimate, because it is frequently overlooked. There is evidence that ectopic ACTH might be produced by as many as 8% of visceral carcinomas. Careful screening of patients with nonpituitary tumors might reveal the production of ectopic ACTH to be the most common cause of hypercortisolism. (2:2152)

85. **B.** Body hair growth in Addison's disease is decreased in both sexes but especially in women in whom axillary hair may be absent. (3:48)

86. **A.** Any hypercalcemic patient with an illness characterized by a few months duration, marked weight loss, and absence of history of renal calculi or peptic ulcer suggests an underlying malignancy. A serum calcium above 14 mg/100 ml, a high serum alkaline phosphatase in the absence of radiographic evidence of subperiosteal bone resorption or bone cysts, a hematocrit below 38%,

and a serum chloride below 102 mEq/liter suggests pseudo-, rather than primary, hyperparathyroidism. If physical examination, intravenous pyelograms, barium enema, upper gastrointestinal series, bronchoscopy, and radioactive liver scan fail to reveal a neoplasm and the serum calcium fails to fall more than 1 to 2 mg/100 ml following one week of corticosteroid administration, neck exploration is indicated. The simultaneous presence of both a parathyroid adenoma and a "parathormone secreting" carcinoma has been described only once.

(*Medicine,* 45:247, 1966)

87. **B.** The commonest form of undiagnosed diabetes occurs with a normal fasting glucose, but undue hyperglycemia develops with a carbohydrate load. (*Res-Int Consult,* 1:12, 1972)

88. **A.** A high concentration of insulin relative to glucagon favors nutrient storage; a low ratio favors mobilization of stored fuels. (1:29)

89. **A.** The hypothalamus and pituitary recover from prolonged hypothalamic-pituitary-adrenal suppression more quickly than the adrenal cortex does. Complete recovery, with normal plasma ACTH and cortisol levels, may require 8 to 12 months. (*Am Fam Physician,* 3:97, 1971)

90. **A.** Orthostatic hypotension and tachycardia are characteristic of Addison's disease. (3:48)

91. **D.** Follicle-stimulating hormone (FSH) stimulates growth of the graffian follicle and estrogen secretion in the female and spermatogenesis in the male; luteinizing hormone (LH) initiates ovulation and luteinization of the mature follicle in the female; in the male, this hormone is the testicular interstitial cell-stimulating hormone (ICSH), responsible for male hormone secretion.

(4.1670–71)

92. **C.** Hypothyroidism sometimes occurs as part of the presentation of Graves' syndrome, with coincident exophthalmos and pretibial myxedema.

(2:2132)

93. **C.** In 19 cases of associated diabetes and Addison's disease seen at the Joslin Clinic, diabetes preceded adrenal insufficiency in all but one instance. The most striking feature of the superimposed adrenal disorder was increased insulin sensitivity, with lower insulin requirement and frequent hypoglycemic reactions.

(*Postgrad Med,* 55:62, 1974)

94. **C.** Medullary carcinomas of the thyroid frequently synthesize and secrete calcitonin. These tumors have also been found to secrete ACTH, serotonin, histaminase, and prostaglandins. Medullary carcinoma of the thyroid may be familial and associated with hyperparathyroidism, multiple pheochromocytomas, and ganglioneuromatosis of the mucous membranes. (1:22)

95. **C.** In hyperinsulinism, there may be prolonged hypoglycemia after tolbutamide administration, and leucine sensitivity. (*JAMA,* 230:1538, 1974)

Textbook References for Chapter 8

1. American College of Physicians (1974): *Medical Knowledge Self-Assessment, Program III: Recent Developments in Internal Medicine,* Petersdorf, R.G., General Editor. American College of Physicians, Philadelphia.

2. Beeson, P.B. and McDermott, W. (1979): *Textbook of Medicine*, Fifteenth Edition, W.B. Saunders Company, Philadelphia.

3. Judge, R.D. and Zuidema, G.D., Editors (1974): *Physical Diagnosis: A Physiologic Approach to the Clinical Examination,* Little, Brown and Company, Boston.

4. Isselbacher, K.J., Editor (1980): *Harrison's Principles of Internal Medicine*, Ninth Edition, McGraw-Hill Book Company, New York.

CHAPTER 9

Gastroenterology

Directions: For each of the incomplete statements below, ONE or MORE of the completions given is correct. In each case, select
A.   if 1, 2, and 3 are correct
B.   if 1 and 3 are correct
C.   if 2 and 4 are correct
D.   if only 4 is correct
E.   if all are correct

1.   Needle biopsy of the liver is of proved value in which of the following situations?

 1. in the differential diagnosis of jaundice, hepatic enlargement, and splenomegaly
 2. in the differential diagnosis of unexplained fever, since a liver biopsy may suggest or establish the diagnosis of miliary tuberculosis, sarcoidosis, brucellosis, or neoplasm
 3. to assess the degree of hepatic fibrosis in chronic hepatitis and cirrhosis, to evaluate the course of hepatitis and acute liver disease, and to estimate hepatic stores of iron in hemochromatosis
 4. in patients with prolonged jaundice which is suspected to be extrahepatic in origin

2.   The barium swallow is one of the most reliable methods for examination of the esophagus; it is useful in detecting a wide variety of lesions, including

 1. diverticula
 2. stricture
 3. carcinoma
 4. achalasia

3.   Chronic relapsing pancreatitis

 1. is characterized by recurrent bouts of moderate to severe pain in the upper abdomen lasting for many hours to days, most frequently associated with alcohol
 2. gradually leads to inadequacy of external secretions of the pancreas
 3. is characterized clinically by steatorrhea and malabsorption, diabetes mellitus (clinical or chemical), and pancreatic calcification
 4. does not affect internal secretions of the pancreas

4.   Which of the following is associated with increased lower esophageal sphincter pressure?

 1. antacids
 2. cigarettes
 3. gastrin
 4. caffeine

5.   Which of the following may be easily visualized with gastroscopy?

 1. lesions along the lesser curvature
 2. lesions in the lower part of the stomach along the greater curvature
 3. lesions in the antrum
 4. lesions in the fundus

6. Medical conditions which may mimic intra-abdominal emergencies include

   1. typhoid fever
   2. pericarditis
   3. lower lobe pneumonia
   4. nephritis

7. Chronic active hepatitis

   1. may occur in the course of Wilson's disease
   2. has occurred as a result of ingestion of laxatives containing phenisatin
   3. may occur as a hypersensitivity reaction to methyldopa (Aldomet)
   4. may be associated with hepatitis B antigen

8. Paraesophageal hiatal hernia

   1. often results in low retrosternal pain and belching, which appear after eating and subsequently can be relieved by walking
   2. may encroach on the lung with dyspnea as a striking symptom
   3. in time has a tendency to "roll up" into the mediastinum
   4. patients may develop macrocytic anemia

9. Plummer-Vinson syndrome

   1. is associated with sideropenic dysphagia
   2. is associated with carcinoma of the esophagus
   3. is associated with mucosal atrophy and formation of a web that encircles the lumen of the upper esophagus
   4. occurs more often in men

10. Which of the following is/are true of alimentary hyperinsulinism?

    1. occurs in patients who have had a gastroenterostomy or subtotal gastrectomy
    2. patients show accelerated absorption of glucose and marked postprandial hyperglycemia with a consequent corresponding accentuation of postprandial insulin release to which hypoglycemia is a response

    3. symptoms of hypoglycemia occur 1½ to 3 hours after ingestion of carbohydrate and should be differentiated from symptoms of dumping that usually are seen within 30 to 60 min of eating
    4. the diagnosis can be confirmed by an oral glucose tolerance test that demonstrates an elevated peak plasma glucose level at ½ or 1 hour (but not an elevation of the 2-hour level) followed by hypoglycemia, plus a history of stomach surgery

11. Endogenous causes of abdominal pain include

    1. uremia
    2. diabetic coma
    3. porphyria
    4. allergic factors (C′ 1 esterase deficiency)

12. Radiographic features which tend to distinguish benign gastric ulcer from gastric cancer include

    1. most benign ulcers extend beyond the confines of the gastric wall, whereas gastric cancers tend to occur within the confines of the gastric wall
    2. benign ulcers tend to be round or ovoid, whereas cancers often are irregular in shape
    3. benign ulcers usually have a smooth base, whereas the base of a cancer may be nodular
    4. the gastric folds radiate to the lip of a benign ulcer, whereas there may be no radiating folds around a cancer, or the folds may be blunted and stop some distance from an ulcerating cancer

Directions: Indicate whether each of the following statements is true or false.

13. Patients with duodenal ulcer, prepyloric ulcer, or gastric plus duodenal ulcer tend to secrete more acid than normal subjects.

14. Absence of bowel sounds suggests paralytic ileus due to diffuse peritoneal irritation.

15. Increased levels of serum carotene may be found in patients with steatorrhea and constitute a useful test for screening purposes.

16. After ingesting 80 to 100 g fat per day, normal fat excretion if 5 g or less per 24 hours.

17. The frequency of lymphoma in patients with adult celiac disease is considerably higher than expected.

18. If a barium study is performed on a patient with gastrointestinal hemorrhage, residual contrast material may prevent angiographic identification of the bleeding point.

19. The most common cause of congestive splenomegaly is cirrhosis of the liver.

20. Malabsorption associated with chronic stasis of the small intestine with bacterial overgrowth in scleroderma and diabetic neuropathy requires continuous administration of broad-spectrum antimicrobials.

21. The presence of a hiatal hernia means that it is clinically significant.

22. Bleeding from gastric ulcers is more likely to stop than is bleeding from duodenal ulcers.

23. Patients with gastric ulcers of the body of the stomach tend to secrete normal amounts of acid.

Directions: For each of the following multiple-choice questions, select the ONE INCORRECT answer.

24. With sliding hiatal hernias,
   A. most patients have symptoms referable to the hernia

   B. symptoms are directly related to the reflux of gastric acid-pepsin secretions and the resultant esophagitis
   C. characteristically, the patients complain of heartburn, sour eructations, postural regurgitation, and even dysphagia
   D. because of the esophagitis, patients are prone to swallow air
   E. temporary relief is usually afforded by drinking water or milk, or taking antacids

25. Regarding α-beta-lipoproteinemia,
   A. it is a very rare disorder
   B. the intestinal cell is unable to invest the reconstituted triglyceride with a protein envelope
   C. chylomicrons are not formed and the lipid is not transported into lacteals
   D. in the fasting state, intestinal mucosa are relatively full of fat, and the serum beta lipoprotein, cholesterol, and plasma total lipid levels are very low
   E. although steatorrhea is noted, fat-balance studies indicate that a considerable percentage of dietary fat can still be absorbed

26. Alpha$_1$-fetoprotein (AFP)
   A. is a normal fetal serum protein, synthesized in large amounts by embryonal liver and yolk-sac cells and secreted into fetal serum and secretions during normal gestation
   B. is a diagnostic test for primary carcinoma of the liver and teratoblastoma
   C. can be detected by sensitive radioimmunoassays in 85 to 95% of patients with hepatoma and in a smaller percentage of gastrointestinal-tract tumors as well as acute viral hepatitis
   D. levels are persistently elevated in almost all children with hepatocellular carcinoma or hepatoblastoma, in approximately one-third of those with

gonadal teratoblastomas, or embryonal carcinoma, and in ataxia telangiectasia

E. decreased levels are found in prenatal amniocentesis fluid in the presence of anencephaly and other neural tube defects

27. Cholesterol gallstone disease is associated with

A. an increase in the total pool of conjugated bile salts
B. a relative decrease in bile salt content of hepatic bile
C. a relative increase in cholesterol content of hepatic bile
D. continually lithogenic bile

28. Adult celiac disease is characterized by

A. gluten enteropathy
B. total or subtotal villous atrophy is not a characteristic histological finding
C. a relative increase in the depth of intestinal mucosa, chronic inflammatory-cell infiltration in the lamina propria and extensive alterations in the surface of epithelial cells
D. severe damage to the microvilli which are short, sparse, and distorted, revealed by electron micrography
E. markedly impaired fat and carbohydrate absorption

29. Nodular lymphoid hyperplasia of the small bowel

A. is described in patients with idiopathic-acquired hypogammaglobulinemia
B. is described in patients with a selective absence of IgA
C. on x-ray shows multiple small filling defects throughout the small intestine
D. on small intestinal biopsy shows large lymphoid nodules
E. is associated, in a minority of patients, with intestinal Giardia infestation

30. Intestinal lymphangiectasia is associated with

A. classic protein-losing enteropathy
B. transudation of plasma proteins due to increased lymphatic pressure
C. circulating plasma cells and lymphocytes and delayed hypersensitivity response which may be diminished
D. signs and symptoms of malabsorption rather than of low plasma proteins
E. chylothorax rarely

31. In Meckel's diverticulum,

A. 1 to 3% of the general population are affected
B. less than 20% become symptomatic
C. approximately one-third of cases occur in the first year of life
D. about 50% contain gastric mucosa and about 5% contain pancreatic tissue
E. diagnosis is usually made by routine gastrointestinal x-rays

32. Regarding biliary cirrhosis,

A. it occurs most frequently in males
B. elevated serum levels of IgM are seen in about 80% of patients
C. antimitochondrial antibodies have been detected in over 95% of patients
D. hyperlipidemia is common early in the disease
E. patients have elevated copper levels in the liver, together with elevated serum and urinary copper levels

33. Fat in the liver after alcohol intake

A. is a precursor of cirrhosis
B. may produce hepatomegaly
C. may produce temporary portal hypertension
D. usually resolves in about 6 weeks

34. The malabsorption syndrome is characterized by

A. weight gain
B. anorexia
C. abdominal distention
D. borborygmus
E. muscle wasting

35. Clinical features of eosinophilic gastroenteritis include

    A. pyloric obstruction
    B. mucosal bleeding
    C. lack of malabsorption
    D. acute peritonitis
    E. protein loss

Directions: For each of the following statements, fill in the correct answer.

36. A _____ hernia, which accounts for about 10% of hiatal hernias, rolls up beside the esophagus and the esophagogastric junction remains in its normal position.

37. Patients with diabetes mellitus, diabetic neuropathy, malabsorption syndrome, and villous atrophy probably have adult _____ disease.

38. Villous atrophy (often responsive to a gluten-free diet), so-called nodular lymphoid hyperplasia (often with giardiasis), and, rarely, granulomatous lesions may be found in the small intestine in congenital or acquired _____ ; plasma levels of Ig— are universally, and those of IgG almost always depressed.

39. _____ resection interrupts the enterohepatic circulation of bile salts by removal of the site of their active reabsorption.

40. Cholestyramine therapy may be complicated by _____ due to vitamin D malabsorption.

41. In pernicious anemia, the hypergastrinemia results from _____ with consequent failure to inhibit the antral release of gastrin.

42. Most cases of celiac disease—childhood and adult—respond to elimination of _____ from the diet. The regimen must be lifelong. Symptoms are alleviated in a matter of a few days, absorption returns to normal over a period of a few weeks, and regeneration of the _____ structure of the mucosa will

ensue in most patients who have adhered strictly to the diet.

43. Malabsorption in patients with dysgammaglobulinemia has been attributed to _____ *lamblia* infestation.

44. Contamination of food by _____ produced by fungi may explain the high incidence of hepatic carcinoma in Africa and Asia.

Directions: For each of the following questions select
    A. if the question is associated with A only
    B. if the question is associated with B only
    C. if the question is associated with both A and B
    D. if the question is associated with neither A nor B

45. The D-xylose tolerance test is diminished in

    A. diseases of the intestinal mucosa
    B. pancreatic insufficiency
    C. both
    D. neither

46. In some cases, *Giardia lamblia* is associated with severe malabsorption by

    A. invasion of the small bowel mucosal cells, without apparent injury
    B. creation of a barrier to normal transport
    C. both
    D. neither

47. At mealtimes, cholecystokinin-pancreozymin released from duodenal mucosa by amino acids, peptides and, to a lesser degree, fat causes

    A. gallbladder relaxation
    B. contraction of the sphincter of Oddi
    C. both
    D. neither

48. The malabsorption associated with diffuse regional enteritis may be alleviated somewhat by the administration of steroids provided the patient does not have bacterial overgrowth due to

A. chronic obstruction
B. fistula
C. both
D. neither

49. In patients with chronic liver disease and ascites, fluid is mobilized into the bloodstream more slowly in those without edema than in those with edema; this disparity is

A. manifest during spontaneous diuresis
B. abolished by administration of diuretics
C. both
D. neither

50. Urinary excretion of indican is elevated in

A. bacterial overgrowth
B. ileal dysfunction
C. both
D. neither

51. Disaccharidase deficiency may

A. be present despite structurally normal microvilli (as a hereditary defect)
B. result from diseases of the small bowel which impair or destroy microvilli
C. both
D. neither

52. Sliding hiatal hernias

A. involves the gastroesophageal junction being displaced into the posterior mediastinum and is followed by a portion of the stomach
B. is a true sliding hernia in the surgical sense, since the anterior portion is formed by a peritoneal sac and the posterior portion consists of the stomach itself
C. both
D. neither

53. Free air from a perforated viscus may be detected by

A. an upright film
B. a lateral decubitus film
C. both
D. neither

54. Tropical sprue

A. does not respond to the administration of a broad-spectrum antimicrobial
B. recovery is hastened by the concomitant administration of vitamin B_{12} parenterally, and folic acid orally
C. both
D. neither

55. In patients with malabsorption after gastrectomy

A. there may be bacterial overgrowth in the afferent limb, which may temporarily be reduced with oral broad-spectrum antimicrobial drugs
B. conversion of the Bilroth II to a Bilroth I anastomosis, even if possible, is not advisable in these cases
C. both
D. neither

56. Lithogenic bile refers to

A. a state of cholesterol supersaturation
B. saturation in the presence of cholesterol microcrystals
C. both
D. neither

57. Chronic pancreatitis may be associated with

A. steatorrhea
B. x-ray evidence of pancreatic calcification
C. both
D. neither

58. Important laboratory features of chronic active hepatitis include

A. changes in serum transaminase levels
B. hypogammaglobulinemia
C. both
D. neither

Directions: For each of the following multiple-choice questions select the ONE CORRECT answer.

59. Antimitochondrial antibodies are detected in about what percentage of patients with primary biliary cirrhosis?

    A. 20%
    B. 40%
    C. 50%
    D. 75%
    E. more than 90%

60. Clinically, duodenal ulcers are how many times as common as gastric ulcers?

    A. 2
    B. 4
    C. 6
    D. 8
    E. 10

61. Sliding hernias comprise what percentage of hiatal hernias?

    A. 5 to 7%
    B. 15 to 23%
    C. 35 to 50%
    D. 60 to 70%
    E. 85 to 90%

62. Liver normally contains how many grams of glycogen?

    A. 5 to 10 g
    B. 20 to 40 g
    C. 50 to 70 g
    D. 80 to 100 g
    E. 200 to 300 g

63. Perforation and gangrene of the colon occur in about what percentage of cases of acute mesenteric ischemia?

    A. 5%
    B. 10%
    C. 20%
    D. 40%
    E. 80%

64. In normal man, the total amount of fluid entering the gut per day is about how many liters?

    A. 1
    B. 3
    C. 5
    D. 10
    E. 20

65. The vagus nerve influences gastric secretion by

    A. direct cholinergic stimulation of parietal cells
    B. release of gastrin
    C. sensitizing the parietal cell to stimulation by gastrin and other stimulants
    D. all of the above
    E. none of the above

66. Sacroiliitis as a feature of colitis and enteritis

    A. is more common in men
    B. differs from ankylosing spondylitis
    C. is helped by radical surgery of the affected bowel
    D. all of the above
    E. none of the above

67. Evidence for an immunological mechanism in celiac disease is its association with

    A. IgG deficiency
    B. IgA deficiency
    C. IgM deficiency
    D. IgD deficiency
    E. IgE deficiency

68. What percentage of patients with acute hepatitis B antigen-positive hepatitis remain positive and develop chronic active hepatitis (chronic aggressive hepatitis)?

    A. less than 5%
    B. 10%
    C. 20%
    D. 40%
    E. 60%

Directions: For each of the following questions select

A. if the question is associated with A only
B. if the question is associated with B only
C. if the question is associated with both A and B
D. if the question is associated with neither A nor B

69. The milk-alkali syndrome is

    A. Burnett's syndrome
    B. associated with hypocalcemia
    C. both
    D. neither

70. Anticholinergics may

    A. suppress the vagal mechanism of acid secretion
    B. delay gastric emptying, which may stimulate the antrum to produce gastrin
    C. both
    D. neither

71. Gastroesophageal reflux may exist

    A. with hiatal hernia
    B. without hiatal hernia
    C. both
    D. neither

72. In chronic gastritis associated with gastric atrophy, there may be

    A. achlorhydria
    B. elevated gastrin levels
    C. both
    D. neither

73. Low-residue diets are presently advocated for

    A. inflammatory bowel disease
    B. diverticulosis
    C. both
    D. neither

74. In alcoholics, hepatic changes frequently include

    A. decreased deposition of fat in the liver
    B. decrease in the drug metabolizing enzymes of the liver endoplasmic reticulum
    C. both
    D. neither

75. Small bowel resections do not predispose to

    A. cholesterol gallstones
    B. oxalate renal stones
    C. both
    D. neither

76. Cholangitis

    A. enteric organisms, often anaerobic, are the usual pathogens
    B. is a rare cause of liver abscess
    C. both
    D. neither

77. Appears necessary to produce alcoholic hepatitis:

    A. intense drinking
    B. malnutrition
    C. both
    D. neither

78. Indicated for hypersplenism in cirrhosis:

    A. splenectomy
    B. shunts
    C. both
    D. neither

79. Patients with dermatitis herpetiformis may exhibit a proximal jejunal mucosal lesion which

    A. is identical with that of celiac disease
    B. does not respond to a gluten-free diet
    C. both
    D. neither

80. Dysgammaglobulinemia with villous atrophy in the absence of giardiasis usually responds to

    A. a gluten-free diet
    B. metronidazole
    C. both
    D. neither

Directions: Indicate whether each of the following statements is true or false.

81. In any patient with normal renal function the urinary excretion of D-xylose after ingestion of a 25 g load will reflect with remarkable accuracy the absorptive capacity of the small intestine for carbohydrate.

82. Patients with celiac disease exhibit an impaired pancreatic secretory response to intraluminal peptides and fat due to a deficient release of pancreozymin-cholecystokinin from the diseased mucosa.

83. The liver scan is not a very useful test in the diagnosis of disease in the right upper quadrant.

84. Hepatitis B antigen appears in the blood during the acute phases of hepatitis B and is cleared in a few weeks except in perhaps 1% of patients who remain positive but clinically well.

85. Calcium-containing antacids may stimulate gastrin production, leading to an acid rebound effect.

86. The incidence of duodenal ulcer in the United States is increasing.

87. With halothane hepatitis, fever within 8 to 14 days of initial exposure, or earlier with recurrent exposure, is accompanied by clinical and chemical evidence of parenchymal cell necrosis.

88. Gallstones may be less common in patients on long-term therapy with clofibrate (Atromid-S) for hypercholesterolemia.

89. Laparotomy in spontaneous peritonitis is frequently indicated.

90. Giardia are best detected in duodenal mucus.

91. Acid injury does not appear to be the basis for alcoholic gastritis.

92. Hypomotility of the small intestine can lead to diarrhea by promoting stasis of intestinal contents and bacterial overgrowth.

93. Gallbladder contrast media requires months for elimination because the media repeatedly pass through the enterohepatic circulation.

94. In cirrhosis, very tense ascites increases portal pressure and should be treated to avoid variceal bleeding.

95. Even sustained hyperglycemia is not felt to lead to atrophic gastritis.

96. Venous hums are at times identified over the cirrhotic liver due to torrential flow through venous collaterals.

97. Diabetics absorb sugar at rates higher than normal.

98. After gastric surgery dumping can often be controlled by restriction of fluids and osmotically active foods, especially sugars, at mealtimes.

99. Inflammation around diverticula in the sigmoid frequently is associated with hemorrhage.

Answers and Commentary

1. **A.** Needle biopsy of the liver is of proved value in all of the situations listed except in patients with prolonged jaundice which is probably extra-hepatic in origin. Other contraindications include: (1) In patients who are uncooperative or who cannot control movements of the diaphragm, e.g., with severe recurrent cough. (2) In patients with bleeding disorders, with clotting defects (prothrombin time elevations greater than 2 to 3 sec over control), or with vascular tumors in the liver. (3) In patients with severe cardiopulmonary disease that would be a contraindication to surgery should a biopsy complication ensue.
(2:1647–48)

2. **E.** The barium swallow is one of the most reliable methods for examination of the esophagus. It is useful in detecting a wide variety of lesions, such as diverticula, stricture, carcinoma, achalasia, or hiatus hernia. (3:214)

3. **A.** Chronic relapsing pancreatitis may lead to internal as well as external secretions of the pancreas. All other statements are true of this disorder. (*N Engl J Med*, 281:1111, 1969)

4. **B.** It has been demonstrated that cigarette smoking may decrease the lower esophageal sphincter pressure, while antacid and gastrin elevate it. Caffeine and fatty foods decrease the pressure. (1:34)

5. **A.** With gastroscopy, lesions along the lesser curvature, in the lower part of the stomach along the greater curvature, and in the antrum may be visualized. Lesions in the fundus are difficult to detect, for this is a "blind spot" with the gastroscope. (3:213)

6. **E.** All the conditions listed may mimic intra-abdominal emergencies, as may tabes dorsalis and tuberculous peritonitis. (3:219)

7. **E.** All the statements are true of chronic active hepatitis. (*Digest Dis*, 18:177, 1973)

8. **E.** All statements are true of paraesophageal hiatal hernias. In addition, patients commonly develop a superficial gastritis secondary to gastric stasis, or a frank gastric ulcer.
(*Am Fam Physician*, 3:107, 1971)

9. **A.** The Plummer-Vinson syndrome occurs more often in women. All other statements are correct.
(*Mod Med*, 41:73, 1973)

10. **E.** All statements are true of alimentary hyperinsulinism. In addition, occasionally alimentary hyperinsulinism and hypoglycemia are observed in patients who have not had gastric surgery. (*Mod Med*, 41:73, 1973)

11. **E.** Endogenous causes of abdominal pain include uremia, diabetic coma, porphyria, and allergic factors (C' l deficiency). (4:35)

12. **E.** All the radiographic features listed tend to distinguish benign gastric ulcer from gastric cancer. In addition, the stomach around a benign ulcer is usually pliable and has normal motility, whereas the wall around a cancer is rigid and has poor motility. (2:1510)

13. **True.** Patients with duodenal ulcer, prepyloric ulcer, or gastric plus duodenal ulcer tend to secrete more acid than normal subjects. (2:1506)

14. **True.** Absence of bowel sounds suggests paralytic ileus due to diffuse peritoneal irritation.
(3:226)

15. **False.** Depressed levels of serum carotene may be found in patients with steatorrhea and

constitute a useful test for screening purposes.
(*N Engl J Med*, 281:1114, 1969)

16. **True.** After ingesting 80 to 100 g fat per day, normal fat excretion is 5 g or less per 24 hours.
(*N Engl J Med*, 281:1114, 1969)

17. **True.** The frequency of lymphoma in patients with adult celiac disease is considerably higher than expected. (*N Engl J Med*, 281:1113, 1969)

18. **True.** If a barium study is performed on a patient with gastrointestinal hemorrhage, residual contrast material may prevent angiographic identification of the bleeding point.
(*New Physician*, 21:308, 1972)

19. **True.** Splenic congestion as a consequence of portal hypertension may be secondary to chronic hepatic disease, chronic congestive heart failure, or occlusion of the splenic or portal veins. The most common cause of congestive splenomegaly is cirrhosis of the liver. (3:236)

20. **True.** Malabsorption associated with chronic stasis of the small intestine with bacterial overgrowth in scleroderma and diabetic neuropathy requires continuous administration of broad-spectrum antimicrobials.
(*N Engl J Med*, 281:1115, 1969)

21. **False.** The mere presence of a hiatal hernia does not necessarily mean that it is clinically significant. Large hiatal hernias may be present without provoking symptoms; conversely, there may be severely symptomatic small hernias. In addition, patients may have heartburn and esophagitis without any hernia at all. One major problem for the clinician is determining if the hernia requires therapy and, if so, whether it can best be managed medically or surgically.
(*Am Fam Physician*, 3:107, 1971)

22. **False.** Bleeding from gastric ulcers is less likely to stop than bleeding from duodenal ulcers.
(*Am Fam Physician*, 3:61, 1971)

23. **False.** Patients with gastric ulcers of the body of the stomach tend to secrete subnormal amounts of acid. (2:1506)

24. **A.** Most patients have no symptoms referable to a sliding hiatal hernia. All other statements are true of sliding hiatal hernias. In addition, the persistence of postural regurgitation of gastric

contents into the esophagus in a nonpregnant patient is virtually diagnostic of this condition.
(*Am Fam Physician*, 3:107, 1971)

25. **A.** A-beta-lipoproteinemia is not a rare disorder. All other statements are correct.
(*N Engl J Med*, 281:1113, 1969)

26. **E.** Increased levels of alpha₁-fetoprotein are found in prenatal aminocentesis fluid in the presence of anencephaly and other neural tube defects. Persistent or rising levels have frequently preceded clinical recognition of tumor recurrence or growth of metastases. During abnormal pregnancies with impending fetal death, AFP can become elevated in maternal serum, presumably by means of fetal-maternal transfusion through a damaged placenta. (*N Engl J Med*, 290:568, 1974)

27. **A.** Cholesterol gallstone disease is associated with a decrease in the total pool of conjugated bile salts. All other statements are true. (1:36)

28. **B.** In adult celiac disease, total or subtotal villous atrophy is the characteristic histological finding. All other statements are true. Additionally, micellar lipid is not taken up normally by the damaged cells, and the material absorbed is transferred suboptimally. In this disease, carbohydrate intolerance results from damage to the microvillous membrane and the deficiency of the disaccharidases, particularly lactase.
(*N Engl J Med*, 281:1111, 1969)

29. **E.** A majority of patients with nodular lymphoid hyperplasia of the small bowel have intestinal Giardia infestation. Treatment of the parasitic infestation with quinacrine may improve the gastrointestinal symptoms and malabsorption syndrome. (*New Physician*, 21:280, 1972)

30. **D.** Patients with intestinal lymphangiectasia most often present with signs and symptoms of low plasma proteins rather than of malabsorption. They may have edema, chylous ascites, and, rarely, chylothorax.
(*N Engl J Med*, 281:1114, 1969)

31. **E.** The diagnosis of Meckel's diverticulum is seldom made by routine gastrointestinal x-rays. All other statements are correct. In addition, Meckel's diverticulum can manifest with bleeding, perforation, obstruction, and inflammation.
(*New Physician*, 21:129, 1972)

32. **A.** Primary biliary cirrhosis occurs almost exclusively (over 90%) in adults, often middle-aged women. All other statements are true. (4:1477–78)

33. **A.** Fat in the liver after alcohol intake is not a precursor of cirrhosis, and though it may produce a large liver with temporary portal hypertension, it usually resolves in about 6 weeks. (1:36)

34. **A.** The malabsorption syndrome is characterized by weight loss and passage of abnormal stools, often more than one stool a day which are usually a light yellow to gray, greasy, and soft and in many cases, bulky, with a tendency to float. When the disorder is more florid, the stools are extremely malodorous. (*N Engl J Med*, 281:1111, 1969)

35. **C.** Clinical manifestations of eosinophilic gastroenteritis include pyloric obstruction, mucosal bleeding, protein loss and malabsorption, and acute peritonitis. (1:39)

36. **Paraesophageal.** A paraesophageal hernia, which accounts for about 10% of hiatal hernias, rolls up beside the esophagus, and the esophagogastric junction remains in its normal position. (*Am Fam Physician*, 3:107, 1971)

37. **Celiac.** Patients with diabetes mellitus, diabetic neuropathy, malabsorption syndrome and villous atrophy probably have adult celiac disease. (*N Engl J Med*, 281:1114, 1969)

38. **Hypogammaglobulinemia; A.** Villous atrophy (often responsive to a gluten-free diet), so-called nodular lymphoid hyperplasia (often with giardiasis) and, rarely, granulomatous lesions may be found in the small intestine in congenital or acquired hypogammaglobulinemia. Plasma levels of IgA are universally, and those of IgG almost always, depressed. (*N Engl J Med*, 281:1113, 1969)

39. **Ileal.** Ileal resection interrupts the enterohepatic circulation of bile salts by removal of the site of their active reabsorption. (1:38)

40. **Osteomalacia.** Cholestyramine therapy may be complicated by osteomalacia due to vitamin D malabsorption; these patients should receive supplements of fat soluble vitamins. (1:38)

41. **Achlorhydria.** In pernicious anemia, the hypergastrinemia results from achlorhydria with consequent failure to inhibit the antral release of gastrin. (1:34)

42. **Gluten, Villous.** Most cases of celiac disease—childhood and adult—respond to elimination of gluten from the diet. This regimen must be lifelong. Symptoms are alleviated in a matter of a few days, absorption returns to normal over a period of a few weeks, and regeneration of the villous structure of the mucosa will ensue in most patients who have adhered strictly to the diet. (*N Engl J Med*, 281:1116, 1969)

43. **Giardia.** Malabsorption in patients with dysgammaglobulinemia has been attributed to *Giardia lamblia* infestation. (1:39)

44. **Aflatoxin.** Contamination of food by aflatoxin produced by fungi may explain the high incidence of hepatic carcinoma in Africa and Asia. (1:43)

45. **A.** After giving 25 g D-xylose orally, normal urinary excretion is 4.5 g or greater per 5 hours. Excretion is diminished in diseases of the mucosa, particularly celiac disease, and in intestinal stasis, but is normal in pancreatic insufficiency. (2:1530)

46. **C.** In some cases, *Giardia lamblia* is associated with severe malabsorption by invasion of the small bowel mucosal cells without apparent injury, and with creation of a barrier to normal transport. (*N Engl J Med*, 281:1113, 1969)

47. **D.** At mealtimes, cholecystokinin-pancreozymin (CCK-PZ) released from duodenal mucosa by amino acids, peptides, and to a lesser degree fat, causes gallbladder contraction with relaxation of the sphincter of Oddi. (1:36)

48. **C.** The malabsorption associated with diffuse regional enteritis may be alleviated somewhat by the administration of steroids provided the patient does not have bacterial overgrowth due to chronic obstruction or fistula. (*N Engl J Med*, 281:1116, 1969)

49. **A.** In patients with chronic liver disease and ascites, fluid is mobilized into the bloodstream more slowly in those without edema than in those with edema. This disparity is manifest during spontaneous diuresis and is enhanced by administration of diuretics. (*Lancet*, 2:596, 1970)

50. **C.** Urinary excretion of indican is elevated in bacterial overgrowth and ileal dysfunction. (2:1531)

51. **C.** Disaccharidase deficiency may be present despite structurally normal microvilli (a hereditary defect); also, a number of diseases of the small bowel impair or destroy the microvilli, thus preventing normal disaccharidase activity. (*N Engl J Med*, 281:1111, 1969)

52. **C.** Both statements are true of sliding hiatal hernia. (*Am Fam Physician*, 3:107, 1971)

53. **C.** Free air from a perforated viscus may be detected by an upright or lateral decubitis film.
(3:309)

54. **B.** Tropical sprue responds dramatically to the administration of broad-spectrum antimicrobial.
(*N Engl J Med*, 281:1116, 1969)

55. **B.** Conversion of the Bilroth II to a Bilroth I anastomosis, if possible, is advisable in patients with malabsorption after gastrectomy.
(*N Engl J Med*, 281:1115, 1969)

56. **C.** Lithogenic bile refers to a state of cholesterol supersaturation or to saturation in the presence of cholesterol microcrystals.
(1:36)

57. **C.** Chronic pancreatitis may be associated with steatorrhea and x-ray evidence of pancreatic calcification.
(*JAMA*, 213:1676, 1970)

58. **A.** The important laboratory features of chronic active hepatitis are changes in serum transaminase levels and hypergammaglobulinemia because it has been shown that these tests reflect the activity of the disease—the extent of liver cell necrosis and the degree of associated round cell infiltration in the liver.
(2:1662)

59. **E.** Antimitochondrial antibodies are detected in more than 90% of patients with primary biliary cirrhosis.
(1:35)

60. **B.** Clinically, gastric ulcers are less common than duodenal ulcers in a ratio of 1:4. (4:1373–74)

61. **E.** In a series of 900 patients undergoing x-ray studies for alimentary tract complaints, Nuzum found hiatal hernias in 12%. Sliding hernias comprise 85 to 90% of the hiatal hernias.
(*Am Fam Physician*, 3:107, 1971)

62. **D.** Normally liver contains only 80 to 100 g glycogen, about one-half day's supply of carbohydrate, should gluconeogenesis not be stimulated to provide the glucose needed by the organism.
(4:453)

63. **B.** Perforation and gangrene of the colon occur in about 10% of cases of acute mesenteric ischemia.
(1:42)

64. **D.** In normal man, the total amount of fluid entering the gut per day is about 10 liters.
(1:39)

65. **D.** The vagus nerve influences gastric secretion in at least three ways: (1) direct cholinergic stimulation of parietal cells, (2) release of gastrin, and (3) sensitization of the parietal cell to stimulation by gastrin and other stimulants.
(2:1505)

66. **B.** Sacroiliitis as a feature of colitis and enteritis is more common in women. It differs from ankylosing spondylitis, and is not helped by radical surgery of the affected bowel.
(1:41)

67. **B.** Celiac disease (gluten enteropathy) has a wide clinical spectrum; evidence for an immunological mechanism is the association with IgA deficiency, the predominant infiltration of the mucosa with plasma cells containing IgM, and changes in serum immunoglobulins.
(1:38)

68. **A.** Less than 5% of patients with acute Australia antigen-positive hepatitis remain positive and develop chronic active hepatitis (chronic aggressive hepatitis) which often evolves into postnecrotic cirrhosis.
(1:35)

69. **A.** The milk-alkali syndrome or Burnett's syndrome describes the hypercalcemia which may occur with ingestion of large amounts of calcium-containing substances, such as dairy products, and antacids containing calcium carbonate.
(*Res-Int Consult*, 1:44, 1972)

70. **C.** Although anticholinergics may suppress the vagal mechanism of acid secretion, they also delay gastric emptying, which may stimulate the antrum to produce gastrin.
(1:34)

71. **C.** Gastroesophageal reflux may exist with or without hiatal hernia.
(1:34)

72. **C.** In chronic gastritis associated with gastric atrophy, there may be achlorhydria and elevated gastrin levels.
(1:34)

73. **D.** Low residue diets are no longer advocated for inflammatory bowel disease or diverticulosis, and low-fat diets are seldom employed in hepatic or gallbladder disease.
(1:43)

74. **D** The most frequent liver changes in alcoholics are increased deposition of fat, often without any abnormality in liver function, and an increase in the drug metabolizing enzymes of the liver endoplasmic reticulum, analogous to the increases after phenobarbital treatment.
(1:36)

75. **D.** Small bowel resections predispose to cholesterol gallstones and oxalate renal stones. (1:43)

76. **A.** Cholangitis may complicate ductal obstruction by stone or stricture and is uncommon with neoplastic obstruction without prior surgery; enteric organisms, often anaerobic, are the usual pathogens. Cholangitis is now the commonest cause of liver abscess (often multiple). (1:36)

77. **C.** Both intense drinking and malnutrition seem necessary to produce alcoholic hepatitis. (1:37)

78. **D.** Splenectomy or shunts are almost never indicated for hypersplenism in cirrhosis. (1:37)

79. **A.** Patients with dermatitis herpetiformis may exhibit a proximal jejunal mucosal lesion which is identical with that of celiac disease; this lesion responds to a gluten-free diet. (1:38)

80. **D.** Dysgammaglobulinemia with villous atrophy in the absence of giardiasis does not usually respond to a gluten-free diet or metronidazole. (1:39)

81. **True.** In any patient with normal renal function the urinary excretion of D-xylose after ingestion of a 25 g load will reflect with remarkable accuracy the absorptive capacity of the small intestine for carbohydrate.
(*N Engl J Med,* 281:1114, 1969)

82. **True.** Patients with celiac disease exhibit an impaired pancreatic secretory response to intraluminal peptides and fat due to a deficient release of pancreozymin-cholecystokinin from the diseased mucosa. Exocrine pancreatic function may be secondarily depressed by protein malnutrition in patients with small bowel disease. (1:38)

83. **False.** The liver scan is one of the most useful tests in the diagnosis of disease in the right upper quadrant. (4:1453)

84. **True.** Hepatitis B antigen appears in blood during the acute phase of the disease and is cleared in a few weeks except in perhaps 1% of patients who remain positive but clinically well. (1:35)

85. **True.** Calcium-containing antacids may stimulate gastrin production, leading to an acid rebound effect. (1:34)

86. **False.** The incidence of duodenal ulcer in England and in the United States is declining sharply, but treatment of peptic ulcer disease has altered little in the past decade. (1:34)

87. **True.** Although the National Halothane Study did not demonstrate an increased frequency of massive fatal hepatic necrosis with the use of halothane compared to other anesthetic agents, the association of hepatic necrosis with halothane use has been well-documented in individual case studies, particularly with recurrent exposure in anesthesiologists. Fever within 8 to 14 days of initial exposure, or earlier with recurrent exposure, is accompanied by clinical and chemical evidence of parenchymal cell necrosis. (1:35)

88. **False.** Gallstones may be more common in patients on long-term therapy with Atromid-S for hypercholesterolemia. (1:36)

89. **False.** Laparotomy in spontaneous peritonitis is rarely indicated. (1:38)

90. **True.** Giardia are best detected in duodenal mucus; their presence may be masked by prior barium studies. (1:39)

91. **False.** Acid injury seems to be the basis for alcoholic gastritis which is observed by gastroscopy or biopsy in the majority of alcoholics. (1:36)

92. **True.** Hypomotility of the small intestine can lead to diarrhea by promoting stasis of intestinal contents and bacterial overgrowth. (1:39)

93. **True.** Gallbladder contrast media requires months for elimination because media repeatedly pass through the enterohepatic circulation.
(*Am Fam Physician,* 3:73, 1971)

94. **True.** In cirrhosis, very tense ascites increases portal pressure and should be treated to avoid variceal bleeding. (1:38)

95. **False.** Fluctuations in blood sugar levels in diabetics may lead to over- or underproduction of gastric acid; sustained hyperglycemia is thought to lead to atrophic gastritis, very common in diabetics. (1:41)

96. **True.** Venous hums are at times identified over the cirrhotic liver due to torrential flow through venous collaterals. (3:170)

97. **True.** Diabetics absorb sugar at rates higher than normal, despite rather irregular motor action of the duodenum and jejunum. (1:41)

98. **True.** Dumping can often be controlled by restriction of fluids and osmotically active foods, especially sugars, at mealtimes, but extreme instances may require corrective operations. (1:42)

99. **False.** Inflammation around diverticula in the sigmoid rarely is associated with hemorrhage, but may lead to perforation, localized peritonitis, and eventually to fistulae, usually between the sigmoid and the adjacent viscera. (1:41)

Textbook References for Chapter 9

1. American College of Physicians (1974): *Medical Knowledge Self-Assessment, Program III: Recent Developments in Internal Medicine,* Petersdorf, R.G., General Editor, American College of Physicians, Philadelphia.

2. Beeson, P.B. and McDermott, W. (1979): *Cecil Textbook of Medicine*, Fifteenth Edition. W.B. Saunders Company, Philadelphia.

3. Judge, R.D. and Zuidema, G.D., Editors (1974): *Physical Diagnosis: A Physiologic Approach to the Clinical Examination,* Little, Brown and Company, Boston.

4. Isselbacher, K.J., Editor (1980): *Harrison's Principles of Internal Medicine*, Ninth Edition, McGraw-Hill Book Company, New York.

CHAPTER 10

Hematology

1. Which drug alters the red cell to produce a typical model of autoimmune hemolytic anemia where an antibody is produced which reacts to the altered red blood cell?

   A. INH
   B. methyldopa (Aldomet)
   C. penicillin
   D. antihistamines
   E. all of the above

2. Under usual circumstances, approximately what percentage of the dietary iron is absorbed?

   A. 1%
   B. 5%
   C. 10%
   D. 26%
   E. over 60%

3. One milliliter blood cells is equivalent to how many milligrams iron?

   A. 1
   B. 2
   C. 3
   D. 4
   E. 5

4. The normal half-life of Cr^{51}-tagged red cells in the circulation is how many days?

   A. 5 to 10
   B. 25 to 30
   C. 60 to 80
   D. 120 to 150
   E. over 300

5. In general, cyanosis becomes apparent when the mean capillary concentration of reduced hemoglobin is about how many grams per 100 milliliters?

   A. 1
   B. 2
   C. 3
   D. 4
   E. 5 or more

6. The immunosuppressed kidney transplant recipient is subject to approximately how many times the normal risk of neoplastic disease?

   A. 4
   B. 10
   C. 20
   D. 200
   E. 2000

7. The most common cause of death in sickle cell anemia is

   A. infection
   B. aplastic crisis

C. renal insufficiency
D. hepatic insufficiency
E. cardiac failure

8. The circulating half-life of the granulocytes is

A. less than 1 hour
B. 6 to 8 hours
C. 24 hours
D. 72 hours
E. 6 days

9. A variety of Hodgkin's disease with the best prognosis is

A. lymphocyte predominant
B. nodular sclerosis
C. mixed cellularity
D. all forms have about the same prognosis

10. In about what percentage of cases of polycythemia vera may patients succumb from acute leukemia?

A. 1%
B. 5%
C. 10%
D. 20%
E. 40%

11. Platelets release an antiheparin factor called platelet Factor

A. 1
B. 2
C. 3
D. 4
E. 5

12. The incidence of "nonsecretory" multiple myeloma in which no abnormal protein can be detected in serum or urine appears to be about what percent?

A. 1 to 2%
B. 5 to 10%
C. 16%
D. 25 to 35%
E. 50%

13. Studies in hemolytic anemia have indicated that the marrow of an adult man appears to be capable of increasing red blood cell production about

A. 2-fold
B. 4-fold
C. 8-fold
D. 16-fold
E. 32-fold

14. Probably about what percentage of patients with nodal Hodgkin's lymphoma, localized at the time of diagnosis, prove to have retroperitoneal lymph node involvement when studies by lymphography or other special x-ray techniques are made?

A. 5%
B. 25%
C. 55%
D. 75%
E. 95%

15. Parahemophilia is associated with a primary defect in

A. Factor II
B. Factor V
C. Factor VII
D. Factor VIII
E. Factor X

16. Sickle cell trait occurs in about what percentage of American blacks?

A. 1%
B. 2%
C. 4%
D. 8%
E. 16%

17. Using the Ann Arbor staging classification for Hodgkin's disease, diffuse involvement of extralymphatic sites with or without lymph node enlargement would be classified as

A. Stage I
B. Stage II
C. Stage III
D. Stage IV
E. Stage V

18. The effect of aspirin on platelet aggregation lasts as long as the platelets are viable, or about

    A. 1 day
    B. 2 days
    C. 4 days
    D. 8 days
    E. 16 days

19. Circulating antibody to intrinsic factor is present in what percentage of patients with pernicious anemia?

    A. less than 1%
    B. 5%
    C. 33%
    D. 50%
    E. 66%

20. The estimated dietary iron requirements of the normal adult male is

    A. less than 4 mg/day
    B. 10 mg/day
    C. 15 to 25 mg/day
    D. 50 to 60 mg/day
    E. 80 to 90 mg/day

21. Fluorescent techniques have shown the Philadelphia chromosome to be derived from

    A. chromosome 17
    B. chromosome 19
    C. chromosome 91
    D. chromosome 22
    E. none of the above

22. Hemoglobin comprises what percentage of the total body iron in man?

    A. 5%
    B. 21%
    C. 44%
    D. 72%
    E. 99%

Directions: For each of the following multiple-choice questions, select the ONE INCORRECT answer.

23. Primary thrombocythemia

    A. has been classified as a myeloproliferative disorder in which the major abnormality is the unregulated production of excessive numbers of platelets
    B. is a clinical syndrome which may be characterized by life-threatening recurrent spontaneous hemorrhages and thromboembolic phenomena
    C. rarely undergoes transition into other myeloproliferative diseases
    D. has been reported to involve an absence of platelet aggregation in response to epinephrine
    E. chemotherapy results in a decrease in platelet count, a decreased incidence of thromboembolic episodes and, occasionally, an improvement in platelet aggregation

24. Ancrod

    A. is snake venom extract
    B. administered intravenously (one dose) will remove all fibrinogen, thus a secondary clot cannot form
    C. results in large amounts of circulating fibrin degradation products as fibrinogen is removed from the body
    D. requires simple dosage adjustment
    E. has more rapid onset of action than heparin

25. Packed red cells as compared to whole blood transfusions

    A. enable transfusion with less increase in circulatory volume
    B. have an increased citrate and ammonia load
    C. have a reduced sodium and potassium load
    D. have a reduced acid load
    E. result in less anaphylactoid reactions to plasma proteins such as immunoglobulin A and beta lipoproteins

26. Regarding eosinophils,

    A. the "Thorn test" uses ACTH for detecting adrenal cortical insufficiency
    B. the lower range is usually 50 to 80 cells per cubic mm and the upper range of normal is between 250 and 500
    C. increased numbers are found in lymph node tuberculosis with marked caseation, erythema multiforme, leprosy, black widow spider bite, iodide and other chemical sensitivities, and Loeffler's syndrome
    D. blood dyscrasias are uncommon causes of eosinophilia
    E. in allergic disorders, eosinophilia is minimal for asthma, hay fever, angioneurotic edema, urticaria and eczema, and is occasionally marked in drug allergy

27. Pure red cell aplasia

    A. is associated with a thymoma in about 20 to 30% of cases
    B. appears to be caused by antibodies directed at the erythroid series
    C. may respond temporarily to large doses of steroids
    D. does not respond to immunosuppressive agents

28. In hereditary nonspherocytic hemolytic anemia,

    A. the clinical course is usually characterized by the occurrence of anemia and jaundice early in life with moderate splenomegaly and the anemia, typically, is normocytic or slightly macrocytic and associated with a reticulocytosis, hyperbilirubinemia, and little or no splenocytosis
    B. signs and symptoms usually become clinically apparent in childhood or early adult life and often a cholecystectomy or splenectomy has been performed at an early age
    C. confirmation of the familial occurrence should be made by examining the kindred, even though they may not have symptoms that suggest hemolytic anemia
    D. chronic hereditary nonspherocytic hemolytic anemias that persist in the absence of oxidant stress are usually caused by enzyme defects that lead to a deficiency in ATP production or, perhaps, ATP utilization
    E. fecal urobilinogen is normal or decreased

29. Hemoglobins associated with cyanosis include

    A. M Boston
    B. M Iwate
    C. M Milwaukee
    D. Chesapeake
    E. Kansas

30. G-6-PD deficiency

    A. is the most frequently recognized human erythrocyte enzyme deficiency
    B. has more than 80 different varients
    C. involves mild to moderately severe hemolytic anemia even in the absence of any known precipitating agent
    D. causes hemolysis which is most often seen in hemizygous males who have received drugs such as primaquine, sulfonamides, nitrofurantoin, nitrofurazone, or acetanilid
    E. involves acute hemolysis occurring in black subjects after ingestion of fava beans (favism)

31. Hemoglobin F

    A. is less resistant to denaturation by alkali than hemoglobin A
    B. normally disappears from the circulating erythrocytes during the first 6 months of life
    C. concentrations are increased in the thalassemia syndrome
    D. high concentration may be seen with hereditary persistence, which is not associated with hemolysis or other clinical symptoms

32. Polycythemia vera involves
    A. increased red cell mass
    B. abnormal arterial oxygen saturation
    C. splenomegaly
    D. elevated leukocyte alkaline phosphatase
    E. elevated serum vitamin B_{12} level

33. Hyperhemolytic sickle cell crisis
    A. is common
    B. involves high serum bilirubin concentrations
    C. involves high fecal urobilinogen values
    D. involves severe anemia

34. The more common, dose-related, reversible bone marrow toxicity that may occur concurrently with chloramphenicol therapy is characterized by
    A. a hypocellular marrow
    B. maturation arrest
    C. vacuolization in erythroid and myeloid cells
    D. reticulocytopenia
    E. ferrokinetic changes indicative of suppressed erythropoiesis

35. In hemophilia,
    A. inheritance is from a sex-linked dominant trait
    B. the degree of clinical severity of the disease roughly corresponds to the degree of clotting factor deficiency and appears to depend upon a series of alternative alleles which replaces the normal gene
    C. when the single X chromosome of a male carries the mutant gene, he will be hemophilic
    D. when the mutant gene occurs on one of the two X chromosomes of a female, she will not usually manifest hemorrhagic symptoms but will be capable of transmitting the gene to her offspring (half of her sons becoming hemophilics, and half of her daughters becoming carriers)
    E. mean concentration of Factor VIII in heterozygous females is lower than that in homozygous normal females

Directions: For each of the incomplete statements below, ONE or MORE of the completions given is correct. In each case, select
    A. if 1, 2, and 3 are correct
    B. if 1 and 3 are correct
    C. if 2 and 4 are correct
    D. if only 4 is correct
    E. if all are correct

36. In iron absorption,
    1. the major site of physiologic control of absorption occurs in the duodenum
    2. iron deficiency acts as a potent stimulus
    3. iron deficiency at the tissue level may impair iron absorption as a result of biochemical derangements of the absorbing epithelium
    4. it is retarded by orange juice

37. The therapeutic options available for treating pulmonary embolism include
    1. inhibition of secondary clot with heparin and warfarin (Coumadin) or its analogs, and use of defibrinating agents such as snake venom extracts
    2. antiplatelet aggregation with aspirin
    3. thrombolysis using urokinase and streptokinase
    4. surgical procedures

38. Haptoglobin levels are invariably low in
    1. autoimmune hemolytic anemia
    2. pernicious anemia
    3. paroxysmal nocturnal hemoglobinuria
    4. sickle cell disease
    5. thalassemia major

39. In iron deficiency anemia, oral intake of 300 mg ferrous sulfate three times daily
    1. is equivalent to 180 mg of elemental iron daily
    2. in the absence of heavy bleeding, in simple iron deficiency should produce a hemoglobin response of 1 to 2 g per week, depending on the initial degree of anemia

3. should effect no appreciable hemoglobin elevation in adults until the second week following the institution of therapy
4. results in the reticulocyte peak occurring anywhere from 7 to 12 days after starting therapy, possibly reaching levels of 15 to 30%

40. In chronic granulocytic leukemia, patients who are Philadelphia chromosome-negative

1. are usually male and are either much older than the typical patients, or are children, usually under the age of 2 years
2. are more frequently thrombocytopenic on presentation, with shorter life span and refractoriness to busulfan and other forms of antileukemic therapy
3. may have elevated levels of fetal hemoglobin in the childhood form of the disease
4. have appreciably higher levels of serum muramidase than chromosome-positive patients and demonstrate muramidasuria

41. Which of the following can be given orally in doses that alter platelet function in man without causing major side effects?

1. phenylbutazone
2. aspirin
3. sulfinpyrazone
4. dipyridamole

42. Which of the following may cause intravascular platelet aggregation?

1. antigen-antibody complexes
2. endotoxin
3. some viruses
4. bacteria

43. In stress erythrocytosis,

1. this term has been applied to the polycythemia seen occasionally in very active, hard-working persons in a state of anxiety
2. subjects appear florid but have none of the characteristic signs of erythremia—

no splenomegaly or leukocytosis with immature cells in the blood
3. plasma volume is below normal
4. total red blood cell mass is increased

44. Heinz body preparation

1. is the simplest test for intracorpuscular abnormalities
2. the presence of Heinz bodies on an appropriately stained blood smear means that oxidatively denatured globin is present. This means that the erythrocyte-reducing system has a deficit or that the globin is unduly susceptible to oxidation, or a high dose of oxidant has overpowered a normal erythrocyte-reducing system
3. may be associated with unstable hemoglobin; e.g., hemoglobin Köln
4. may be associated with glucose-6-phosphate dehydrogenase deficiency and with thalassemia

45. Platelet inhibitors include

1. dextran
2. aspirin
3. dipyridamole
4. mini-dose heparin

46. Eosinophils

1. form Charcot-Leyden crystals
2. have high levels of leukocyte alkaline phosphatase
3. possess diurnal variation, with highest levels at midnight
4. exist mainly in the peripheral blood

47. Immune hemolytic anemia is

1. an uncommon cause of "extrinsic" red cell defects
2. occasionally associated with systemic lupus erythematosus, chronic lymphocytic leukemia and other lymphoproliferative disorders

3. not improved by adrenocorticosteroids
4. associated with an IgG antibody which is often specific for the Rh system

48. Which of the following is/are capable of mitosis and constitute the proliferating portion or "metabolic pool" of the granulocyte series?

    1. myeloblasts
    2. promyelocytes
    3. myelocytes
    4. metamyelocytes

49. Hemoglobin CC disease is associated with

    1. chronic hemolytic anemia
    2. splenic enlargement
    3. target cells
    4. a hemoglobin electrophoresis pattern of Hb CC which establishes the diagnosis

50. Hypochromia and microcytosis may occur in

    1. inflammatory disease such as infections and rheumatoid arthritis
    2. sideroblastic and sideroachrestic anemias
    3. hemoglobin C and unstable hemoglobin
    4. lead poisoning

51. Patients with large numbers of thrombi in their body generally, but not always, tend to resist heparin therapy. One possible explanation for this involves platelet Factor 4 which is

    1. a membrane surface activating factor
    2. antiheparin in its action
    3. released from the surface of the platelets, leukocytes, and red cells
    4. increased in patients with massive clotting

52. Thrombocytosis may provide a clue to the presence of certain underlying disease states such as

    1. myeloproliferative disorders
    2. inflammation
    3. infection
    4. iron deficiency

53. Which of the following is/are true of unstable hemoglobins?

    1. include hemoglobins Geneva, Zurich, and Seattle
    2. characteristically, hemolysis, inclusion bodies in the red blood cells, and hemoglobin precipitation at 50°C are observed and the spleen is usually enlarged
    3. in some patients, hemolysis may become more severe with the ingestion of certain drugs
    4. electrophoretic differences are always observed

54. Thalassemia major is characterized by

    1. childhood tolerance of the condition
    2. hepatic and splenic enlargement
    3. infrequent incidence of jaundice
    4. marked hypochromic, microcytic anemia

55. Pseudolymphomas

    1. are malignant lymphoid collections
    2. may be confused with lymphomas
    3. require laparotomies and splenectomies which are usually done for staging
    4. may occur in the gastrointestinal tract, lungs, skin, and conjunctivae

56. The intestinal absorption of physiologic amounts of vitamin B_{12}—about 1 μg daily—depends on a complex sequence of events in the gastrointestinal tract. Major steps in this sequence include the

    1. secretion of intrinsic factor (IF) by gastric parietal cells
    2. formation of intrinsic factor vitamin B_{12} complex (IF-B_{12}) in the intestinal lumen
    3. binding of IF-B_{12} by specific "receptors" on the microvilli of distal small bowel epithelial cells
    4. transfer of vitamin B_{12} across the epithelium

57. Evidence of intravascular hemolysis includes

    1. hemoglobinemia
    2. methemalbuminemia
    3. decreased serum hemopexin
    4. hemoglobinuria

58. Heinz bodies

   1. are discrete erythrocyte inclusions, demonstrable by supravital staining with methyl violet or under phase microscopy
   2. probably represent denatured intracellular hemoglobin
   3. may be seen in blood smears from patients with some of the unstable hemoglobin syndromes, especially if the patient has had a splenectomy; may be observed during hemolytic episodes associated with G-6-PD deficiency
   4. can be brought out after incubation of blood with acetylphenylhydrazine if the erythrocytes have a defect in the hexose monophosphate shunt pathway related to the metabolism of reduced glutathione

Directions: Use the key below to answer questions 59 through 62. Select
   A. if the statement is characteristic of urokinase
   B. if the statement is characteristic of streptokinase

59. Plasmin excess is common

60. Plasminogen depletion is common

61. Adjusting of dose is simple

62. Higher antigenicity

Directions: Use the key below to answer questions 63 and 64. Select
   A. if the biologic half-life is 31 hours
   B. if the biologic half-life is 6 days

63. Factor XIII

64. Factor IX

Directions: Use the key below to answer questions 65 and 66. Select
   A. if the test detects pyruvate kinase deficiency
   B. if the test detects glucose-6-phosphatase deficiency

65. Type I abnormal autohemolysis test

66. Type II abnormal autohemolysis test

Directions: Use the key below to answer questions 67 through 69. Select
   A. if the protein listed binds hemoglobin but not heme
   B. if the protein listed binds free heme but not hemoglobin

67. Hemopexin

68. Haptoglobin

69. Albumin

Directions: Indicate whether each of the following statements is true or false.

70. In general, disseminated intravascular coagulation is clinically evident only in hypertensive patients.

71. A thalassemic disorder can be classified as alpha-, beta-, gamma- or delta-thalassemia, depending on the particular globin polypeptide chain associated with defective synthesis.

72. Iron loss is characteristic of chronic hemosiderinuria, which may be the result of intravascular hemolysis.

73. The majority of patients with megaloblastic anemia have splenomegaly.

74. Appearance of hemolytic anemia after many years of good health usually, but not always, implies the development of an acquired extracorpuscular process.

75. Electrophoresis may reveal an increased concentration of hemoglobin A_2 in many cases of thalassemia.

76. Nutritional deficiencies of vitamin B_{12}, folate, or iron can result in the production of

erythrocytes of such poor quality that they have shortened survival.

77. In patients with hemolysis, frank anemia is probably more frequent than compensated hemolysis.

78. The uncontrovertible diagnosis of the presence of a hemolytic process requires the demonstration of a decreased survival of erythrocytes in the circulation.

79. Burkitt's lymphomas respond poorly to cyclophosphamide.

80. In the peripheral smear, polychromatophilia suggests reticulocytosis.

81. Cells which are in extended G_1 phase (or G_0) and do not engage in DNA synthesis are not affected by antileukemic therapy.

82. The presence of normoblasts suggests hemolysis, but it almost always indicates some type of marrow distress (e.g., tumor or myelofibrosis) as well, since normoblasts are rarely seen in uncomplicated hemolytic disorders.

83. There is considerable evidence that reversible bone marrow suppression and aplastic anemia from chloramphenicol are related.

84. Diphenylhydantoin (Dilantin) enhances the absorption of folate.

85. The relationship between coagulation and platelets is probably responsible for the characteristic layered structure of arterial thrombi consisting of successive layers of platelets and fibrin.

86. In Hodgkin's disease, positive liver biopsies are frequently found in the absence of splenic involvement.

87. Erythrocytes from patients with paroxysmal nocturnal hemoglobinuria (PNH) hemolyze when incubated in isotonic solutions of low ionic strength provided a small amount of serum is present in the reaction mixture.

88. In hereditary spherocytosis, the osmotic fragility of erthyrocytes is increased

89. Some of the unstable hemoglobins move normally on routine electrophoresis.

Directions: Use the key below to answer questions 90 and 91. Select
  A. **if the type of amyloid protein involved is protein A**
  B. **if the type of amyloid protein involved is Ig-light chain**

90. Amyloidosis Pattern I

91. Amyloidosis Pattern II

Answers and Commentary

1. **B.** Methyldopa (Aldomet) alters the red cell to produce a typical model of autoimmune hemolytic anemia where an antibody is produced which reacts to the altered red blood cell. (1:50)

2. **C.** Iron tends to complex with ligands in the intestinal milieu. Some, such as phytate or oxalate, form insoluble complexes with iron, thus decreasing its availability. Others, such as certain amino acids, may form soluble complexes which are readily absorbed. Hence iron in vegetables in general is less available, while iron in meat is more readily absorbed. Under usual circumstances, approximately 10% of the dietary iron is absorbed. (4:1514)

3. **A.** One milliliter blood cells is equivalent to one milligram iron. (1:49)

4. **B.** The normal half-life of Cr^{51}-tagged red cells in the circulation is 25 to 30 days.
(*Postgrad Med*, 47:45, 1970)

5. **E.** In general, cyanosis becomes apparent when the mean capillary concentration of reduced hemoglobin exceeds 5 g/100 ml. (4:166)

6. **D.** The immunosuppressed kidney transplant recipient is subject to approximately 200 times the normal risk of neoplastic disease, with one-third being malignant lymphoma. (1:57)

7. **A.** Sickle cell anemia in the past has had a high mortality rate in early childhood, few patients reaching adult life. Recent decades have seen progressively increasing longevity, and increasing numbers of patients survive beyond the age of 50. This improvement in outlook is not attributable to advances in specific therapy, but is largely the result of better nutrition and more adequate prevention and treatment of infections. Infection remains the most common cause of death. Aplastic crises are a serious threat to life if not treated promptly. Death may result from renal or hepatic insufficiency, cardiac failure, or vascular occlusions in the nervous system. Widespread intravascular sickling is found in some patients dying suddenly or during a painful crisis. The clinical spectrum of the disease is broad, and mild cases of sickle cell anemia are increasingly recognized. Some older patients have chronic anemia but have not had the characteristic symptoms associated with the disease. (2:1775)

8. **B.** The circulating half-life of granulocytes is low—only 6 to 8 hours. (1:54)

9. **A.** Patients with lymphocyte predominant Hodgkin's disease have the best prognosis. However, this constitutes only about 5% of cases. (1:57)

10. **C.** In about 10% of cases of polycythemia vera, patients may succumb from acute leukemia. (1:48)

11. **D.** Platelets release an antiheparin factor called platelet Factor 4. (*Hosp Practice*, 7:115, 1972)

12. **A.** The incidence of "nonsecretory" multiple myeloma in which no abnormal protein can be detected in serum or urine, appears to be about 1 to 2%. (*Blood*, 40:204, 1972)

13. **C.** The essential feature of a hemolytic disorder is shortening of the life span of the red blood cells. The patient may have a compensated hemolytic state without anemia if the bone marrow responds

adequately. As the marrow of adult man appears to be capable of increasing red blood cell production about 8-fold and as the normal life span of human red cells is about 120 days, anemia may not develop in some cases even if the average life span of the red cells is reduced to 15 to 20 days. The reserve capacity may likewise result in maintenance of a normal concentration of bilirubin in the blood plasma. In a large proportion of the hemolytic states recognized clinically, however, patients are either anemic or mildly icteric, or both, so that the terms hemolytic anemia and hemolytic icterus are applicable. (2:1751)

14. **E.** Probably about 95% of patients with nodal Hodgkin's lymphoma which is apparently localized at the time of diagnosis prove to have retroperitoneal lymph node involvement when studies by lymphography or other special x-ray techniques are made. (1:58)

15. **B.** Parahemophilia is associated with a primary defect in Factor V. (2:1888)

16. **D.** Sickle cell anemia, the clinical expression of homozygosity for Hb S, is a serious disease characterized by unrelenting hemolytic anemia, recurrent episodes of pain and fever, and pathologic involvement of many organs. Affected persons are predominately blacks who have obtained the mutant gene from both parents. Since sickle cell trait occurs in about 8% of American blacks, about 15/10,000 are expected to be homozygous at the time of conception; the actual incidence of sickle cell anemia is lower because of its high mortality rate. (2:1773)

17. **D.** The Ann Arbor staging classification for Hodgkin's disease is as follows: Stage I: Involvement of a single lymph node region (I) or a single extra-lymphatic site (IE). Stage II: Involvement of two or more lymph node regions on the same side of the diaphragm (II) or a solitary extralymphatic site and one or more of lymph node areas on the same side of the diaphragm (IIE). Stage III: Involvement of lymph node regions on both sides of the diaphragm (III) accompanied by spleen involvement (IIIS), or by solitary involvement of an extralymphatic organ or site (IIIE) or both (IIISE). Stage IV: Diffuse involvement of extralymphatic sites with or without lymph node enlargement. Clinical stage and pathologic state are defined for each patient; extranodal sites are designated by specific denominators; presence or absence of symptoms is designated B or A, respectively. (2:1834)

18. **D.** The effect of aspirin on platelet aggregation lasts as long as the platelets are viable, or about eight days. (*Chest*, 63:1006, 1973)

19. **E.** Circulating antibody to intrinsic factor is present in two-thirds of patients with pernicious anemia and, when found, is essentially diagnostic. Less than 10% saturation of serum vitamin B_{12} binding capacity is also essentially diagnostic. (2:1726)

20. **B.** Assuming 10% absorption, the estimated dietary iron requirements of normal adult males is 10 mg/day. (2:1671)

21. **D.** Fluorescent techniques have shown the Philadelphia chromosome to be derived from chromosome 22. (*Mod Med*, 41:104, 1973)

22. **D.** In man, hemoglobin comprises approximately 72% of total body iron. (2:1743)

23. **C.** Transition between primary thrombocythemia and other myeloproliferative diseases is common. All other statements are true. (*J Lab Clin Med*, 80:385, 1972)

24. **E.** The rapidity of onset of ancrod is 4 to 6 hours; heparin acts immediately. All other statements are true. In addition, ancrod is safe to use 48 hours after surgery. (*Chest*, 63:1006, 1973)

25. **B.** Packed red cells have a decreased citrate and ammonia load; all other statements are true of packed red cells as compared to whole blood transfusions. (*Am Fam Physician*, 3:82, 1971)

26. **D.** Blood dyscrasias are common causes of eosinophilia. All other statements are correct. In addition, destructive skin diseases may produce marked elevations in eosinophils. (*Am Fam Physician*, 5:61, 1972)

27. **D.** Pure red cell aplasia is associated with a thymoma in about 20 to 30% of cases and appears to be caused by antibodies directed at the erythroid series. Like other autoimmune disorders, it may respond temporarily to large doses of prednisone and more permanently to immunosuppressive agents such as Cytoxan or Imuran. (1:48)

28. **E.** Fecal urobilinogen is increased in patients with hereditary nonspherocytic hemolytic anemia. All other statements are true. (*JAMA*, 216:5, 1971)

29. **D.** All the hemoglobins listed are associated with cyanosis except Chesapeake. Also, M Saskatchewan, M Hyde Park, and Freiburg are hemoglobins associated with cyanosis. (*Am Fam Physician*, 2:87, 1970)

30. **E.** Acute hemolysis after ingestion of fava beans may occur in G-6-PD deficient Caucasian or Chinese males, but has not been reported in black subjects. All other statements are true.
(*Res Staff Phys*, 19:24, 1973)

31. **A.** Hemoglobin F is more resistant to denaturation by alkali than hemoglobin A. All other statements are correct.
(*Res Staff Phys*, 19:24, 1973)

32. **B.** Normal arterial oxygen saturation is present in patients with polycythemia vera. All other statements are true. (1:48)

33. **A.** Hyperhemolytic crises are probably quite rare. All other statements are true.
(*Am Fam Physician*, 2:87, 1970)

34. **A.** The more common, dose-related, reversible bone marrow toxicity which may occur concurrently with chloramphenicol therapy is characterized by a normally cellular marrow. All other statements are correct. (*JAMA*, 213:1183, 1970)

35. **A.** Hemophilia is inherited as a sex-linked recessive trait. All other statements are true.
(*Am J Med*, 38:119, 1965)

36. **A.** Some foods such as orange juice appear to enhance iron uptake, probably owing to the presence of ascorbic acid, while others, such as wheat, contain phytates and appear to retard this process. (*Med Clin North Am*, 54:1399, 1970)

37. **E.** All methods listed are therapeutic options available for treating pulmonary embolism.
(*Chest*, 63:1006, 1973)

38. **E.** Haptoglobin levels are invariably low in all the disorders listed.
(*N Engl J Med*, 283:1090, 1970)

39. **E.** All the statements are true of an oral intake of ferrous sulfate in the treatment of iron deficiency anemia.
(*Med Clin North Am*, 54:1399, 1970)

40. **E.** All the statements are true of chronic granulocytic leukemia patients who are Philadelphia chromosome-negative.
(*N Engl J Med*, 283:456, 1970)

41. **E.** Any of the drugs listed, as well as chloroquine, can be given orally in doses that alter platelet function in man without causing major side effects. (*Hosp Practice*, 7:115, 1972)

42. **E.** Any of the factors listed may cause intravascular platelet aggregation.
(*Hosp Practice*, 7:115, 1972)

43. **A.** The term stress erythrocytosis has been applied to the polycythemia seen occasionally in very active, hard-working persons in a state of anxiety, who appear florid but who have none of the characteristic signs of erythremia—no splenomegaly or leukocytosis with immature cells in the blood. In such persons the total red blood cell mass is normal and the plasma volume is below normal. (4:170)

44. **E.** All the statements are true of Heinz body preparation. (*Postgrad Med*, 47:45, 1970)

45. **E.** All the drugs listed are platelet inhibitors.
(*JAMA*, 228:757, 1974)

46. **B.** Eosinophils form Charcot-Leyden crystals and possess diurnal variation, with highest levels at midnight. (*J Allergy*, 49:142, 1972)

47. **C.** Immune hemolytic anemia is a common cause of "extrinsic" red cell defects, and adrenocorticosteroids are usually effective. (1:50)

48. **A.** Myeloblasts, promyelocytes, and myelocytes are capable of mitosis and constitute the proliferating portion or "metabolic pool" of the granulocyte series. (*N Engl J Med*, 286:262, 1972)

49. **A.** An electrophoretic pattern of Hb CC does not necessarily establish the diagnosis of Hb CC disease. (*Am Fam Physician*, 2:87, 1970)

50. **E.** Hypochromia and microcytosis are the major findings in advanced iron deficiency anemia but may also occur with inflammatory disease such as occurs with infections, rheumatoid arthritis and various malignancies, unstable hemoglobin, hemoglobin C, sideroblastic and sideroachrestic anemias, and as a result of certain poisons such as lead. (1:50)

51. **E.** All the statements are true of platelet Factor 4. (*Chest*, 63:1006, 1973)

52. **E.** Thrombocytosis may provide a clue to the presence of certain underlying disease states, including malignancies, iron deficiency infection, inflammation, or a myeloproliferative disorder. (1:52)

53. **E.** In unstable hemoglobins, electrophoretic differences may or may not be present, depending on the amino acid substitution.
(*Am Fam Physician*, 2:87, 1970)

54. **E.** All statements are true of thalassemia major.
(*Am Fam Physician*, 2:87, 1970)

55. **C.** Pseudolymphomas are lymphoid collections that may be confused with lymphomas but are benign and occur in the gastrointestinal tract, lungs, skin, and conjunctivae. In general, laparotomies and splenectomies are not done for staging. (1:58)

56. **E.** All statements are true of the intestinal absorption of vitamin B_{12}.
(*N Engl J Med*, 284:666, 1971)

57. **E.** All the disorders listed are evidence of intravascular hemolysis.
(*Res Staff Phys*, 19:24, 1973)

58. **E.** All statements are true of Heinz bodies.
(*Res Staff Phys*, 19:24, 1973)

59. **B.**   (*Chest*, 63:1006, 1973)

60. **B.**   (*Chest*, 63:1006, 1973)

61. **A.**   (*Chest*, 63:1006, 1973)

62. **B.**   (*Chest*, 63:1006, 1973)

63. **B.**   (*JAMA*, 212:2256, 1970)

64. **A.**   (*JAMA*, 212:2256, 1970)

65. **B.**   (*Postgrad Med*, 47:45, 1970)

66. **A.**   (*Postgrad Med*, 47:45, 1970)

67. **B.**   (*N Engl J Med*, 283:1090, 1970)

68. **A.**   (*N Engl J Med*, 283:1090, 1970)

69. **A.**   (*N Engl J Med*, 283:1090, 1970)

70. **False.** In general, disseminated intravascular coagulation is clinically evident only in hypotensive patients.   (3:54)

71. **True.** A thalassemic disorder can be classified as alpha-, beta-, gamma- or delta-thalassemia, depending on the particular globin polypeptide chain associated with defective synthesis.
(*Am Fam Physician*, 2:87, 1970)

72. **True.** Iron loss is characteristic of chronic hemosiderinuria, which may be the result of intravascular hemolysis. This condition can develop in patients with leaking prosthetic heart valves.
(*Int Med News*, 5:27, 1972)

73. **False.** About one-third of patients with megaloblastic anemia have splenomegaly, but this may be observable only on abdominal radiography, because the spleen exceeds two to three times normal size in less than 10% of cases. Moderate hepatomegaly may also be present.   (2:1725)

74. **True.** Appearance of hemolytic anemia after many years of good health usually, but not always, implies the development of an acquired extracorpuscular process.   (*Res Staff Phys*, 19:24, 1973)

75. **True.** Electrophoresis may reveal an increased concentration of hemoglobin A_2 which is seen in many, but not all, cases of thalassemia.
(*Res Staff Phys*, 19:24, 1973)

76. **True.** Nutritional deficiencies of vitamin B_{12}, folate, or iron can result in the production of erythrocytes of such poor quality that they have shortened survival.
(*Res Staff Phys*, 19:24, 1973)

77. **False.** Compensated hemolysis, where the bone marrow can keep up with increased destruction, is probably more frequent than frank anemia.
(*Res Staff Phys*, 19:24, 1973)

78. **True.** The uncontrovertible diagnosis of the presence of a hemolytic process requires the demonstration of a decreased survival of erythrocytes in the circulation.
(*Res Staff Phys*, 19:24, 1973)

79. **False.** The Burkitt lymphomas respond well to cyclophosphamide.   (1:58)

80. **True.** In the peripheral smear, polychromatophilia suggests reticulocytosis.
(*Postgrad Med*, 47:45, 1970)

81. **True.** Cells which are in extended G_1 phase (or G_0) and do not engage in DNA synthesis are not affected by antileukemic therapy.   (1:56)

82. **True.** The presence of normoblasts suggests hemolysis, but it almost always indicates some type of marrow distress as well, since normoblasts are rarely seen in uncomplicated hemolytic disorders.   (*Postgrad Med*, 47:45, 1970)

83. **False.** There is no evidence that reversible bone marrow suppression and aplastic anemia from chloramphenicol are related.
(*JAMA*, 213:1183, 1970)

84. **False.** Dilantin blocks the absorption of folate.
(*Mod Med*, 41:69, 1973)

85. **True.** The relationship between coagulation and platelets is probably responsible for the characteristic layered structure of arterial thrombi consisting of successive layers of platelets and fibrin. (*Hosp Practice*, 7:115, 1972)

86. **False.** In Hodgkin's disease positive liver biopsies are not found without splenic involvement. (1:57)

87. **True.** Erythrocytes from patients with paroxysmal nocturnal hemoglobinuria hemolyze when incubated in isotonic solutions of low ionic strength provided a small amount of serum is present in the reaction mixture.
(*Blood*, 35:462, 1970)

88. **True.** In hereditary spherocytosis, the osmotic fragility of erythrocytes is usually abnormally increased. (4:1542)

89. **True.** Some of the unstable hemoglobins move normally on routine electrophoresis.
(*Postgrad Med*, 47:45, 1970)

90. **B.** (2:1863)

91. **A.** (2:1863)

Textbook References for Chapter 10

1. American College of Physicians (1974): *Medical Knowledge Self-Assessment, Program III: Recent Developments in Internal Medicine,* Petersdorf, R.G., General Editor, American College of Physicians, Philadelphia.

2. Beeson, P.B. and McDermott, W. (1979): *Cecil Textbook of Medicine*, Fifteenth Edition. W.B. Saunders Company, Philadelphia.

3. Lauler, D.P. et al. (1971): *Gram Negative Sepsis,* Medcom, Clifton, New Jersey.

4. Isselbacher, K.J., Editor (1980): *Harrison's Principles of Internal Medicine*, Ninth Edition, McGraw-Hill Book Company, New York.

CHAPTER 11

Immunology

Directions: Indicate whether each of the following statements is true or false.

1. In allergic subjects, IgE antibodies contribute to the elimination of allergenic materials from the gastrointestinal tract via vomiting and diarrhea, and respiratory tract via coughing.

2. Mucosal surfaces cannot secrete certain immunoglobulins independent of their production in the rest of the body.

3. Atopic individuals with pollen hay fever do not have a significantly greater total peripheral eosinophil count during the pollen season than at other times.

4. In man, there is evidence that cell-mediated reactivity toward renal antigens may accompany the humoral autoantibody response that accounts for the glomerular lesions in anti-glomerular-basement-membrane antibody disease.

5. Most patients with extrinsic asthma have depression of serum levels of immune globulin.

6. Linear, irregular thickening of the glomerular basement membrane may be seen in Type II autoimmune nephritis.

Directions: For the following statements, fill in the blank(s) with the correct answer(s).

7. IgD levels are more than 100 times those of IgE, and Ig__ levels in turn are a 100-fold greater than those of IgD.

8. Fractions __, __, and __ of complement attract polymorphonuclear leukocytes and cause them to release lysosomes, which in turn induce inflammation or necrosis in blood vessels or adjacent structures.

9. Induction of asthma by allergens is related to the presence of IgE antibodies fixed to _____ cells and _____ .

10. Saline isoagglutinin titers of anti-A or anti-B or both are a measure of Ig__ antibodies.

11. Immunotherapy is often considered an attempt to stimulate preferentially the production of blocking antibodies, largely of the Ig__ class. It is believed that these antibodies will compete for _____ and foster its elimination without blocking allergy symptoms.

12. In extrinsic asthma,

 1. washed leukocytes will release histamine when challenged with appropriate allergens
 2. serum will passively sensitize the skin of nonallergic recipients to the offending allergens
 3. lymphocytes demonstrate a blastogenic response to antigen in tissue culture
 4. serum will agglutinate tanned red cells whose surfaces have been coated with antigen

13. Conditions often associated with increased serum IgE include

 1. atopic (extrinsic) asthma and atopic dermatitis
 2. severe food sensitivities and parasitic infestations
 3. hypersensitivity pulmonary aspergillosis
 4. Laennec's cirrhosis

14. Allergic reactions responsible for hypersensitivity diseases of the lungs include

 1. Type I (IgE dependent)
 2. Type II (cytotoxic; tissue specific antibody)
 3. Type III (immune complex disease)
 4. Type IV (cell-mediated, delayed hypersensitivity)

15. T cells

 1. are resistant to irradiation
 2. have a longer life than B cells
 3. are primarily responsible for humoral antibody release
 4. are constantly recirculating through the thoracic duct and systemic circulation

16. Depressed delayed hypersensitivity has been associated with

 1. viral infections
 2. carcinoma
 3. cirrhosis
 4. lymphomas and lymphatic leukemia

17. Which of the following bind(s) complement?

 1. IgG
 2. IgA
 3. IgM
 4. IgD
 5. IgE

18. Secondary acquired hypogammaglobulinemia occurs with

 1. exfoliative dermatitis
 2. renal disorders
 3. gastrointestinal disorders
 4. Hodgkin's disease

19. Nodular deposits of electron-dense proteinaceous material projecting from the epithelial surface of glomerular basement membrane occur in

  A. systemic lupus erythematosus
  B. poststreptococcal glomerulonephritis
  C. both
  D. neither

20. Immune complexes that are formed when there is antibody excess are

    A. apt to be soluble
    B. not removed from the circulation by the reticuloendothelial system
    C. both
    D. neither

21. Associated with humoral antibody deficiency:

    A. trouble with recurrent viral or fungal infections
    B. great susceptibility to hepatitis virus
    C. both
    D. neither

22. Frequently present in patients with hypogammaglobulinemia:

    A. diarrhea
    B. malabsorption
    C. both
    D. neither

23. Commercial gamma globulin contains only trace amounts of

    A. IgA
    B. IgM
    C. both
    D. neither

24. Which of the following is/are true of measurement of thyroid antibodies?

    A. a high titer is useful in the diagnosis of hyperthyroidism due to Hashimoto's disease
    B. it is of limited value in the initial diagnosis of hyperthyroidism as antibodies are also found in a small percentage of normal people as well as in patients with other, nontoxic, thyroid disorders
    C. both
    D. neither

25. In the lungs, Type I allergic reactions begin within minutes of the union of inhaled or circulating antigens and

    A. tissue mast cells located beneath the respiratory mucosa
    B. circulating leukocytes whose surface has been sensitized to these antigens by IgE antibodies
    C. both
    D. neither

Directions: For the following questions, select the ONE INCORRECT answer.

26. Immune complex glomerulonephritis may include

    A. lupus nephritis
    B. nephritis with anaphylactoid purpura
    C. nephritis in periarteritis nodosa
    D. nephritis in idiopathic mixed cryoglobulinemia
    E. Goodpasture's syndrome

27. Regarding idiopathic mixed cryoglobulinemia,

    A. serum contains cryoglobulins composed of IgM and IgG
    B. IgM components possess rheumatoid activity
    C. patients exhibit a characteristic clinical picture with purpura, weakness, arthralgia, and anemia
    D. fatal, diffuse, proliferative glomerulonephritis is associated
    E. there is a distinctive serum electrophoretic pattern

28. Bruton's disease includes the following characteristics:

    A. defective immunoglobulin synthesis
    B. found in boys, inherited as an x-linked recessive characteristic
    C. pyogenic infections frequently occur
    D. anti-A and anti-B isohemagglutinins are low or absent
    E. inability to reject homografts

Directions: Use the key below to answer questions 29 through 37. Select

A. if the disorder listed is a clinical prototype of Type I allergic reaction
B. if the disorder listed is a clinical prototype of Type II allergic reaction
C. if the disorder listed is a clinical prototype of Type III allergic reaction
D. if the disorder listed is a clinical prototype of Type IV allergic reaction

29. Transfusion reaction

30. Tuberculin reaction

31. Hemolytic anemia

32. Anaphylaxis

33. Delayed serum sickness

34. Acute nephritis

35. Graft rejection

36. Asthma

37. Arthus reaction

Directions: Use the key below to answer the following question.

A. if both the statement and reason are true and are related as to cause and effect
B. if both the statement and reason are true, but are not related as to cause and effect
C. if the statement is true, but the reason is false
D. if the statement is false, but the reason is true
E. if both the statement and reason are false

38. Allergic symptoms occur commonly in the respiratory tract because mast cells are abundant beneath the respiratory mucosa, where they may come in contact with inhaled antigens.

Directions: For each of the incomplete statements below, ONE or MORE of the completions given is correct. In each case, select

A. if 1, 2, and 3 are correct
B. if 1 and 3 are correct
C. if 2 and 4 are correct
D. if only 4 is correct
E. if all statements are correct

39. Tuberculin sensitivity, which may endure for many months, may be conferred upon a nonsensitive recipient by

1. blood transfusions
2. injection of leukocytes
3. injection of leukocyte extracts
4. injection of transfer factor

40. Regarding immune complex glomerular disease,

1. histologic forms may include acute proliferative disease or chronic disease with membranous, proliferative, or sclerosing features
2. all forms are characterized to some extent by accumulation of immunoglobulins, complement components, and antigen within glomeruli, as seen by immunofluorescence
3. although a number of patterns of staining are seen, the accumulation is always granular or irregular
4. may be associated with bacterial infections (streptococcal and pneumococcal), bacterial endocarditis, secondary syphilis, and malaria

41. Delayed hypersensitivity

1. was the first immune reaction to be identified by a specific test (the tuberculin test)
2. is the least understood of the four main types of immune reactions
3. probably occurs during the course of all infections
4. the characteristic lesion in a reaction is composed of mononuclear cells often located near venules

42. Arthus reaction

    1. takes 2 to 8 hours to begin
    2. lasts 12 to 24 hours
    3. occurs in walls of small blood vessels as a result of antibody from the circulation meeting antigen diffusing inward from the extravascular space
    4. has a gross appearance of hemorrhage and edema with a polymorphonuclear infiltrate, microscopically

43. Histamine is found in

    1. tissue mast cells
    2. basophils
    3. circulating leukocytes
    4. platelets

44. Mediators of cytotoxic (Type II) allergic reactions include

    1. histamine and slow reacting substance of anaphylaxis
    2. sensitized lymphocytes
    3. antigen plus antibodies (IgG and IgM) and, at times, complement
    4. circulating tissue-specific antibodies in high titer

45. A group of patients with selective IgA deficiency followed for a long period have been found to have a greater incidence of autoimmune disease, especially

    1. rheumatoid arthritis
    2. systemic lupus erythematosus
    3. thyroiditis
    4. pernicious anemia

Directions: Use the key below to answer questions 46 through 49.
   A. **if the reaction listed is a Type I allergic reaction**
   B. **if the reaction listed is a Type II allergic reaction**
   C. **if the reaction listed is a Type III allergic reaction**
   D. **if the reaction listed is a Type IV allergic reaction**

46. Delayed hypersensitivity (cell-mediated)

47. Cytotoxic tissue-specific antibody

48. Immediate (IgE-dependent)

49. Delayed (immune complex disease)

Directions: For the following multiple-choice questions, select the ONE CORRECT answer.

50. About what percentage of the population shows evidence of clinical allergy during life?

    A. 3 to 5%
    B. 10 to 15%
    C. 25 to 30%
    D. 40 to 50%
    E. 70 to 80%

51. Which of the following has the longest half-life?

    A. IgG
    B. IgA
    C. IgM
    D. IgD
    E. IgE

Directions: Indicate whether each of the following statements is true or false.

52. The anergy of miliary tuberculosis has been thought to be due to extreme antigen excess, which may bind all available lymphocyte receptors, preventing interaction with intradermal antigen.

53. If the thymus is removed in animals in early neonatal life, this will enable development of cellular immunity.

54. Acute systemic atopic antigen-antibody reactions have an initial eosinopenic phase.

Answers and Commentary

1. **True.** In allergic subjects, IgE antibodies contribute to the elimination of allergenic materials from the gastrointestinal tract via vomiting and diarrhea, and respiratory tract via coughing. (*Ann Intern Med*, 78:401, 1973)

2. **False.** Mucosal surfaces can secrete certain immunoglobulins independent of their production in the rest of the body. (*Ann Intern Med*, 78:401, 1973)

3. **False.** Atopic individuals with pollen hay fever have a significantly higher total peripheral eosinophil count during the pollen season than at other times. (*J Allergy*, 49:142, 1972)

4. **True.** In man, there is evidence that cell-mediated reactivity toward renal antigens may accompany the humoral autoantibody response that accounts for the glomerular lesions in anti-glomerular-basement-membrane antibody disease. (*N Engl J Med*, 288:564, 1973)

5. **False.** Most patients with extrinsic asthma have elevation of serum levels of immune globulin. (*N Engl J Med*, 286:1166, 1972)

6. **True.** Linear, irregular thickening of the glomerular basement membrane may be seen in Type II autoimmune nephritis. (*N Engl J Med*, 286:1166, 1972)

7. **A.** IgD levels are more than 100 times those of IgE, and IgA levels in turn are a 100-fold greater than those of IgD. (*Ann Intern Med*, 78:401, 1973)

8. **5, 6, 7.** Fractions 5, 6, and 7 of complement attract polymorphonuclear leukocytes and cause them to release lysosomes, which in turn induce

inflammation or necrosis in blood vessels or adjacent structures. (*N Engl J Med*, 286:1166, 1972)

9. **Mast, Basophils.** Induction of asthma by allergens is related to the presence of IgE antibodies fixed to mast cells and basophils. (*Ann Intern Med*, 78:405, 1973)

10. **M.** Saline isoagglutinin titers of anti-A or anti-B or both are a measure of IgM antibodies. (*Lahey Clinic Found Bull*, 22:68, 1973)

11. **G, Antigen.** Immunotherapy is often considered an attempt to stimulate preferentially the production of blocking antibodies, largely of the IgG class. It is believed that these antibodies will compete for antigen and foster its elimination without producing allergy symptoms. (*Ann Intern Med*, 78:401, 1973)

12. **D.** All the statements are true of extrinsic asthma. (*N Engl J Med*, 286:1166, 1972)

13. **D.** All the conditions listed are often associated with increased serum IgE. Additionally, the Wiscott-Aldrich syndrome and nephrotic syndrome are associated with increased serum IgE. (*Ann Intern Med*, 78:401, 1973)

14. **D.** Allergic reactions responsible for hypersensitivity diseases of the lungs include all the reactions listed. (*N Engl J Med*, 286:1166, 1972)

15. **C.** T cells are susceptible to irradiation. T cells are involved in cellular immunity, and lymphocytes believed to be independent of thymus control (B cells) are primarily responsible for humoral antibody release. All other statements are correct. (*Lahey Clinic Found Bull*, 22:68, 1973)

16. **D.** Depressed delayed hypersensitivity has been associated with all the disorders listed, as well as with bacterial infections.
(*Int Arch All Appl Immunol*, 42:583, 1972; *Ann Intern Med*, 56:323, 1974)

17. **B.** Only IgG and IgM bind complement.
(*Lahey Clinic Found Bull*, 22:68, 1973)

18. **D.** Secondary acquired hypogammaglobulinemia occurs in all the diseases listed, as well as in chronic lymphatic leukemia and lymphosarcoma. (*Lahey Clinic Found Bull*, 22:68, 1973)

19. **C.** Nodular deposits of electron-dense proteinaceous material projecting from the epithelial surface of glomerular basement membrane occur in systemic lupus erythematosus and poststreptococcal glomerulonephritis.
(*N Engl J Med*, 286:1166, 1972)

20. **C.** Immune complexes formed when there is antibody excess are apt to be soluble. These complexes are not removed from the circulation by the reticuloendothelial system.
(*N Engl J Med*, 286:1166, 1972)

21. **B.** There is no trouble with recurrent viral or fungal infections but one is very susceptible to hepatitis virus with humoral antibody deficiency.
(*Lahey Clinic Found Bull*, 22:68, 1973)

22. **C.** Both diarrhea and malabsorption are frequently present in patients with hypogammaglobulinemia. (*New Physician*, 21:280, 1972)

23. **C.** Commercial gamma globulin contains only trace amounts of IgA and IgM and is made from a pool of donor plasmas so that antibodies to many infectious agents will be present in adequate titer. (*Lahey Clinic Found Bull*, 22:68, 1973)

24. **C.** Both statements are true of the measurement of thyroid antibodies.
(*Br Med J*, 2:5809:337, 1972)

25. **C.** In the lungs, Type I allergic reactions begin within minutes of the union of inhaled or circulating antigens and tissue mast cells located beneath the respiratory mucosa or circulating leukocytes whose surface has been sensitized to these antigens by IgE antibodies.
(*N Engl J Med*, 286:1166, 1972)

26. **E.** `All the disorders listed except Goodpasture's syndrome are classified under immune-complex glomerulonephritis. Also included are membraneous and membranoproliferative glomerulonephritis and IgA-IgG nephropathy (Berger).
(*N Engl J Med*, 288:564, 1973)

27. **E.** There is no distinctive serum electrophoretic pattern in patients with idiopathic mixed cryogobulinemia. All other statements are true.
(*N Engl J Med*, 288:564, 1973)

28. **E.** In Bruton's disease, the ability to reject homografts is maintained. All other statements are true. In addition, disabling collagen disorders are found in high frequency.
(*Lahey Clinic Found Bull*, 22:68, 1973)

29. **B.** (*Curr Med Digest*, 39:1117, 1972)

30. **D.** (*Curr Med Digest*, 39:1117, 1972)

31. **B.** (*Curr Med Digest*, 39:1117, 1972)

32. **A.** (*Curr Med Digest*, 39:1117, 1972)

33. **C.** (*Curr Med Digest*, 39:1117, 1972)

34. **B.** (*Curr Med Digest*, 39:1117, 1972)

35. **D.** (*Curr Med Digest*, 39:1117, 1972)

36. **A.** (*Curr Med Digest*, 39:1117, 1972)

37. **C.** (*Curr Med Digest*, 39:1117, 1972)

38. **A.** Allergic symptoms occur commonly in the respiratory tract because mast cells are abundant beneath the respiratory mucosa, where they may come in contact with inhaled antigens.
(*N Engl J Med*, 286:1166, 1972)

39. **E.** Tuberculin sensitivity, which may endure for many months, may be conferred upon a nonsensitive recipient by blood transfusions or injections of leukocytes, leukocyte extracts, or transfer factor. (*N Engl J Med*, 286:1166, 1972)

40. **E.** All statements are true of immune complex glomerular disease.(*N Engl J Med*, 288:564, 1973)

41. **E.** All statements are true of delayed hypersensitivity. (*N Engl J Med*, 286:1166, 1972)

42. **E.** All statements are true of the arthus reaction. (*Lahey Clinic Found Bull*, 22:68, 1973)

43. **E.** Histamine is found in tissue mast cells, basophils, circulating leukocytes, and platelets.
(*N Engl J Med*, 286:1166, 1972)

44. **D.** Circulating tissue-specific antibodies in high titer are the only mediators of cytotoxic (Type II) allergic reactions.
(*Curr Med Digest*, 39:1117, 1972)

45. **E.** A group of patients with selective IgA deficiency followed for a long period were shown to have a greater incidence of autoimmune disease, especially rheumatoid arthritis, systemic lupus erythematosus, thyroiditis, and pernicious anemia. Many of these patients had recurrent sinus and upper respiratory tract infections.
(*Lahey Clinic Found Bull*, 22:68, 1973)

46. **D.**   (*Curr Med Digest*, 39:1117, 1972)

47. **B.**   (*Curr Med Digest*, 39:1117, 1972)

48. **A.**   (*Curr Med Digest*, 39:1117, 1972)

49. **C.**   (*Curr Med Digest*, 39:1117, 1972)

50. **C.** About 25 to 30% of the population shows evidence of clinical allergy during life.
(*Ann Intern Med*, 78:401, 1973)

51. **A.** IgG has the longest half-life.
(*Lahey Clinic Found Bull*, 22:68, 1973)

52. **True.** The anergy of miliary tuberculosis has been thought to be due to extreme antigen excess which may bind all available lymphocyte receptors, preventing interaction with intradermal antigen.   (*Am J Med*, 56:323, 1974)

53. **False.** If the thymus is removed in animals in early neonatal life, this will not enable development of cellular immunity.
(*Lahey Clinic Found Bull*, 22:68, 1973)

54. **True.** Acute systemic atopic antigen-antibody reactions have an initial eosinopenic phase.
(*J Allergy*, 49:142, 1972)

CHAPTER 12

Infectious Diseases

Directions: For each of the following multiple-choice questions, select the ONE CORRECT answer.

1. Of common helminth infections, which of the following has the highest world incidence?

    A. *Schistosoma mansoni*
    B. *Diphyllobothrium latum*
    C. *Taenia saginata*
    D. *Ascaris lumbricoides*
    E. *Trichinella spiralis*

2. Every gram of carbenicillin contains

    A. 1 mEq sodium
    B. 2.5 mEq sodium
    C. 4.5 mEq sodium
    D. 8.5 mEq sodium
    E. 12.5 mEq sodium

3. The fatality rate of gram-negative bacteremia is about

    A. below 1%
    B. 5%
    C. 20 to 50%
    D. 70%
    E. 90%

4. After gram-negative sepsis is controlled, antibiotics should be continued for

    A. 1 to 3 days
    B. 4 to 6 days
    C. 7 to 10 days
    D. 14 to 21 days
    E. 2 months

5. The earliest nervous system manifestation of diphtherial polyneuropathy is usually

    A. paralysis of accommodation
    B. paralysis of the palate
    C. generalized polyneuritis
    D. none of the above

6. Most drug resistance of gram-negative bacteria has been shown to be due to

    A. transformation (DNA from one organism is induced into another organism)
    B. transduction (a bacteriophage carries into an organism the code to produce resistance)
    C. conjugation or sexual recombination
    D. A. and B.
    E. none of the above

Directions: For each of the following multiple-choice questions, select the ONE INCORRECT answer.

7. Predominantly renal excretion is associated with

    A. penicillin G
    B. cephalothin

C. chloramphenicol
D. nalidixic acid
E. isoniazid

8. The combination of trimethoprim (80 mg) and sulfamethoxazole (400 mg)

A. has been found effective in infections of the skin and soft tissues, septicemias, acute and subacute bacterial endocarditis, enteric fever, brucellosis, prostatitis, and gonorrhea
B. penetrates particularly efficiently into the central nervous system in synergistic concentrations
C. clinically has had low emergence of strains resistant to it, and cross-resistance between the combination and other anti-infective agents has not been reported
D. is rapidly and almost completely absorbed following oral administration and peak plasma levels are achieved in 2 to 4 hours
E. may be maintained in effective concentrations for 6 to 8 hours following a single dose

9. Mechanism of action by inhibition of protein synthesis is characteristic of

A. amphotericin B
B. chloramphenicol
C. clindamycin
D. erythromycin
E. gentamicin

10. Regarding *Mycoplasma pneumoniae* infections,

A. they are most often nasopharyngeal or respiratory
B. they may be associated with bullous myringitis
C. antibodies and immunity develop concurrently
D. immunization with inactivated vaccines is fully effective
E. immunity persists for years

11. Cytomegalovirus mononucleosis is characterized by

A. marked tonsillopharyngeal involvement
B. minimal or no lymphadenopathy
C. slow rising cytomegalovirus complement fixation antibody titers with maximal levels achieved some 6 weeks after onset
D. acute febrile illness
E. abnormal liver function tests common

12. Regarding involvement of the nervous system in infectious mononucleosis,

A. generally accepted incidence is around 20%
B. neurological manifestations may be the presenting, or indeed the only clinical feature of the disease
C. the more common neurologic complications include lymphocytic meningitis, encephalomyelitis, polyneuritis, and mononeuritis
D. ophthalmoplegia, optic neuritis, and facial palsy have been described
E. the disease may present as an acute cerebellar syndrome

13. In infectious mononucleosis,

A. restriction of physical activity should be maintained until the acute febrile phase is well over, until splenic enlargement or tenderness has been absent for at least a week, and until the patient feels energetic enough to participate in sports
B. the return to activity should be gradual, over a couple of weeks
C. the major concern in early resumption of play activity is possible rupture of the spleen from abdominal trauma
D. the Paul-Bunnell test, the degree of lymphocytosis, and abnormal results from tests for levels of serum enzymes (SGOT and LDH) are useful as a guide for restriction of physical activity
E. if actual jaundice is present, which occurs in about 5% of cases, activity

should be restricted until the serum bilirubin value has returned to normal

14.   For infection with atypical mycobacteria,

A.   do not isolate patients, though it must be presumed that the infection is typical until cultures prove otherwise
B.   treatment may be given in the physician's office and hospitalization is advised only for complications
C.   a successful outcome occurs in less than 50% of infections with atypical mycobacteria
D.   the patient may be advised to continue work and to remain active

15.   In acute epiglottitis,

A.   total airway obstruction may occur
B.   published studies indicate a mortality of greater than 50%
C.   the main organism that is involved is *Hemophilus influenzae*, which may be demonstrated either by pharyngeal or blood culture
D.   steroids are contraindicated
E.   tentative diagnosis is made by laryngoscopy and confirmed by a lateral soft tissue x-ray of the neck

16.   Regarding endotoxins,

A.   they are found only within the cell wall
B.   they are excreted only during the cell's death and autolysis
C.   molecular biology has definitely implicated lipid A as the major toxic component
D.   most adult animals and many newborns have antibodies to some determinant within the endotoxin molecule
E.   a primary toxicity does not occur independent of hypersensitivity reactions

17.   Carbenicillin

A.   has shown *in vitro* effectiveness against nonpenicillinase-producing *Staphylococcus albus, Staphylococcus aureus*, and several other gram-positive organisms
B.   when heated degenerates into penicillin G and carbon dioxide
C.   does not induce spheroplast formation in *Pseudomonas aeruginosa*
D.   may be given in high doses to patients with a normal creatinine clearance, regardless of their hepatic function
E.   in large doses is accompanied by a heavy sodium load (108 mg/g)

18.   R factor bacteria

A.   are resistant to high levels of antibiotics
B.   because resistance is due to enzymes which inactivate the antibiotics, as the number of bacteria increases, so does the resistance
C.   like mutants, usually do not grow as well as nonresistant bacteria
D.   may synthesize a penicillinase (beta-lactamhydrolase) active against penicillins and cephalosporins
E.   may inactivate tetracycline and sulfonamides by changes in the permeability of the bacterial cell wall which prevent the antibiotics from entering the cell

Directions: For each of the incomplete statements below, ONE or MORE of the completions given is correct. In each case, select

A.   **if 1, 2, and 3 are correct**
B.   **if 1 and 3 are correct**
C.   **if 2 and 4 are correct**
D.   **if only 4 is correct**
E.   **if all are correct**

19.   In acute pyelonephritis,

1.   the patient may be extremely ill
2.   there is tenderness to deep palpation or percussion in the costovertebral angle, and the entire flank region may be tender
3.   when the peritoneum overlying the kidneys is affected by the inflammatory reaction, signs of peritonitis are present

with abdominal distention, muscle spasm, rebound tenderness, and hypoactive bowel sounds
4. fever is seldom present

20. Early cases of gram-negative septicemia typically have

1. hyperventilation and respiratory alkalosis
2. high cardiac index
3. a response to therapy with higher cardiac indices
4. high peripheral vascular resistance

21. In infectious endocarditis,

1. 80% of the bacterially induced disease is subacute and has an insidious onset and, untreated, has a 100% mortality
2. the organisms most likely to be involved in orally engendered endocarditis are the viridans streptococci, against which penicillin is the drug of choice
3. enterococci are most often involved in endocarditis following surgery or instrumentation of either the GU or GI tract and an aminoglycoside plus penicillin are usually effective prophylactically
4. subacute bacterial endocarditis often occurs in previously healthy hearts

22. Regarding chronic granulomatous disease of childhood,

1. it usually affects young females
2. it is a recurrent infection with streptococci
3. PMN from these patients are unable to ingest bacteria normally
4. recurrent infection occurs with gram-negative enteric bacteria and staphylococci

23. Advantages of carbenicillin over ampicillin include

1. significantly more active against indole-positive *Proteus* species
2. bactericidal against most strains of *P. aeruginosa*
3. frequently has a synergistic effect with gentamicin sulfate against *P. aeruginosa*
4. inexpensive

24. Atypical mycobacteria

1. account for only 5% of acid-fast infections
2. skin infections, which rarely disseminate, come from direct inoculation of the skin with strains such as *M. marinum*—swimming pool or fish tank granuloma
3. may be ingested by children, and a subclinical infection gives rise to nonspecific tuberculin hypersensitivity which is very common in children in the southeastern United States, where *M. intracellulare* is prevalent
4. can be transmitted from one person to another

25. Defects in both humoral and cellular immunity occur with

1. chronic lymphocytic leukemia
2. lymphosarcoma
3. "Swiss type" agammaglobulinemia
4. Hodgkin's disease

26. Regarding infectious mononucleosis,

1. it spreads readily by ordinary contact
2. households frequently have multiple cases
3. heterophil-negative patients with EBV-associated infectious mononucleosis are mainly adults
4. the causative agent appears to be one that spreads early in life especially under low socioeconomic conditions, when the infection might not lead to a characteristic disease but might leave permanent immunity

27. Candidiasis may be seen in

1. Addison's disease
2. diabetes mellitus
3. hypoparathyroidism
4. Hashimoto's disease

28. Renal causes of hypertension include

1. acute and chronic glomerulonephritis
2. pyelonephritis
3. diabetic kidney
4. polyarteritis nodosa

29. Regarding 5-fluorocytosine,

    1. cerebrospinal fluid levels are approximately two-thirds of serum levels
    2. it is not effective orally
    3. *Candida neoformans* and *Candida albicans* are uniformly susceptible
    4. antifungal activity is less restricted than amphotericin B

30. Regarding Pseudomonas pneumonias,

    1. the victim usually harbors an underlying disease, is debilitated, and has been subjected to the use of respiratory equipment or manipulation
    2. symptoms are severe dyspnea and copious sputum
    3. fever is not usually in proportion to the amount of pulmonary involvement and ranges from 101° to 105° F
    4. chills are common

31. Defects in humoral immunity

    1. occur in sex-linked congenital agammaglobulinemia
    2. occur in multiple myeloma
    3. usually involve initial infection of the patient with organisms such as *Diplococcus pneumoniae* and *Haemophilus influenzae*
    4. usually allow preservation of type-specific opsonizing antibody

32. Delayed hypersensitivity is an important factor in the development of immunity to

    1. certain viruses (vaccinia, varicella, mumps, and lymphogranuloma)
    2. some bacteria (brucella and possibly tuberculosis)
    3. most fungi
    4. most parasites

33. Indications for the use of chloramphenicol include

    1. typhoid fever or other Salmonella infections
    2. an alternative drug for ampicillin in *Hemophilus influenzae,* pneumococcal, and meningococcal meningitis
    3. severe anaerobic infections for which clindamycin is not effective
    4. gram-negative bacillary infections that do not respond to other antimicrobial agents

34. In perinephric abscess,

    1. there is often a low-grade or septic elevation in temperature
    2. there is frequently a bulging mass in the flank
    3. edema of the skin over the abscess may occur
    4. the affected side is seldom tender

35. *Giardia lamblia*

    1. can cause diarrhea and/or malabsorption
    2. may be found in patients with lymphoid nodular hyperplasia and associated immunoglobulin deficiency
    3. diagnosis is confirmed by small bowel biopsy and duodenal aspiration and demonstration of trophozoites
    4. patients with protracted diarrhea respond promptly to quinacrine hydrochloride or metronidazole

36. Pyrantel pamoate is useful against which of the following intestinal nematode(s)?

    1. *Ascaris lumbricoides* (roundworm)
    2. *Enterobius vermicularis* (pinworm)
    3. *Necator americanus* (hookworm)
    4. *Ancylostoma duodenale* (hookworm)

37. A mononuclear pleocytosis may occur in

    1. neurosyphilis
    2. tuberculous meningitis
    3. multiple sclerosis during acute exacerbations
    4. cerebral abscess and subarachnoid hemorrhage

Directions: Use the key below to answer questions 38 to 41. Select
  A. if the statement describes intermittent fever
  B. if the statement describes remittent fever
  C. if the statement describes continuous fever
  D. if the statement describes relapsing fever

38. Diurnal fluctuations occur but normal levels are never attained

39. There is a return to normal or subnormal levels one or more times daily

40. Only minor variations are recorded

41. Periods of fever for several days' duration are punctuated by spontaneous periods of normal temperature

Directions: Use the key below to answer questions 42 through 46. Select
  A. if the statement is characteristic of M. tuberculosis
  B. if the statement is characteristic of atypical mycobacteria

42. Guinea pig inoculation is fatal

43. Grows slowly in culture

44. Does not produce niacin

45. May produce a pigmented colony

46. Forms colonies of a creamy buff color

Directions: Use the key below to answer questions 47 and 48. Select
  A. if the disease is transmitted by the mite
  B. if the disease if transmitted by the tick

47. Rocky Mountain spotted fever

48. Scrub typhus

Directions: Indicate whether each of the following statements is true or false.

49. Foul or putrid odor of discharges is a major clue to anaerobic infection and is invariably present.

50. In chronic syphilitic meningitis and other forms of late syphilis, particularly tabes dorsalis, the pupils are usually small, irregular, and unequal.

51. Resistance to most antibiotics is widespread among members of the Enterobacteriaceae: *E. coli,* klebsiella, proteus, enterobacter, and serratia.

52. Surgical drainage is frequently required in amebic liver abscess.

53. Most strains of Pseudomonas isolated in the United States produce a penicillinase with a specific affinity for carbenicillin.

54. While the polymyxins are quite active against Pseudomonas *in vitro*, they have proven to be only minimally effective *in vivo*.

55. Anaerobes associated with pleuropulmonary disease usually are derived from the oropharynx.

56. There is considerable difference in the bacterial flora found during acute exacerbations and that noted during stable stages of chronic bronchitis.

57. Many of the strains of Bacteroides that are resistant to chloramphenicol are sensitive to tetracycline.

58. With *Pneumocystis carinii* infection, open-lung biopsy with impression or touch smears of the cut fresh specimen which can be stained with methenamine silver offers the best opportunity for a diagnosis.

59. Anterior cervical node enlargement is characteristic of clinical toxoplasmosis in adults.

60. In the absence of urinary obstruction, the radiographic changes of pyelonephritis in adults are usually the residua of childhood infection.

61. The most important site of antibiotic drug inactivation is the kidney.

62. *Streptococcus viridans* is usually the organism responsible for acute infective endocarditis.

63. Vancomycin is an unacceptable substitute for patients allergic to penicillin in the treatment of enterococcal endocarditis.

64. The epidemiology of infectious mononucleosis resembles that of several other viral diseases such as polio; in lower socioeconomic groups where EBV antibodies appear early in life, there is little clinical infectious mononucleosis.

65. The doses of penicillin recommended for gonorrhea will cure incubating syphilis whereas the tetracycline and spectinomycin regimens may be ineffective.

66. Patients sensitive to penicillin generally do not have allergic reactions to cephalothin; when they do, it is probably not a true cross-reaction but a manifestation of hyperreactive sensitivity in a very allergic individual.

67. Hepatitis B infection is of importance in a significant number of patients with chronic active hepatitis.

68. Production of IgA and IgE is linked; absence of either may be associated with sinopulmonary infections.

69. Renal failure is a common complication of urinary tract infection, even in the absence of anatomic abnormalities.

70. In patients with acid urine, sulfonamides are known to form microcrystalline deposits and result in obstruction or hematuria.

71. Courses of amphotericin B of less than 5 g total dose do not produce significant residual changes in renal function.

72. Bacteremias caused by *E. coli* are acquired in the hospital slightly more often than in the community.

73. Septic thrombophlebitis and abscess formation are common features of anaerobic infection and account for the chronicity of these infections, their refractoriness to therapy, and the tendency for relapse.

74. About 5 to 8% of patients meeting the criteria for fever of obscure origin appear to recover completely without ever having a diagnosis established.

75. The frequency of resistant enteric bacteria is much less in "highly civilized" countries than in less developed nations.

76. When daily gentamicin is given intrathecally, cerebrospinal fluid antibacterial activity can be achieved and maintained.

77. Antibiotics are the treatment of choice for salmonella gastroenteritis.

78. Pseudomonas may be present in sputum cultures as part of the residual flora after treatment with other antibiotics and not be pathogenic.

79. Drugs which markedly reduce the meningococcal carrier state will abort an epidemic of meningococcal disease.

80. The most frequent source of gram-negative bacteremia is the gastrointestinal tract.

81. Recent studies of host responses to endotoxin suggest that the pathophysiology of gram-negative bacteremia is best explained as a result of the influences of the complement, kinin, and coagulation systems on the function of the microcirculation.

82. Antibiotic treatment does not prolong the excretion rate of viable Salmonella bacilli in uncomplicated gastroenteritis.

83. The phagocytic function of the reticuloendothelial system is compromised in sickle cell disease.

84. Tetracycline is a poor choice for the empirical treatment of pulmonary infections because 5 to 10% of *D. pneumoniae*, 30 to 40% of group A Streptococci, and many strains of *S. aureus* are resistant to this antibiotic.

85. Syphilitic aortitis is common in all forms of neurosyphilis.

86. Chloramphenicol does not penetrate cerebral spinal fluid very well.

87. A majority of those infected with *Treponema pallidum* subsequently show evidence that the organism has invaded the nervous system.

88. Preexisting valve damage is usually present in acute infective endocarditis.

89. Cephalothin is adequate in the treatment of meningococcal meningitis.

90. Polymyxins directly damage the bacterial cell membrane of many gram-negative bacilli; essential cell constituents then leak out and the cell dies.

91. The cerebrospinal fluid and nervous tissue levels of clindamycin are good.

92. Even when patients are operated upon within 48 hours of the onset of acute cholecystitis, bacteria are usually grown from the bile.

Directions: For each of the following statements, fill in the blank.

93. Relapses of upper urinary tract infection in males are usually related to chronic _____ .

94. When a combination of two antibiotics is at least four times as effective as either one alone, they are considered to have a(n) _____ effect.

95. Anterior perforation of the nasal septum occurs with tuberculosis, while posterior perforation is more common with _____ .

Answers and Commentary

1. **D.** It has been estimated that approximately 25% of the world's population is infected with *Ascaris lumbricoides*. (3:626)

2. **C.** Every gram of carbenicillin contains 4.5 mEq sodium. (*Emerg Med*, 5:71, 1973)

3. **C.** The fatality of gram-negative bacteremia ranges from 20 to 50%. Assuming an average fatality rate midway between these values, as many as 84,000 deaths per year may result from gram-negative bacteremia. (5:18)

4. **C.** Antibiotics should always be continued for 7 to 10 days after the septicemia has been controlled. (5:96)

5. **B.** Paralysis of the palate, usually the earliest nervous system manifestation of diphtherial polyneuropathy, develops during the third or fourth week after infection. (2:373)

6. **C.** Most drug resistance of gram-negative bacteria has been shown to be due to conjugation. (5:26)

7. **C.** Chloramphenicol is mainly excreted or metabolized by nonrenal routes. It must be given in normal dosage for therapeutic effect. With the other antibiotics listed, some dosage reduction is desirable from the start. Normal sized doses should be spaced more widely than usual, but not more than 24 hours apart. In addition, cephaloridine, lincomycin, clindamycin, cotrimoxazole, ethambutol, and rifampicin are also predominantly excreted by renal mechanisms. (3:562)

8. **B.** Penetration of the combination of trimethoprim and sulfamethoxazole into the central nervous system in synergistic concentrations is not particularly efficient. (*JAMA*, 231:635, 1974)

9. **A.** Mechanism of action of amphotericin B is by interaction with sterols of cell membrane. The other antibiotics listed interfere with protein synthesis. Other antibiotics which interfere with protein synthesis include lincomycin, kanamycin, and tetracyclines. (3:556)

10. **D.** Immunization with inactivated vaccines is only partially effective against *Mycoplasma pneumoniae* infections. All other statements are correct. (1:67)

11. **A.** In one study, five patients with cytomegalovirus mononucleosis were compatible hematologically with infectious mononucleosis but lacked the tonsillopharyngeal involvement of that entity. All other statements are true of this disorder.

12. **A.** Involvement of the nervous system in infectious mononucleosis is rare, with a generally accepted incidence of around 1%. All other statements are correct. (*Lancet 2*, 7831:707, 1973)

13. **D.** The Paul-Bunnell test, the degree of lymphocytosis, and abnormal results from tests for levels of serum enzymes (SGOT and LDH) are not useful guides for restriction of physical activity in patients with infectious mononucleosis. All other statements are correct. (*JAMA*, 229:847, 1974)

14. **C.** A successful outcome in the treatment of atypical mycobacteria infection may be expected in 80 to 90% of cases. All other statements are correct. (*Res-Int Consult*, 2:22, 1973)

15. **D.** In severe, early epiglottitis, a single pharmacologic dose of 500 to 1000 mg hydrocortisone may be given. Steroids are not felt to be indicated beyond the first 24 hours, however. All other statements are correct. Ampicillin is the drug of choice. (*Emerg Med*, 5:235, 1973)

16. **E.** There is a primary toxicity independent of hypersensitivity reactions. All other statements are true of endotoxins. (5:40, 43, 44)

17. **C.** Carbenicillin induces spheroplast formation in *Pseudomonas aeruginosa* as early as 90 min after initial exposure to the drug. All other statements are true of carbenicillin. (5:73, 75, 77, 79, 88)

18. **C.** R factor bacteria, unlike mutants, are resistant bacteria which usually grow as well as nonresistant bacteria. All other statements are true of R factor bacteria. They have enzymes located at the surface of the bacterial cell that inactivate antibiotics. Thus they can destroy the antimicrobial agents before they can even enter the bacteria (5:27)

19. **A.** Acute pyelonephritis usually produces fever. All other statements are true. (4:247)

20. **A.** Patients with hyperventilation and respiratory alkalosis, high cardiac index, and low peripheral vascular resistance typify early cases of gram-negative sepsis. With therapy, these patients generally respond with higher cardiac indices, and their prognosis is good. (5:56)

21. **A.** Unlike the subacute variety, acute bacterial endocarditis often occurs in previously healthy hearts. All other statements are true. (*Emerg Med*, 5:128, 1973)

22. **D.** Patients with chronic granulomatous disease of childhood are usually young males who suffer from recurrent infection with gram-negative enteric organisms and staphylococci. PMN from these patients are able to ingest bacteria normally, but do not show normal postphagocytic metabolic alterations. Abnormal amounts of hydrogen peroxide are produced. (1:62)

23. **A.** The chief disadvantage of disodium carbenicillin is its high cost. All other statements are true. (*Hosp Physician*, 9:20, 1973)

24. **A.** Atypical mycobacteria are not transmitted from one person to another. All other statements are true. (*Res-Int Consult*, 2:22, 1973)

25. **A.** Some diseases are associated with defects in both humoral and cellular immunity. Examples include chronic lymphocytic leukemia and lymphosarcoma in adults; the "Swiss type" of agammaglobulinemia is an example of an inheritable form of combined immunodeficiency appearing in childhood. The importance of a competent cellular immune system is seen in infants with thymic dysgenesis or in adults with Hodgkin's disease or sarcoidosis. (1:62)

26. **D.** Infectious mononucleosis does not spread readily by ordinary contact, and households infrequently have multiple cases. Heterophil-negative patients with EBV-associated infectious mononucleosis are mainly children. The causative agent appears to be one that spreads early in life, especially under low socioeconomic conditions when the infection might not lead to a characteristic disease but might leave permanent immunity. (*Hosp Prac*, 5:33, 1970)

27. **E.** Candidiasis may be seen in any of the disorders listed as well as pernicious anemia. (*Postgrad Med*, 55:62, 1974)

28. **E.** Practically all renal diseases known have been associated with hypertension. Important examples are acute and chronic glomerulonephritis, pyelonephritis, diabetic kidney, polyarteritis nodosa, and polycystic disease. Hemangiopericytoma (renin-producing tumor) is also known to produce hypertension. (3:1210)

29. **B.** 5-fluorocytosine is effective orally; cerebrospinal fluid levels approximate two-thirds of serum levels. Its activity is more restricted than amphotericin B. *Candida neoformans* and *Candida albicans* are uniformly susceptible. (1:57)

30. **A.** In Pseudomonas pneumonias, chills are rare. In addition, there is little correlation between bacteriologic and clinical course. All other statements are true. (5:82)

31. **A.** Patients with defects in humoral immunity, e.g., sex-linked congenital agammaglobulinemia and multiple myeloma, are infected initially with organisms such as *Diplococcus pneumoniae* and *Haemophilus influenzae*, immunity being dependent upon the presence of type-specific opsonizing antibody. (1:62)

32. **E.** Delayed hypersensitivity is an important factor in the development of immunity to certain viruses (vaccinia, varicella, mumps, and lymphogranuloma), some bacteria (brucella and possibly tuberculosis), and most fungi and parasites. (*N Engl J Med*, 286:1166, 1972)

33. **E.** Chloramphenicol has a broad spectrum of activity against the rickettsiae, gram-positive bacteria, gram-negative bacteria including Salmonella and Shigella, and anaerobic bacteria. The drug is well absorbed from the gastrointestinal tract. It is metabolized by the liver and can therefore be used in patients with renal insufficiency. Adequate levels in the cerebrospinal fluid are present after intravenous injection. Chloramphenicol causes bone marrow aplasia and fatal pancytopenia in one of every 40,000 or more courses of therapy or in one of every 25,000 to 50,000 people exposed. This severe toxic reaction is a form of hypersensitivity or idiosyncratic reaction which cannot be predicted before therapy. For this reason, chloramphenicol should be used only for certain specific, severe infections. These indications include all of those listed as well as severe rickettsial infections when tetracycline is not effective. (3:562)

34. **A.** Perinephric abscess may be associated with a low-grade or septic elevation in temperature. There usually is exquisite tenderness on the affected side, and frequently a bulging mass may be felt in the flank. Edema of the skin may occur over the abscess. In addition, scoliosis of the spine with the concavity pointing toward the affected side occurs because of irritation of the psoas major and quadratus lumborum muscles. The diaphragm is elevated and somewhat fixed on the affected side; because of inflammatory reaction, basilar rales may be present. (4:247–48)

35. **E.** All statements are true of *Giardia lamblia*. (1:68)

36. **E.** Pyrantel pamoate is useful against all the intestinal nematodes listed. Thiabendazole is effective against *Trichuris trichiura* (whipworm). (3:625, 627, 629)

37. **E.** A mononuclear pleocytosis may occur in any of the disorders listed. (2:133)

38. **B.** (4:36)

39. **A.** (4:36)

40. **C.** (4:36)

41. **D.** (4:36)

42. **A.** (*Res-Int Consult*, 2:22, 1973)

43. **A.** (*Res-Int Consult*, 2:22, 1973)

44. **B.** (*Res-Int Consult*, 2:22, 1973)

45. **B.** (*Res-Int Consult*, 2:22, 1973)

46. **A.** (*Res-Int Consult*, 2:22, 1973)

47. **B.** (*Res Staff Physician*, 20:82, 1974)

48. **A.** (*Res Staff Physician*, 20:82, 1974)

49. **False.** Foul or putrid odor of discharges is a major clue to anaerobic infection, but may be absent. (1:66)

50. **True.** In chronic syphilitic meningitis and other forms of late syphilis, particularly tabes dorsalis, the pupils are usually small, irregular, and unequal; they do not dilate properly in response to mydriatic drugs and fail to react to light, although they do constrict on accommodation. In some cases, there is an associated atrophy of the iris with Argyll Robertson pupil. (7:720)

51. **True.** Resistance to most antibiotics is widespread among members of the *Enterobacteriaceae: Escherichia coli*, klebsiella, proteus, enterobacter, and serratia. (5:26)

52. **False.** Surgical drainage rarely is required in amebic liver abscess. (1:67)

53. **False.** Most strains of Pseudomonas isolated in the United States do *not* produce a penicillinase with a specific affinity for carbenicillin. Although the Pseudomonas may be able to destroy penicillin or ampicillin, it is ineffective against carbenicillin. (5:89)

54. **True.** While the polymyxins are quite active against pseudomonas *in vitro*, they have proven to be only minimally effective *in vivo*. (5:81)

55. **True.** Anaerobes associated with pleuropulmonary disease usually are derived from the oropharynx. (*Lancet*, 1:338, 1974)

56. **False.** There is little difference in the bacterial flora found during acute exacerbations and that noted during stable stages of chronic bronchitis. (*Ann Intern Med*, 77:993, 1972)

57. **True.** Many of the strains of Bacteroides that are resistant to chloramphenicol are sensitive to tetracycline. (*Emerg Med*, 5:71, 1973)

58. **True.** Some controversy exists regarding the proper classification of *Pneumocystis carinii*; identification of various stages of maturation found in the lung suggest a parasitic etiology. Open-lung biopsy with impression or touch smears of the cut fresh specimen which can be stained with methenamine silver offers the best opportunity for diagnosis. (1:68)

59. **False.** Posterior cervical node enlargement is characteristic of clinical toxoplasmosis in adults.
(*Am J Pathol*, 69:349, 1972)

60. **True.** In the absence of urinary obstruction, the radiographic changes of pyelonephritis in adults are usually the residua of childhood infection. These changes result from lack of growth of renal tissue due to infection usually in the presence of vesicoureteral reflux. Reflux tends to disappear with elimination of bacteriuria or with increasing age. (1:64)

61. **False.** Since the most important site of drug inactivation is the liver, particular care should be taken in the treatment of gram-negative infections in uremic patients with serious liver disease. Patients in shock should be included in this category, since their blood flow is decreased in both the kidneys and the liver. (5:68)

62. **False.** Streptococcus viridans, normally noninvasive, is usually the organism responsible for subacute infective endocarditis. Organisms capable of primary invasion, e.g., *Staphylococcus aureus*, are responsible for acute infectious endocarditis. (3:386)

63. **False.** Vancomycin is an acceptable substitute for patients allergic to penicillin in the treatment of enterococcal endocarditis. (1:63)

64. **True.** The epidemiology of infectious mononucleosis resembles that of several other viral diseases, such as polio. In lower socioeconomic groups where EBV antibodies appear early in life, there is little clinical infectious mononucleosis.
(*Hosp Prac*, 5:33, 1970)

65. **True.** The doses of penicillin recommended for gonorrhea will cure incubating syphilis, whereas the tetracycline and spectinomycin regimens may be ineffective. (1:64)

66. **True.** Patients sensitive to penicillin generally do not have allergic reactions to cephalothin; when they do, it is probably not a true cross-reaction but a manifestation of hyperreactive sensitivity in a very allergic individual. (5:66)

67. **True.** It is now evident that the clinical and pathologic spectrum of chronic active hepatitis is a syndrome of diverse etiology. In a large percentage of patients, the primary etiologic factor has not been identified. Hepatitis B infection is of importance in a significant number of patients. (3:1661)

68. **True.** Production of IgA and IgE is linked. Absence of either may be associated with sinopulmonary infections.
(*N Engl J Med*, 286:1166, 1972)

69. **False.** Renal failure is a rare complication of urinary tract infection in the absence of anatomic abnormalities. Although there are trends suggesting an association between urinary tract infection and hypertension, no cause and effect relationship has been demonstrated. (1:64)

70. **True.** In patients with acid urine, sulfonamides are known to form microcrystalline deposits and result in obstruction or hematuria.
(*N Engl J Med*, 287:975, 1972)

71. **True.** Courses of amphotericin B of less than 5 g total dose do not produce significant residual changes in renal function. (1:67)

72. **False.** Bacteremias caused by *E. coli* are acquired in the community slightly more often than in the hospital, while those due to pseudomonas, klebsiella-enterobacter-serratia (KES group), herellea-mima, and proteus are usually nosocomial in origin. (5:23)

73. **True.** Septic thrombophlebitis and abscess formation are common features of anaerobic infection and account for the chronicity of these infections, their refractoriness to therapy, and the tendency for relapse. (1:66)

74. **True.** About 5 to 8% of patients meeting the criteria for fever of obscure origin appear to recover completely without ever having a diagnosis established. (*N Engl J Med*, 289:1407, 1973)

75. **False.** Sanitation does not seem a factor, since the frequency of resistant enteric bacteria is as great in "highly civilized" countries as in less developed nations. (5:27)

76. **True.** When daily gentamicin is given intrathecally, cerebrospinal fluid antibacterial activity can be achieved and maintained.
(*Johns Hopkins Med J*, 133:51, 1973)

77. **False.** Antibiotics are not the treatment of choice for salmonella gastroenteritis.
(*N Engl J Med*, 287:975, 1972)

78. **True.** Pseudomonas may be present in sputum cultures as part of the residual flora after treatment with other antibiotics and not be pathogenic. (5:82)

79. **True.** It has been shown that drugs which markedly reduce the meningococcal carrier state will abort an epidemic of meningococcal disease. (1:65)

80. **False.** The most frequent source of gram-negative bacteremia is the urinary tract. (5:21)

81. **True.** Recent studies of host responses to endotoxin suggest that the pathophysiology of gram-negative bacteremia is best explained as a result of the influences of the complement, kinin, and coagulation systems. (5:48)

82. **False.** Antibiotic treatment can prolong the excretion rate of viable Salmonella bacilli in uncomplicated gastroenteritis. (1:66)

83. **True.** The phagocytic function of the reticuloendothelial system is compromised in sickle cell disease. (*N Engl J Med*, 288:845, 1973)

84. **True.** Tetracycline is a poor choice for the empirical treatment of pulmonary infections because 5 to 10% of *D. pneumoniae*, 30 to 40% of group A Streptococci, and many strains of *S. aureus* are resistant to this antibiotic.
(*Hosp Physician*, 9:20, 1973)

85. **True.** Syphilitic aortitis is common in all forms of neurosyphilis. (2:430)

86. **False.** Chloramphenicol penetrates into cerebrospinal fluid very well. (1:65)

87. **False.** Only a small proportion, perhaps 10%, of persons infected with the *Treponema pallidum*, subsequently show evidence that the organism has invaded the nervous system. (2:428)

88. **False.** Preexisting valve damage is usually present in subacute infective endocarditis. Such damage is not usually present in acute infective endocarditis. (3:386)

89. **False.** Cephalothin is not adequate in the treatment of meningococcal meningitis. (1:65)

90. **True.** Polymyxins directly damage the bacterial cell membrane of many gram-negative bacilli. Essential cell constituents then leak out and the cell dies. (5:36)

91. **False.** Clindamycin is very effective against most anaerobes, the chief exceptions being certain strains of *Fusobacterium varium* and several species of Clostridium other than *C. perfringens*. The cerebrospinal fluid and nervous tissue levels of clindamycin are poor. (1:66)

92. **False.** It has been shown that no bacteria are grown from the bile of patients operated upon within 48 hours of the onset of acute cholecystitis, but when operation was delayed until 6 days after the onset of symptoms, about three-fourths of patients showed positive bile cultures. (6:939)

93. **Prostatitis.** Relapses of upper urinary tract infection in males are usually related to chronic prostatitis. (1:64)

94. **Synergistic.** When a combination of two antibiotics is at least four times as effective as either one alone, they are considered to have a synergistic effect. (5:85)

95. **Syphilis.** Perforation of the nasal septum may be on a traumatic or infectious basis. Anterior perforation occurs with tuberculosis, while posterior perforation is more common with syphilis. (4:100)

Textbook References for Chapter 12

1. American College of Physicians (1974): *Medical Knowledge Self-Assessment, Program III: Recent Developments in Internal Medicine,* Petersdorf, R.G., General Editor. American College of Physicians, Philadelphia.

2. Bannister, Roger (1978): *Brain's Clinical Neurology*, Fifth Edition, Oxford Medical Publications, New York.

3. Beeson, P.B. and McDermott, W. (1979): *Cecil Textbook of Medicine*, Fifteenth Edition, W.B. Saunders Company, Philadelphia.

4. ·Judge, R.D. and Zuidema, G.D., Editors (1974): *Physical Diagnosis: A Physiologic Approach to the Clinical Examination,* Little, Brown and Company, Boston.

5. Lauler, D.P., Editor-in-Chief (1971): *Gram Negative Sepsis,* Medcom, Incorporated, Clifton, New Jersey.

6. Spiro, Howard M. (1977): *Clinical Gastroenterology*, Second Edition, Collier-Macmillan Limited, Toronto, Ontario.

7. Isselbacher, K.J. Editor (1980): *Harrison's Principles of Internal Medicine*, Ninth Edition McGraw-Hill Book Company, New York.

CHAPTER 13

Medical Malpractice Law

Directions: Indicate whether each of the following statements is true or false.

1. Simple medical negligence in diagnosis with the result that a patient is involuntarily hospitalized supports an action for false imprisonment.

2. When a patient is reasonably believed to have a communicable disease, the physician is usually liable if he discusses the problem with those who are in close contact with the patient.

3. The admission of nonessential persons during treatment without the specific consent of the patient constitutes a violation of privacy.

4. The plaintiff in a malpractice suit is required to prove that the physician was negligent; in most cases, the physician is not expected to prove that he was not negligent.

5. Standard medical malpractice insurance policies usually cover deliberate torts.

6. Failure to abide by a physician's instructions to take proper medication is usually a good defense against an action for negligence against the physician.

7. When two or more physicians create a partnership for the purpose of practicing medicine, each is liable not only for his own negligence, but also, under general principles of partnership law, for the negligence of any of his partners and for any of the employees of the partnership.

8. Under no circumstance does the physician have the right to render treatment without attempting to explain or inform the patient of any risks.

9. A physician who refers a patient to a specialist and then withdraws from the case is usually liable for any negligence committed by the specialist.

10. The Uniform Anatomical Gift Act empowers a person to execute a written instrument which is legally binding on the next of kin at death.

11. In matters involving routine nursing care, a physician is not liable if hospital employee nurses carry out his orders negligently.

12. The hospital may be held liable for a private duty nurse's negligence.

13. When physicians volunteer to take each other's calls on occasion, any negligence by the substitute imposes liability on the first physician.

Directions: For each of the following multiple-choice questions, indicate the ONE CORRECT answer.

14. In a malpractice suit, hospital records are considered the property of the

    A. hospital
    B. physician
    C. patient or the patient's guardian
    D. patient's attorney
    E. county medical society

15. The most frequent cause of suits against a hospital for nonemployee physician liability is

    A. assault on a patient
    B. making unwarranted promises to the patient
    C. negligence during one's turn on call in the emergency room
    D. failing to obtain patient consent
    E. abandonment

16. A tort action is an action instituted in a court of law which, to be maintained, must allege that

    A. a legal duty was owed to the plaintiff by the defendant
    B. the defendant breached that duty
    C. the plaintiff was damaged as a result of that breach
    D. all of the above
    E. none of the above

17. The most common ground for revocation of physicians' licenses is

    A. releasing privileged information
    B. conviction of a crime
    C. negligence
    D. breach of contract
    E. failure to join the American Medical Association

18. One of the most important duties a physician owes a patient under the general concept of due care is an obligation to

    A. join the American Medical Association
    B. obtain board certification
    C. keep abreast of new developments in medicine
    D. attend national medical conferences at least twice a year
    E. always obtain a second medical opinion

19. About what percentage of malpractice cases actually go to trial?

    A. less than 10%
    B. 20%
    C. 40%
    D. 60%
    E. 80%

Directions: For each of the following questions select
    A. if the question is associated with A only
    B. if the question is associated with B only
    C. if the question is associated with both A and B
    D. if the question is associated with neither A nor B

20. The right to determine the times and frequency of appointments is held by the

    A. physician
    B. patient
    C. both
    D. neither

21. Failure to see a patient when necessary may

    A. constitute abandonment
    B. be negligence in terms of the standard of care of both diagnosis and treatment
    C. both
    D. neither

22. When a physician refers a patient to a second physician, the first physician can be held liable for

    A. abandonment
    B. any negligence committed by the physician to whom he referred the patient
    C. both
    D. neither

23. A physician whose policy is not to make house calls

   A. may be obliged to do so
   B. is justified in telling the patient to come to the office or see him at the hospital
   C. both
   D. neither

24. Any information in hospital records which applies solely to the patient who requests the information or on whose behalf the information is requested must be made available to the

   A. patient
   B. patient's attorney
   C. both
   D. neither

25. Medical records which have been altered for any reason should always include

   A. notation of the date
   B. reason for the change
   C. both
   D. neither

26. Assault and battery is

   A. wrongful, harmful or offensive contact with another's body
   D. putting another in fear of an offensive physical attack
   C. both
   D. neither

27. Allowing a layman to perform medical treatment may result in an action for

   A. negligence against the physician
   B. invasion of privacy against the physician
   C. both
   D. neither

28. Assuring a patient that no risk is involved when he knows that proposed treatment carries a potential of serious harm may make the physician liable for

   A. fraud
   B. any problems arising from the foreseeable consequence of the therapy
   C. both
   D. neither

Directions: For each of the following statements, fill in the correct answer.

29. To _____ means to give oral evidence, under oath, as a witness in a judicial inquiry in order to prove a fact.

30. Even if a patient can prove that a physician or surgeon did not meet the required standard of care, he cannot recover damages unless he can also prove that the negligence caused him injuries which would not have occurred in its absence; this requirement of proof between cause and effect is known as the legal concept of " _____ cause."

31. The term " _____ liability" is legal shorthand for a doctrine which involves the responsibility of one person who is not negligent for the wrongful conduct of another.

32. The _____ rule is a doctrine which permits the filing of an appropriate case after the statute of limitations has expired, if the injured party could not have known of possible negligence at the time it occurred.

33. _____ consent is the primary consideration in situations in which medical experimentation takes place.

34. _____ has been defined as "the unilateral severance by the physician of the professional relationship between himself and a patient without reasonable notice, at a time when there is still the necessity of continuing medical attention."

35. The doctrine of " _____ of risk" means that the patient understands the possibility of all risks of untoward, unpreventable results of treatment and knowingly consents to that treatment.

Directions: Indicate whether each of the following statements is true or false.

36. Most medical school deans believe that their students could not be held liable for medical malpractice for activities during the regular course of medical education.

37. Discharging a patient from the hospital prior to the time when his condition justifies is not abandonment if the discharge results from an honest mistake as to his condition and need for further medical care.

38. If physicians who practice together see each other's patients on a rotating basis, none of them can be held to have abandoned a patient if another member of the group or partnership has been to see him.

39. In most jurisdictions today, the local standard of practice is considered the only determining factor presented to the jury and is in and of itself determinative of the presence or absence of negligence.

40. A physician who carefully follows standard and accepted procedures will not be held negligent whatever the outcome of the case.

41. Most courts hold that a public hospital may require membership in the local medical society before a physician may be admitted to the staff if he is otherwise qualified.

42. As long as the patient is told about inherent and unavoidable risks prior to administration of treatment, in the absence of negligence, he cannot recover damages if an unfortunate result occurs.

43. A doctor may be liable for an error of judgment in diagnosis, even if he has complied with recognized medical standards and used due care.

44. A physician may be liable for negligence if he is remiss in his obligation to realize that he is not capable of treating the patient and should therefore send him to a specialist.

45. A physician can be subject to prosecution for practicing without a license or to disciplinary action if he treats an emergency patient in a state where he is not licensed, even though he has a valid license in another state.

46. Physicians who withdraw from cases in which patients still require medical treatment on the grounds that the patient has not paid a past due bill have a good defense in an abandonment case.

47. A physician is legally bound to guarantee to keep his patients safe from all harm while they are on his premises.

Answers and Commentary

1. **False.** Generally speaking, simple medical negligence in diagnosis with the result that a patient is involuntarily hospitalized does not support an action for false imprisonment. However, if a psychiatrist or other physician certifies that he has examined a patient for commitment when he has not, a civil action for false imprisonment will lie and criminal penalties may also result. (1:291)

2. **False.** In any situation in which a patient is reasonably believed to have a communicable disease, the physician is not liable if he advises those who are in close contact with the patient. In fact, there have been several decisions in recent years holding that a physician has a duty to warn either the patient or his family if there is a possibility that those living in the house with the patient might contract the disease. (1:275)

3. **True.** A patient has the right to privacy in the course of medical treatment. Most states have established such a right either by court decision or statute and the Supreme Court has recognized it as a constitutional right. The admission of nonessential persons during treatment without the specific consent of the patient constitutes a violation of his right of privacy. (1:277)

4. **True.** The plaintiff in a malpractice suit is required to prove that the physician was negligent; in most cases, the physician is not expected to prove that he was not negligent, although there are some unusual factual situations which are so obviously unlikely to occur in the absence of negligence (such as leaving a sponge in a patient's body) that courts hold that these do raise an inference of negligence. Once the patient proves that such an act occurred, it is incumbent on the physician to rebut that presumption by a defense of his own. (1:298)

5. **False.** All physicians should be aware that standard medical malpractice insurance policies do not usually cover deliberate torts. The physician is protected only from accidents and good faith mistakes and errors of judgment. He is not protected against deliberate actions which harm his patients for the very simple reason that he could have avoided them. (1:266)

6. **True.** Failure to abide by a physician's instructions to take proper medication is usually a good defense against an action for negligence. Other good defenses include violation of instructions to exercise or undergo other forms of rehabilitation therapy and failure to comply with instructions pertaining to one's activities in the hospital. (1:306)

7. **True.** When two or more physicians create a partnership for the purpose of practicing medicine, each is liable not only for his own negligence but also, under general principles of partnership law, for the negligence of any of his partners and for any of the employees of the partnership. Where a partnership exists and is sued, however, assets of the partnership and of the physician who was himself negligent must usually be exhausted before any of the other partners may be asked to contribute from his personal funds to the judgment obtained by the plaintiff. (1:202)

8. **False.** The doctrine of informed consent does not apply in a genuine emergency. When a patient is unconscious or sufficiently ill to be unable to comprehend what is being said to him, the physician has the right to render necessary treatment without attempting to explain or inform the patient of any risks. (1:228)

9. **False.** A physician who refers a patient to a specialist and then withdraws from the case is not usually liable for any negligence committed by the specialist unless the patient can show that the specialist was unqualified or incompetent and that the referring physician should have known it.
(1:203)

10. **True.** The Uniform Anatomical Gift Act empowers a person to execute a written instrument which is legally binding on the next of kin at death. There is a uniform donation card which has been prepared by the American Medical Association and which is available to physicians for distribution to their patients who may wish to make use of them, indicating the desire for the person's body, or as much of it as he wishes, to be used for transplantation or research.
(1:242)

11. **True.** In matters involving routine nursing care, a physician is not liable if hospital employee nurses carry out the orders negligently. The general rule is that the only time a physician is liable for a hospital nurse's negligence in the course of routine nursing care is when the nurse acts under the direct and personal control of the physician or the physician knows or should know that the nurse is incompetent.
(1:204)

12. **False.** Private duty nurses are generally considered to be employees of the patient even when they are hired through the hospital's registry and, therefore, if a private duty nurse is negligent, the hospital is not liable.
(1:211)

13. **False.** Where physicians volunteer to take each other's calls on occasion, it is quite clear that any negligence by the substitute does not impose liability on the first physician. These physicians are clearly independent practitioners. If a substitute is chosen with due care and is not paid a salary but bills directly for his services, it is unlikely that the first physician will be found liable for his negligence. If, on the other hand, the substitute physician is on salary from the treating physician, the employer is liable for his negligence. A physician must make all reasonable efforts to insure that the substitute is adequately qualified and if he has failed to use due care in the selection process, he may well be liable for the substitute's negligence.
(1:201)

14. **A.** Hospital records are normally considered the property of the hospital. However, a patient, his guardian, or his attorney, with written permission from the patient, has the right to inspect and to copy any of these records if they are relevant to any legal proceedings.
(1:390)

15. **C.** The most frequent cause of suits against a hospital for nonemployee physician liability is one in which a staff physician who is taking his turn on call in the emergency room is negligent. If he is assigned to the patient by a rotating system and the patient has no choice in his selection, the question of whether or not the hospital is liable is a major issue in medical law at the present time.
(1:214)

16. **D.** All the conditions listed must be present to signify a tort action. (*J Leg Med,* 4:36, 1976)

17. **B.** Conviction of a crime is the most common ground for revocation of physicians' licenses. It is quite clear that the crime charged does not necessarily have to involve the practice of medicine. For example, there are probably more license revocation proceedings after physicians have been convicted of violation of income tax laws than on any other grounds. Other physicians have recently had their licenses revoked after convictions for counterfeiting and carrying an unregistered firearm. In short, conviction of any felony is generally considered sufficient to revoke a medical license even if the physician is convicted on a charge which is not a crime in the state of license.
(1:342)

18. **C.** One of the most important duties a physician owes his patient under the general concept of due care is his obligation to keep abreast of new developments in medicine. This can be done by postgraduate study, meetings, etc. (1:52)

19. **A.** Only about 8% of malpractice cases actually go to trial; 24% are settled before suit is filed and 68% are settled before trial.
(*Res Staff Phys,* 20:111, 1974)

20. **A.** The physician, not the patient, has the right to determine the times and frequency of appointments. He certainly has the right to reasonable time off as long as an adequate, competent substitute is available. (1:35)

21. **C.** Simple failure to see a patient when necessary may constitute abandonment, and it may also be negligence in terms of the standard of care of both diagnosis and treatment owed to the patient in the sense that if the physician had been properly attentive, he might well have known what was wrong with the patient and treated it properly. Thus, even if a physician comes back to see the patient, if he has unreasonably refused to come at the time when the patient needs him, he may well have been so negligent as to be held to have abandoned his patient. The longer the delay, of course, the more likely that a court will find abandonment.
(1:377)

22. **D.** When a physician refers a patient to a second physician, the first physician obviously cannot be held liable for abandonment. He is also not liable for any negligence committed by the physician to whom he referred the patient as long as he used due care in selecting him. (1:387)

23. **B.** A physician has the right to make reasonable limitations on his practice. He is under no legal obligation whatever to treat any patient who wishes him to exceed the stated limitations of that practice. A physician whose policy is not to make house calls is not obliged to do so and is perfectly justified in telling the patient to come to the office or to see him at the hospital. (1:388)

24. **C.** Any information in the hospital records which applies solely to the patient who requests the information or on whose behalf the information is requested must be made available to the patient or to his attorney. In some states, the patient does not have the right to read his records himself, but his attorney in all states does have the right as long as he has the written permission of his client. (1:391)

25. **C.** Records which disclose negligent treatment will materially benefit the patient's case. Records which have been altered for any reason, even the most innocent, should always include notations of the date and reason for change. If a negligence suit is filed subsequent to alteration of a record, and that alteration is apparent, it will undoubtedly be construed as a dishonest attempt to avoid liability. (1:298)

26. **C.** Assault and battery is wrongful, harmful, or offensive contact with another's body or putting the other person in fear of such an attack; in other words, a deliberate attack of some type upon the patient. (1:266)

27. **C.** Allowing a layman to perform medical treatment may not only result in an action for negligence, but may involve an action for invasion of privacy. (1:278)

28. **C.** Assuring a patient that no risk is involved when he knows that proposed treatment carries a potential of serious harm may make the physician liable for fraud as well as for any problems arising from the foreseeable consequence of the therapy. (1:283)

29. **Testify.** To testify means to give oral evidence, under oath, as a witness in a judicial inquiry in order to prove a fact. (*J Leg Med*, 3:50, 1975)

30. **Proximate.** Even if a patient can prove that a physician or surgeon did not meet the required standard of care, he cannot recover damages unless he can also prove that the negligence caused him injuries which would not have occurred in its absence; this requirement of proof between cause and effect is known as the legal concept of "proximate cause." No matter how negligent the physician may have been harm must be shown to have resulted before damages may be awarded. (1:62)

31. **Vicarious.** The term "vicarious liability" is legal shorthand for a doctrine which involves the responsibility of one person who is not negligent for the wrongful conduct or negligence of another. Thus, the concept of vicarious liability in the context of medical malpractice law involves at least three persons: First, the patient who is injured by negligent treatment; second, the person, such as a nurse, who is actually the negligent party; and third, the physician who may or may not be financially responsible for the nurse's negligence. (1:200)

32. **Discovery.** The discovery rule is a doctrine which permits the filing of an appropriate case after the statute of limitations has expired, if the injured party could not have known of possible negligence at the time it occured.
(*Res Staff Phys*, 20:110, 1974)

33. **Informed.** Informed consent is the primary consideration in situations in which medical experimentation takes place. (1:254)

34. **Abandonment.** Abandonment has been defined as the "unilateral severance by the physician of the professional relationship between himself and a patient without reasonable notice, at a time when there is still the necessity of continuing medical attention." (1:374)

35. **Assumption.** The doctrine of "assumption of risk" means that the patient understands the possibility of all risks of untoward, unpreventable results of treatment and knowingly consents to that treatment. Where it applies, this is usually a good defense to an action for negligence on the part of the physician. (1:310)

36. **False.** Over 80% of medical school deans in one survey believed that their students could be held liable for medical malpractice for activities during the regular course of medical education.
(*Am Med News*, 4, 1976)

37. **False.** Discharging a patient from the hospital prior to the time when his condition justifies it is abandonment, whether the discharge is because

the patient cannot pay his bill or results from an honest mistake as to his condition and need for further medical care. (1:382)

38 **True.** If physicians who practice together see each other's patients on a rotating basis, none of them can be held to have abandoned a patient if another member of the group or partnership has been to see him. (1:386)

39. **False.** Until quite recently, as a matter of law, comparison was made of the due care exercised by the particular physician in reference to that of other physicians in his geographical area. The standard test was "that degree of care which other physicians exercise in the same or similar communities." The skill and knowledge of a physician were compared only to other physicians in the same geographical area on the theory that physicians practicing in isolated rural areas, for example, should not be expected to be as well trained and up-to-date as a physician in an urban area. This rule does remain strictly adhered to in some states, but it has been completely abrogated in others and, in general, even where it is still theoretically accepted it has been modified. In most jurisdictions today, the local standard of practice is considered only one factor presented for the jury's determination and is not in and of itself determinative of the presence or absence of negligence. (1:58)

40. **True.** Most medical treatment which is held to be negligent involves one of two situations: either the physician does not follow the standard practice in treating the condition, meaning that he administers incorrect treatment, or he undertakes to administer proper treatment, but does it in an inadequate or incorrect manner. A physician who carefully follows standard and accepted procedures will not be held negligent whatever the outcome of the case. (1:04)

41. **False.** Most courts hold that a public hospital may not require membership in the local medical society before a physician may be admitted to the staff if he is otherwise qualified. In many cases in which physicians were arbitrarily excluded from county or state medical societies for racial reasons and were thereafter denied staff memberships in public hospitals, courts held that their constitutional rights had been violated. (1:356)

42. **True.** As long as the patient is told about inherent and unavoidable risks prior to administration of treatment, in the absence of negligence, he cannot recover damages if an unfortunate result occurs. When a patient undergoes x-ray treatment for example, he assumes the risk of x-ray burns as long as no negligence is present. (1:104)

43. **False.** A physician is not negligent simply because he has not made a correct diagnosis of his patient's illness or injury. The general rule is that a doctor is not liable for an error of judgment in diagnosis as long as he has complied with recognized medical standards and used due care. If he has performed or ordered all the accepted tests and procedures which a reasonably careful physician would consider appropriate, has taken into consideration all the relevant symptoms, and has made a careful evaluation of the patient's past and present illness history, he is not legally negligent simply because he is wrong. (1:89)

44. **True.** A physician may be liable either for failure to know what he is doing, if a reasonably prudent physician would have known, or he may be liable if he knows what to do, but for some reason does not do it carefully or omits doing it at all. "Skill and knowledge" usually include the former, "diligence" the latter. A physician may, for example, be liable of negligence if he is remiss in his obligation to realize that he is not capable of treating the patient and should therefore send him to a specialist. (1:45)

45. **False.** A physician who has a valid license in one state is not subject to prosecution for practicing without a license or to disciplinary action if he treats an emergency patient in another state. A physician, for example, who is on vacation in a state where he is not licensed and who is summoned to help a person who has had a heart attack or who delivers a baby on an airline is not subject to any form of penalty. (1:342)

46. **False.** The financial question is absolutely irrelevant to the question of a patient's care. Physicians who withdraw from cases in which patients still require medical treatment on the grounds that the patient has not paid a past due bill do not have a good defense in an abandonment case. (1:378)

47. **False.** For example, if the reasonably careful physician or assistant did not realize and should not have realized that a machine was not functioning as usual at the time an accident occurred, he is not liable. The occupier of business premises does not guarantee to keep invitees safe from harm. He merely is held to the standard of protecting them from injuries which they cannot foresee or avoid, but the possibility of which the occupier has noticed. In the use of office equipment, the physician is only liable for injuries which result from those mechanical problems of which he either knew or about which, on the basis of reasonable observation, he should have known. (1:176–77)

Textbook Reference for Chapter 13

1. Holder, Angela R. (1978): *Medical Malpractice Law*, Second Edition, John Wiley and Sons, New York.

CHAPTER 14

Metabolism

Directions: For each of the following multiple-choice questions, select the ONE INCORRECT answer.

1. Hypovolemic disorders with urinary sodium concentration greater than 10 mEq/liter include

    A. adrenal insufficiency
    B. use of diuretics
    C. renal salt wastage (chronic renal failure and renal tubular acidosis, Type 11)
    D. vomiting with metabolic alkalosis and bicarbonaturia
    E. extrarenal sodium losses (as with excessive sweat losses and gastrointestinal losses without bicarbonaturia)

2. Fat-soluble vitamins include vitamin

    A. A
    B. B
    C. D
    D. E
    E. K

3. In vitamin D intoxication,

    A. hypercalcemia occurs as a result of excessive absorption of calcium from the gastrointestinal tract and of increased bone resorption
    B. hypercalciuria is an unusual finding
    C. the serum iPTH value is low or undetectable
    D. serum phosphorus concentration tends to be normal or high

4. In sick-cell syndrome,

    A. hyponatremia is seen due to cells having acquired excess intracellular sodium at the expense of the extracellular compartment
    B. hyponatremia is a side-effect of underlying illness
    C. direct correction of hyponatremia is usually required
    D. tissue hypoxia may be at the root of some cases

5. In metabolic acidosis, an increase in unmeasured anions would be expected in

    A. diarrhea
    B. diabetic ketoacidosis
    C. alcoholic ketoacidosis
    D. salicylate poisoning
    E. ethylene glycol poisoning

6. Wilson's disease is associated with

    A. hepatolenticular degeneration
    B. autosomal recessive inheritance
    C. increased ceruloplasmin
    D. decreased serum copper with a high urinary copper
    E. increased muscular rigidity and tremor

7. Metabolic alkalosis may be caused by

    A. vomiting or gastric drainage
    B. diuretic therapy

C. Addison's disease
D. primary aldosteronism
E. Bartter's syndrome

8. Regarding Wernicke's encephalopathy,

A. its causes, prognosis, and treatment are the same as those of beriberi
B. congestion and hemorrhages in the thalamus and hypocampus and in the hypothalamus and gray matter of the upper brainstem are present
C. difficulty in concentrating, disturbed sleep, confusion and, finally, stupor and coma occur
D. nystagmus and ophthalmoplegia are important signs
E. polyneuropathy is always present

Directions: For each of the following statements, fill in the correct answer.

9. With the exception of _____ acid, there are no carbohydrates known to be essential in the human diet.

10. Primary water retention in the absence of fluid volume deficit overexpands the body water and results in _____ hyponatremia.

11. The administration of cyanide and several other similarly acting poisons leads to a paradoxic state in which the tissues are unable to utilize oxygen and as consequence the venous blood tends to have a high oxygen tension; this condition has been termed _____ hypoxia.

12. In correcting metabolic acidosis with sodium bicarbonate, the ratio of ionized to protein bound calcium _____ as the pH increases.

13. " _____ gap" is defined as the difference between the concentration of sodium and the sum of measured anions (chloride plus bicarbonate).

14. The stupor caused by hyperosmolarity may be secondary to _____ of brain tissue.

15. Low-density lipoprotein (LDL) is the principal carrier of _____ .

16. In Wilson's disease corneal pigmentation, the _____ ring, consists of a zone of golden brown granular pigmentation about 2 mm in diameter on the posterior surface of the cornea towards the limbus.

Directions: Use the key below to answer questions 17 through 19.
A. if the statement describes asthenic (ectomorph) body type
B. if the statement describes the asthenic (mesomorph) body type
C. if the statement describes the pyknic (endomorph) body type

17. Heavy, soft, and rounded, due to an accumulation of body fat

18. Slender and may appear to be underweight

19. Relatively square and athletic

Directions: For each of the following multiple-choice questions, select the ONE CORRECT answer.

20. Regarding lactose tolerance tests,

A. failure to split lactose (lactase deficiency) may be detected by oral administration of 50.0 g lactose followed by serial determinations of reducing substance as in a glucose tolerance test
B. failure of capillary blood glucose to rise at least 20.0 mg/100 ml above the baseline indicates lactase deficiency provided the subject is capable of absorbing glucose
C. interpretation of a positive test does not require an oral glucose tolerance test
D. A. and B.
E. all of the above

21. Vitamin D increases serum calcium levels by

    A. enhancing intestinal absorption of calcium
    B. increasing resorption of calcium from bone
    C. decreasing urinary phosphate excretion
    D. A. and B.
    E. all of the above

Directions: For each of the following questions, select
  A. **if the question is associated with A only**
  B. **if the question is associated with B only**
  C. **if the question is associated with both A and B**
  D. **if the question is associated with neither A nor B**

22. The initial therapy in patients with hypercalcemia should be rehydration with normal saline; this usually produces

    A. a decrease in serum calcium by hemodilution
    B. an increase in urine calcium excretion
    C. both
    D. neither

23. Phosphate depletion by low dietary intake combined with the administration of aluminum hydroxide gels can produce hypercalcemia in patients with

    A. primary hyperparathyroidism
    B. secondary hyperparathyroidism
    C. both
    D. neither

24. Dilutional hyponatremia is found when water excretion is defective as in

    A. acute renal failure
    B. inappropriate secretion of antidiuretic hormone (ADH)
    C. both
    D. neither

25. Hypomagnesemia

    A. is most frequently seen in patients with gastrointestinal disorders (malabsorption) or alcoholism

    B. manifestations include tetany, positive Chvostek's sign, negative Trousseau's sign, absent muscle cramps, tremor, changes in personality, muscle weakness, and seizures
    C. both
    D. neither

26. Hypervolemia and edema associated with urinary sodium concentration less than 10 mEq/liter may occur in

    A. congestive heart failure
    B. hepatic cirrhosis
    C. both
    D. neither

27. Generally, hyperkalemia should be treated immediately if

    A. the serum potassium level exceeds 6.5 mEq/liter
    B. cardiac arrhythmia is present
    C. both
    D. neither

28. In congenital lymphangiectasia, the protein loss, which is moderate, will be reduced considerably by the administration of

    A. medium chain triglycerides
    B. a high fat diet
    C. both
    D. neither

29. A metabolic or toxic abnormality such as barbiturate poisoning or hypoglycemia may produce unconsciousness by affecting the

    A. cerebral hemispheres
    B. ascending reticular activating system
    C. both
    D. neither

30. Hypothermia may occur in

    A. hypoglycemia
    B. extensive exfoliative dermatitis
    C. both
    D. neither

31. Hypochloremic alkalosis is a common complication of chronic obstructive pulmonary disease because

    A. the kidneys lose chloride when bicarbonate is retained to compensate for carbon dioxide retention
    B. diuretic therapy, frequently used in patients with chronic obstructive pulmonary disease, produces hypochloremia along with hypokalemic alkalosis
    C. both
    D. neither

32. Chlorpromazine may be used in the treatment of overdose with

    A. amphetamines
    B. methylphenidate
    C. both
    D. neither

Directions: Indicate whether each of the following statements is true or false.

33. Quantitatively, the principal extracellular cation is potassium.

34. Mithramycin is the most rapidly acting of drugs used to treat hypercalcemia.

35. The finding of systemic metabolic alkalosis, i.e., elevated blood pH and normal or elevated pCO_2 in a hypercalcemic patient who has no other cause to be alkalotic, can be accepted as evidence against hyperparathyroidism and emphasizes the need for a search for other causes of hypercalcemia.

36. On a normal potassium intake of 40 to 100 mEq, the urinary potassium excretion varies between 40 and 90 mEq/24 hours.

37. Patients with gram-negative sepsis who have metabolic acidosis on initial determinations have an extremely poor prognosis which is further worsened if the central venous pressure is low.

38. The seizures associated with alcoholic intoxication, i.e., withdrawal seizures, usually appear within 48 hours after cessation of drinking.

39. Slowly developing changes in the serum potassium level may be compensated by potassium fluxes across the cellular membranes, thus maintaining a normal extracellular to intracellular ratio.

40. In most persons, there is a diurnal (occurring every day) variation in body temperature of one-half to two degrees.

41. The abnormality of calcium metabolism in sarcoidosis closely resembles that of vitamin D intoxication.

42. The level of very low-density lipoprotein (VLDL) triglyceride is increased by a diet restricted in carbohydrates to approximately 40% of the daily calories.

43. The lactate-pyruvate ratio of blood has been closely associated with the state of oxygenation of tissues, being depressed in situations of insufficient oxygenation.

44. Impaired intestinal absorption of calcium has been documented in patients with chronic renal failure.

45. The obese subject's thermal dissipation of energy is more marked than the normal subject's, so that more fat is laid down.

Directions: For each of the following multiple-choice questions, select the ONE CORRECT answer.

46. A serum potassium of 2.5 to 3 mEq/liter suggests that the potassium deficit may be in the range of

A. 25 mEq
B. 80 mEq
C. 140 mEq
D. 200 mEq
E. 300 mEq

47. In a normal man, fat stores represent 90% of available stored energy, enough to last him for how many months total starvation?

    A. 1
    B. 2
    C. 4
    D. 8
    E. 16

48. In normal patients doing light exercise, such as light housework or office work, caloric expenditure is about how many calories/kg body weight/day?

    A. 10 to 25
    B. 30 to 35
    C. 45
    D. 50 to 60
    E. 75 to 100

49. In a normal 70 kg man, fat comprises what percentage of body weight?

    A. less than 1%
    B. 2 to 5%
    C. 10%
    D. 15 to 25%
    E. 50%

50. Normal B_{12} body stores last

    A. 1 month
    B. 6 months
    C. 1 year
    D. 3 to 6 years
    E. greater than 10 years

Directions: For each of the incomplete statements below, ONE or MORE of the completions given is correct. In each case, select
A. **if 1, 2, and 3 are correct**
B. **if 1 and 3 are correct**
C. **if 2 and 4 are correct**
D. **if all are correct**
E. **if all are incorrect**
F. **if another combination is correct**

51. Anion gap (greater than 15 mmol/liter) may occur with

    1. uremia
    2. ketonemia
    3. salicylate poisoning
    4. lactic acidosis

52. Dilutional hyponatremia

    1. occurs as a consequence of water retention and is characterized by a low plasma osmolality with a concentrated urine
    2. is characterized by weakness, confusion, disorientation, convulsions, and muscle cramps
    3. when due to congestive heart failure, cirrhosis of the liver, or myxedema, patients are unable to excrete solute-free water, probably related to decreased delivery of glomerular filtrate to the diluting segment of the nephron. This results in decreased urinary sodium excretion
    4. when due to congestive heart failure, cirrhosis of the liver, or myxedema, there is a clear-cut relationship to excessive antidiuretic hormone

Directions: Each of the incomplete statements is followed by a numbered list of three factors. Arrange these factors in their correct order of frequency or incidence, from the most to the least frequent. Select
A. **if the correct order is 1, 2, 3**
B. **if the correct order is 1, 3, 2**
C. **if the correct order is 2, 1, 3**
D. **if the correct order is 2, 3, 1**
E. **if the correct order is 3, 1, 2**
F. **if the correct order is 3, 2, 1**

53. Serum calcium exists in the following forms:

    1. calcium ion
    2. protein-bound, largely to albumin
    3. complexed with citrate and similar ions

Directions: Use the key below to answer questions 54 through 57.
A. **if A is greater than or more appropriate than B**
B. **if B is greater than or more appropriate than A**
C. **if A and B are equal or approximately equal**

54. Plasma acetone is a crude measure largely of
    A. acetoacetic acid
    B. hydroxybutyric acid

55. The more severe form of mucopolysaccharidosis is
    A. Hunter's syndrome
    B. Hurler's syndrome

56. Hypercalciuria occurs in
    A. sarcoidosis
    B. tuberculosis

57. Which of the following usually responds to weight reduction?
    A. low-density lipoprotein cholesterol
    B. very low-density lipoprotein triglyceride

Directions: For each of the incomplete statements below, ONE or MORE of the completions given is correct. In each case, select
    A. if 1, 2, and 3 are correct
    B. if 1 and 3 are correct
    C. if 2 and 4 are correct
    D. if only 4 is correct
    E. if all statements are correct

58. Which of the following is associated with multiple endocrine adenomatosis syndromes?
    1. pituitary disorders
    2. pancreatic disorders (insulin or gastrin secretion)
    3. pheochromocytoma
    4. medullary carcinoma of thyroid

59. Naloxone may be used in the treatment of overdose with
    1. heroin
    2. morphine
    3. Demerol
    4. methadone

60. Respiratory alkalosis may be secondary to
    1. central neurogenic hyperventilation
    2. severe hypoglycemia
    3. acute anoxia
    4. hepatic coma

61. Protein-calorie deficiency disease may be associated with
    1. edema
    2. muscle wasting
    3. low body weight
    4. psychomotor change

Directions: Use the key below to answer questions 62 and 63.
    A. if the findings indicate a probable diagnosis of methyl alcohol poisoning
    B. if the findings indicate a probable diagnosis of ethylene glycol poisoning

62. Oxalate crystals in urine

63. Hyperemic optic discs, dilated sluggish pupils

Directions: For each of the following questions, select
    A. if the question is associated with A only
    B. if the question is associated with B only
    C. if the question is associated with both A and B
    D. if the question is associated with neither A nor B

64. Homocystinuria may be
    A. pyridoxine-responsive
    B. pyridoxine-unresponsive
    C. both
    D. neither

65. Avitaminosis A results in
    A. skin and eye lesions
    B. increased resistance to infection
    C. both
    D. neither

Answers and Commentary

1. **E.** States with urinary sodium concentrations less than 10 mEq/liter include extrarenal sodium losses, as with excessive sweat losses, and gastrointestinal losses without bicarbonaturia. All other conditions are examples of hypovolemic disorders with urinary sodium concentration greater than 10 mEq/liter.
(*Ann Intern Med*, 82:64, 1975)

2. **B.** Food fat serves as a vehicle for absorption of the fat-soluble vitamins; notably, vitamins A, D, E, and K. Thus, when the diet remains very low in fat or when steatorrhea is chronically present, deficiencies of the fat-soluble nutrients, particularly of vitamin A and carotenes, are much more likely to occur.
(6:1395)

3. **C.** In vitamin D intoxication, hypercalciuria is a common finding.
(*Med Clin North Am*, 56:941, 1972)

4. **C.** Treatment of underlying disease usually corrects hyponatremia in the sick-cell syndrome.
(*Lancet*, 1:342, 1974)

5. **A.** Diarrhea may cause metabolic acidosis without increase in unmeasured anions. The other disorders listed can increase unmeasured anions. Similarly, methyl alcohol poisoning, paraldehyde (rarely), lactic acidosis, and renal failure can increase anion gap.
(2:1961)

6. **C.** Wilson's disease is caused by a disturbance of copper metabolism, though the metabolic disorder is complex and also includes aminoaciduria. It is believed that ceruloplasmin, which normally contains almost the whole of the copper in the blood, is deficient. This leads to a low serum copper level. The copper is carried loosely bound to albumin. Hence, it is deposited in the tissues and excreted in the urine. All other statements are true of this disorder.
(1:296)

7. **C.** Cushing's syndrome may be associated with metabolic alkalosis. Other causes include adrenal steroid therapy, relief of chronic hypercapnia, vomiting or gastric drainage, diuretic therapy with ethacrynic acid, thiazides or furosemide, primary aldosteronism, and Bartter's syndrome.
(2:1965)

8. **E.** Polyneuropathy may or may not be present in Wernicke's encephalopathy. All other statements are true of this disorder.
(1:447)

9. **Ascorbic.** With the exception of ascorbic acid, there are no carbohydrates known to be essential in the human diet. However, the body requires carbohydrate as an energy source for the brain and for other specialized purposes. If these needs are not met by carbohydrate from the diet, the body must draw first on its very limited stores of liver glycogen and then use protein from dietary and endogenous sources to maintain glucose homeostasis.
(6:429)

10. **Dilutional.** Primary water retention in the absence of fluid volume deficit overexpands the body water and results in dilutional hyponatremia. The dilutional hyponatremia syndromes may be subdivided into at least two categories based on the source of the ADH. Those due to tumor production of ADH are referred to as the ectopic ADH syndrome. The nontumorous causes of dilutional hyponatremia are of diverse etiology and involve multiple systems. They fall within the persistent pituitary ADH syndrome and may be subdivided further according to the

specific pathways involved as more knowledge accrues. In the main, the central neural receptors provide the dominant drive for ADH secretion in these diseases. Secretion of ADH in the face of dilutional hyponatremia has heretofore been considered inappropriate. With further knowledge, it may be shown to be quite appropriate and homeostatic in nature.
(*Mod Med*, 41:39, 1973)

11. **Histotoxic.** The administration of cyanide and several other similarly acting poisons leads to a paradoxic state in which the tissues are unable to utilize oxygen and as a consequence the venous blood tends to have a high oxygen tension. This condition has been termed histotoxic hypoxia.
(6:168)

12. **Decreases.** In correcting metabolic acidosis with sodium bicarbonate, the ratio of ionized to protein-bound calcium decreases as pH increases.
(*Ann Intern Med*, 82:64, 1975)

13. **Anion.** "Anion gap" is defined as the difference between the concentration of sodium and the sum of measured anions (chloride plus bicarbonate).
(*Emerg Med*, 4:91, 1972)

14. **Dehydration.** The stupor caused by hyperosmolarity may be secondary to dehydration of brain tissue. (*Lancet*, 1, 7853:635, 1973)

15. **Cholesterol.** Low-density lipoprotein is the principal carrier of cholesterol and elevated levels of this lipoprotein are primarily responsible for increased serum cholesterol levels.
(*JAMA*, 233:275, 1975)

16. **Kayser-Fleischer.** In Wilson's disease corneal pigmentation, the Kayser-Fleischer ring, consists of a zone of golden brown granular pigmentation about 2 mm in diameter on the posterior surface of the cornea towards the limbus. (1:297)

17. **C.** (3:40–41)

18. **A.** (3:40–41)

19. **B.** (3:40–41)

20. **D.** In the lactose tolerance test, interpretation of a positive test requires an oral glucose tolerance test. (*N Engl J Med*, 281:1114, 1969)

21. **D.** Vitamin D increases serum calcium levels by enhancing intestinal absorption, increasing resorption of calcium from bone, and increasing urinary phosphate excretion.
(*Ann Intern Med*, 82:64, 1975)

22. **C.** In patients with hypercalcemia, rehydration with normal saline usually decreases serum calcium levels by hemodilution and increases urinary calcium excretion. (*Ann Intern Med*, 82:64, 1975)

23. **C.** Phosphate depletion by low dietary intake combined with the administration of aluminum hydroxide gels can produce hypercalcemia in patients with primary or secondary hyperparathyroidism. Phosphate depletion also results in hypercalciuria, which is undesirable in patients with renal damage or stones.
(*N Engl J Med*, 285:1006, 1971)

24. **C.** In both acute renal failure and inappropriate secretion of antidiuretic hormone, dilutional hyponatremia is found and water excretion is defective. (*Lancet*, 1, 7853:342, 1974)

25. **C.** Both statements are true of hypomagnesemia. (*Ann Intern Med*, 82:64, 1975)

26. **C.** Hypervolemia and edema with urinary sodium concentration less than 10 mEq/l may occur in both congestive heart failure and hepatic cirrhosis. (*Ann Intern Med*, 82:64, 1975)

27. **C.** Generally, hyperkalemia should be treated immediately if the serum potassium level exceeds 6.5 mEq/liter or if cardiac arrhythmia is present.
(*JAMA*, 231:631, 1975)

28. **A.** In congenital lymphangiectasia, the protein loss, which is moderate, will be reduced considerably by the administration of medium chain triglycerides or a low fat diet.
(*N Engl J Med*, 281:1116, 1969)

29. **C.** A metabolic or toxic abnormality such as barbiturate poisoning or hypoglycemia may produce unconsciousness by affecting the cerebral hemispheres or the ascending reticular activating system. (*Med Clin North Am*, 57:1363, 1973)

30. **C.** Hypothermia may occur in both hypoglycemia and extensive exfoliative dermatitis. (*N Engl J Med*, 289:920, 1973)

31. **C.** Both statements are true of the association between hypochloremic alkalosis and chronic obstructive pulmonary disease.
(*Mod Med*, 41:32, 1973)

32. **C.** Patients with an overdose of amphetamines or methylphenidate may be hyperactive, aggressive, sometimes paranoid with repetitive behavior. Dilated pupils, tremor, hyperactive reflexes, hyperthermia, tachycardia, arrhythmia, and acute torsion dystonia may also be noted. Treatment includes reassurance if symptoms are

mild, and chlorpromazine, if intense. Signs of severe overdose include agitation, assaultive and paranoid excitement, occasionally convulsions, hypothermia, and circulatory collapse. (2:701–02)

33. **False.** Quantitatively, potassium is the principal intracellular cation. Within the cell, it is mostly bound to proteins including various enzymes whose reactions it facilitates. It also influences the osmotic equilibrium of the cell and is in part responsible for the transmembrane resting potential. The uptake of glucose and amino acids by cells requires its presence and simultaneous entry. Thus, the requirement for potassium is related to those processes which maintain the intracellular milieu and affect anabolism.

34. **False.** A limitation to the use of mithramycin has been the fact that the decrease in serum calcium often has not been rapid enough to consider the drug sufficiently dependable for use in emergencies. Rebound in serum calcium usually occurs on cessation of therapy, but the drug can be given repeatedly as long as hemorrhagic complications do not occur. Some workers feel that this agent should be reserved for hypercalcemia due to malignant tumors, although its use in other circumstances may sometimes be warranted. The use of this drug almost uniformly causes a reduction in serum calcium during the usual course of its administration. Side effects have varied from mild (nausea and vomiting) to severe (hemorrhagic tendency), depending on dosage and frequency. (*Med Clin North Am*, 56:951, 1972)

35. **True.** Several workers have shown that patients with nonparathyroid hypercalcemia (hypercalcemia due to carcinomatosis, vitamin D overdose, myelomatosis, sarcoidosis, or Paget's disease) have elevated blood pH and metabolic alkalosis and are clearly separable from hyperparathyroid subjects based on the blood pH values. The presence of alkalosis in these subjects is particularly striking inasmuch as they tend to have some degree of renal impairment in which acidosis would be more likely to occur. (*Ann Intern Med*, 76:826, 1972)

36. **True.** On a normal potassium intake of 40 to 100 mEq, the urinary potassium excretion varies between 40 and 90 mEq/24 hours. (*JAMA*, 231:631, 1974)

37. **True.** Patients with gram-negative sepsis who have metabolic acidosis on initial determinations have an extremely poor prognosis which is further worsened if the central venous pressure is low. (4:56)

38. **True.** The seizures associated with alcoholic intoxication, i.e., withdrawal seizures, usually appear within 48 hours after cessation of drinking. (5:847)

39. **True.** Slowly developing changes in the serum potassium level may be compensated by potassium fluxes across the cellular membranes thus maintaining a normal extracellular to intracellular ratio. (*JAMA*, 231:631, 1975)

40. **True.** In most persons, there is a diurnal variation in body temperature of one-half to two degrees. (3:35)

41. **True.** In sarcoidosis, hypercalcemia is generally thought to be due to hypersensitivity to vitamin D. The hypercalcemia, therefore, is presumably due primarily to excessive absorption of calcium from the gastrointestinal tract. (*Med Clin North Am*, 56:941, 1972)

42. **False.** The level of very low-density lipoprotein (VLDL) triglyceride is lowered by a diet restricted in carbohydrates to approximately 40% of the daily calories. (*JAMA*, 233:275, 1975)

43. **False.** The lactate-pyruvate ratio of blood has been closely associated with the state of oxygenation of tissues, being elevated in situations of insufficient oxygenation. (*N Engl J Med*, 283:968, 1970)

44. **True.** Many investigators have documented impaired intestinal absorption of calcium in patients with chronic renal failure. However, it apparently is not an invariable finding and, according to one study, severe uremia may coexist with supernormal calcium absorption. (*Med Clin North Am*, 56:961, 1972)

45. **False.** Thin and obese subjects differ in the extent of their thermogenesis after taking food. In normal subjects, overeating leads to a 25 to 50% increase of heat production which tends to dissipate the excess intake. This energy dissipation is potentiated by exercise in persons with good energy equilibrium. In obese subjects, thermal dissipation of energy is less marked, so that more fat is laid down. (*N Engl J Med*, 291:178, 1974)

46. **E.** A serum potassium of 2.5 to 3.0 mEq/liter suggests that the potassium deficit may be in the range of 300 mEq. (*Ann Intern Med*, 82:64, 1975)

47. **B.** In a normal man fat stores represent 90% of available stored energy, enough to last him for 2 months total starvation.
(*N Engl J Med*, 291:178, 1974)

48. **B.** In normal patients, doing light exercise such as light housework or office work, expends 30 to 35 calories/kg body weight/day. (2:1704)

49. **D.** In a normal 70 kg man, fat comprises 15 to 25% of body weight. (2:1703)

50. **D.** Normal B12 body stores last 3 to 6 years.
(6:1519)

51. **D.** Anion gap may occur with any of the disorders listed. (*Lancet*, 2, 7819:27, 1973)

52. **A.** When dilutional hyponatremia is due to congestive heart failure, cirrhosis of the liver, or myxedema, there is no clear-cut relationship to excessive antidiuretic hormone. All other statements are true. (*Postgrad Med*, 52:232, 1972)

53. **C.** Serum calcium exists in three forms. Approximately 45% occurs as calcium ion. This is the physiologically active portion. Approximately 50% is protein-bound, largely to albumin, and approximately 5% is complexed with citrate and similar ions. In hyperproteinemia such as occurs with sarcoidosis or multiple myeloma, the total plasma calcium may be elevated, largely as a result of an increase in the protein-bound portion. The physiologically active ionized portion, however, may be elevated only minimally with correspondingly mild symptoms. Conversely, hyperparathyroidism may occur with increased ionic calcium, but normal total calcium levels.
(*Int. Cons*, p. 44, June 1972)

54. **A.** Plasma acetone is a crude measure largely of acetoacetic acid. (*JAMA*, 223:1348, 1973)

55. **B.** Hunter's syndrome, or mucopolysaccharidosis II, is the only mucopolysaccharidosis known to be inherited in an X-linked recessive fashion.

This disease is similar to but clinically less severe than classic Hurler's syndrome. (2:2052)

56. **A.** Hypercalciuria occurs in sarcoidosis, but not in tuberculosis. (2:215)

57. **B.** Reduction to ideal body weight is one of the most important factors in successfully treating elevated levels of very low-density lipoprotein triglyceride. On the other hand, low-density lipoprotein cholesterol usually does not respond to weight reduction. (*JAMA*, 233:275, 1975)

58. **E.** All of the endocrine gland disorders listed may be associated with multiple endocrine adenomatosis syndromes.
(*Med Clin North Am*, 56:941, 1972)

59. **E.** Signs of overdose with the drugs listed include coma, pinpoint pupils, slow irregular respiration or apnea, hypotension, hypothermia, or pulmonary edema. Naloxone, given intravenously, has been used in the treatment of such overdoses. (2:712)

60. **E.** Respiratory alkalosis can be produced by all the conditions listed as well as salicylate poisoning, and can cause hyperpnea with stupor or even coma. Central neurogenic hyperventilation may be due to brainstem infarcts or secondary brainstem compression. Sepsis may also cause respiratory alkalosis. (2:1969)

61. **E.** All the findings listed may be associated with protein-calorie deficiency disease. Other findings that may be noted include hair dyspigmentation, thin, sparse hair, moon face, "flaky paint dermatosis," and areas of hyperpigmentation.
(2:1681–83)

62. **B.** (2:1434)

63. **A.** (2:75)

64. **C.** Homocystinuria may be pyridoxine-responsive or pyridoxine-unresponsive. (2:41)

65. **A.** Avitaminosis A results in skin and eye lesions and reduced resistance to infection.
(2:1684–85)

Textbook References for Chapter 14

1. Bannister, Roger (1978): *Brain's Clinical Neurology*, Fifth Edition, Oxford Medical Publications, New York.

2. Beeson, P.B. and McDermott, W. (1979): *Cecil Textbook of Medicine*, Fifteenth Edition, W.B. Saunders Company, Philadelphia.

3. Judge, R.D. and Zuidema, G.D., Editors (1974): *Physical Diagnosis: A Physiologic Approach to the Clinical Examination,* Little, Brown and Company, Boston.

4. Lauler, D.P., Editor-in-Chief (1971): *Gram Negative Sepsis,* Medcom, Incorporated, Clifton, New Jersey.

5. Merritt, H. Houston (1979): *A Textbook of Neurology*, Sixth Edition, Lea and Febiger, Philadelphia.

6. Isselbacher, K.J., Editor (1980): *Harrison's Principles of Internal Medicine*, Ninth Edition, McGraw-Hill Book Company, New York.

CHAPTER 15

Miscellaneous Topics

Directions: For each of the following multiple-choice questions, select the ONE CORRECT answer.

1. The frequency of malignancy with pheochromocytomas is about

   A. less than 1%
   B. 6%
   C. 20%
   D. 40%
   E. over 60%

2. Stomatocytes

   A. are cup- or bowl-shaped erythrocytes
   B. occur in hereditary stomatocytosis, in cation-leaking erythrocytes, and in alcoholic liver disease
   C. cells have central clefts or slits, rather than the normal, round central pallor
   D. all of the above
   E. none of the above

3. Ticks

   A. can be removed by either kerosene or by heat
   B. may cause urticaria
   C. may cause a paralysis which disappears when the tick is removed
   D. all of the above
   E. none of the above

Directions: Indicate whether each of the following statements is true or false.

4. The patient with aortic stenosis tolerates atrial fibrillation surprisingly well.

5. Patients who die from pulmonary embolism usually do so 6 to 12 hours from the appearance of the clinical signs.

6. Prostatic calculi are usually clinically significant.

7. Arsenic is carcinogenic but only in the inorganic form, such as exemplified by Fowler's solution.

8. Experimental evidence suggests that there are antigenic similarities between alveolar and glomerular basement membranes.

9. Blood should always be withdrawn with the aid of a tourniquet if it is being analyzed for serum calcium content.

194 / *Miscellaneous Topics*

Directions: Use the key below to answer questions 10 and 11
- **A. if the statement is characteristic of Type IIa hyperlipoproteinemia**
- **B. if the statement is characteristic of Type IIb hyperlipoproteinemia**

10. Elevation of low-density lipoprotein (LDL) with no elevation of very low-density lipoprotein (VLDL)

11. Elevation of low-density lipoprotein (LDL) and very low-density lipoprotein (VLDL)

Directions: For each of the following questions, select
- **A. if the question is associated with A only**
- **B. if the question is associated with B only**
- **C. if the question is associated with both A and B**
- **D. if the question is associated with neither A nor B**

12. An opacified gallbladder does not prevent the radiologist from obtaining a satisfactory urogram since he can separate the kidney and opacified gallbladder with
    - A. oblique projections
    - B. the use of nephrotomography
    - C. both
    - D. neither

13. Large amounts of potassium are normally excreted through
    - A. sweating
    - B. fecal excretion
    - C. both
    - D. neither

14. Phimosis
    - A. occurs when it is impossible to retract the prepuce
    - B. is usually secondary to recurrent balanoposthitis
    - C. both
    - D. neither

15. Which do not concentrate nuclide on brain scans because of the blood-brain barrier between intracranial vessels and the brain?
    - A. cerebral hemispheres
    - B. cerebellar hemispheres
    - C. both
    - D. neither

Directions: For each of the incomplete statements below, ONE or MORE of the completions given is correct. In each case, select
- **A. if 1, 2, and 3 are correct**
- **B. if 1 and 3 are correct**
- **C. if 2 and 4 are correct**
- **D. if only 4 is correct**
- **E. if all statements are correct**

16. Norepinephrine
    1. will increase coronary flow by beta receptor action
    2. will increase arterial pressure by alpha action
    3. can produce arrhythmias
    4. can produce renal shutdown

17. Intermittent positive pressure breathing may
    1. promote bronchial drainage
    2. open up areas of microatelectasis when present
    3. provide effective breathing exercise
    4. improve alveolar ventilation, increase carbon dioxide elimination, and permit oxygen to be given safely in cases with carbon dioxide retention

18. Production of murmurs is favored by a number of basic factors which tend to promote turbulence, including
    1. lowering the viscosity of the fluid
    2. decreasing the diameter of the tube (vessel)
    3. changing the caliber of a tube abruptly
    4. decreasing the velocity of flow

19. On the normal brain scan, areas of radionuclide concentration include

1. scalp
2. salivary glands
3. choroid plexus
4. temporalis muscle, neck muscle

Directions: For each of the following multiple-choice questions, select the ONE INCORRECT answer.

20. Isoproterenol produces

    A. an increase in sinus heart rate
    B. an increase in force of myocardial contraction
    C. a decrease in atrioventricular conduction velocity
    D. relaxation of bronchial smooth muscle, spleen capsule, gut, and myometrium
    E. increased blood flow in skeleton muscle

21. The alpha receptor is associated with

    A. vasoconstriction
    B. mydriasis
    C. contraction of spleen capsule
    D. contraction of myometrium
    E. contraction of gut

22. In Von Recklinghausen's disease,

    A. neurofibromatosis is based on a genetic defect
    B. neurofibroma are always multiple
    C. lesions are soft and elevated
    D. café au lait spots on the trunk may be present
    E. involvement of the acoustic and other nerves may lead to deafness, paralysis and sensory disturbances

Directions: For each of the incomplete statements below, ONE or MORE of the completions given is correct. In each case, select

    A. if 1, 2, and 3 are correct
    B. if 1 and 3 are correct
    C. if 2 and 4 are correct
    D. if all statements are correct
    E. if all statements are incorrect
    F. if another combination is correct

23. Methysergide therapy has been associated with retroperitoneal fibrosis and other fibrotic lesions involving the

    1. heart valves
    2. lungs
    3. pleura
    4. great vessels

24. Cyclic 3′ 5′-AMP

    1. formed from adenosine triphosphate (ATP) under the induction of the enzyme adenyl cyclase and magnesium ions
    2. mediates the alpha-adrenergic effects on effector tissue
    3. under the influence of phosphodiesterase, is broken down to inactive 5′-AMP
    4. its available level is decreased by methylxanthines which pharmacologically block the action of phosphodiesterase

Directions: Use the key below to answer questions 25 and 26.
    A. **if A is greater than or more appropriate than B**
    B. **if B is greater than or more appropriate than A**
    C. **if A and B are equal or approximately equal**

25. Scrotal hernia
    A. indirect type
    B. direct type

26. Second heart sound results from
    A. aortic and pulmonary valve closure
    B. rapid filling of the ventricles

Directions: Indicate whether each of the following statements is true or false.

27. Care must be exercised when adding calcium to intravenous solutions with other electrolytes such as bicarbonate, since they may precipitate out as the calcium salt.

28. The most effective measure for emergency treatment of heat stroke is to immerse the patient in an ice-water bath.

29. Widened pulse pressure indicates a decrease in cardiac stroke volume.

30. It has become clear that the level of blood pressure is not necessarily an indicator of effective microcirculation; more emphasis must be placed on urinary output and arterial pO_2, which reflect blood flow to very sensitive capillary beds.

Directions: For each of the following statements, fill in the correct answer.

31. Adenyl cyclase is found in all animal cells except the mature _____ .

32. _____ and germinal-cell neoplasms constitute most of the masses that occur in the anterior mediastinum.

33. _____ is a state of masculinization in the female.

Directions: For each of the following questions, select
A. if the question is associated with A only
B. if the question is associated with B only
C. if the question is associated with both A and B
D. if the question is associated with neither A nor B

34. Very low-density lipoprotein (VLDL)

A. elevations are associated with increases of serum triglyceride levels
B. levels, if very high, can elevate serum cholesterol levels because some cholesterol is present in the VLDL molecule
C. both
D. neither

35. Evidence of increased erythrocyte production includes

A. reticulocytosis, usually greater than 5%
B. erythroid hypoplasia of the bone marrow
C. both
D. neither

36. With the use of aspirin, tinnitus and hearing loss are

A. dose-related
B. irreversible
C. both
D. neither

37. Blood pressure is dependent upon

A. cardiac output
B. peripheral vascular resistance
C. both
D. neither

Directions: For each of the incomplete statements below, ONE or MORE of the completions given is correct. In each case, select
A. if 1, 2, and 3 are correct
B. if 1 and 3 are correct
C. if 2 and 4 are correct
D. if only 4 is correct
E. if all statements are correct

38. Hyponatremic patients who are volume-contracted may have

1. diarrhea
2. vomiting
3. been on diuretic therapy
4. Cushing's syndrome

39. Contrast media used for

1. cholecystography require months for elimination because they repeatedly pass through the enterohepatic circulation
2. bronchography are poorly absorbed from the lungs and may release organic iodinated compounds into the blood for years
3. myelograms may persist for years

4. pyelography are eliminated by the kidneys very slowly

40. Stimulators of cyclic AMP accumulation in the cell include

1. prostaglandin E_1 and E_2
2. epinephrine and isoproterenol
3. theophylline
4. propranolol

Directions: For the following multiple-choice questions, select the ONE INCORRECT answer.

41. An estimate of serum osmolality may be obtained by multiplying the serum sodium concentration by 2 and adding 10; this approximation holds true in the absence of significant

A. hyperglycemia
B. azotemia
C. hyperlipemia
D. alkalosis
E. blood alcohol levels

42. Ringer's lactate solution

A. contains 130 mEq/liter sodium
B. contains 4 mEq/liter potassium
C. contains 111 mEq/liter chloride
D. contains 27 mEq/liter lactate which is metabolized to an equivalent amount of bicarbonate
E. is indicated in patients with hyperkalemia, hypercalcemia, and metabolic alkalosis

Directions: Use the key below to answer questions 43 and 44.
A. if the subdivision of the beta adrenergic system causes lipolysis and cardiac stimulation
B. if the subdivision of the beta adrenergic system causes bronchodilation and vasodepression

43. Beta 1

44. Beta 2

Answers and Commentary

1. **B.** The frequency of malignancy with pheochromocytomas is about 6%.
(*N Engl J Med*, 288:1010, 1973)

2. **D.** All statements are true of stomatocytes.
(*Res Staff Phys*, 19:24, 1973)

3. **D.** All statements are true of ticks.
(*Hosp Med*, 7:9, 1971)

4. **False.** The patient with aortic stenosis does not tolerate atrial fibrillation very well because he misses the atrial "kick."
(*Emerg Med*, 5:157, 1973)

5. **False.** Patients who die from pulmonary embolism usually do so within 1 or 2 hours from the appearance of clinical signs.
(*Arch Intern Med*, 133:372, 1974)

6. **False.** Prostatic calculi are seldom of clinical importance. They may often be palpated at rectal examination and mistaken for carcinoma. (1:251)

7. **True.** Arsenic is carcinogenic but only in the inorganic form, such as exemplified by Fowler's solution. (*Hosp Med*, 7:9, 1971)

8. **True.** Experimental evidence suggests that there are antigenic similarities between alveolar and glomerular basement membranes.
(*N Engl J Med*, 286:1166, 1972)

9. **False.** It has been suggested that blood should be withdrawn without the aid of a tourniquet if it is being analyzed for serum calcium. It has been shown that if a tourniquet is applied for 2 min before phlebotomy, an elevation in serum calcium to 12 mg/100 cu ml may occur in normocalcemic subjects. (*Geriatrics*, 27:100, 1972)

10. **A.** (*JAMA*, 233:275, 1975)

11. **B.** (*JAMA*, 233:275, 1975)

12. **C.** An opacified gallbladder does not prevent the radiologist from obtaining a satisfactory urogram since he can separate the kidney and opacified gallbladder with oblique projections and the use of nephrotomography.
(*New Phys*, 20:308, 1972)

13. **D.** Large amounts of potassium are not excreted through sweating or fecal excretion.
(*JAMA*, 231:631, 1975)

14. **C.** Phimosis occurs when it is impossible to retract the prepuce, and is usually secondary to recurrent balanoposthitis. There may be local signs of infection. (1:250)

15. **C.** Neither the cerebral hemispheres nor the cerebellar hemispheres concentrate nuclide on brain scans because of the blood-brain barrier between intracranial vessels and the brain.
(*New Phys*, 21:729, 1973)

16. **E.** All statements are true of norepinephrine.
(*Am Heart J*, 86:149, 1974)

17. **E.** All statements are true of intermittent positive pressure breathing. Additionally it provides a more effective administration and distribution of bronchodilator aerosols, especially in poorly ventilated areas. (*Hosp Med*, 9:8, 1973)

18. **B.** Production of murmurs is favored by a number of basic factors which tend to promote turbulence, including: (1) lowering the viscosity of the fluid, (2) increasing the diameter of a tube, (3) changing the caliber of a tube abruptly, and (4) increasing the velocity of flow. (1:183)

19.   **E.**   All the areas listed are areas of radionuclide concentration on the normal brain scan.
(*New Physician,* 21:729, 1973)

20.   **C.**   Isoproterenol produces an increase in atrioventricular conduction velocity.
(*Am Heart J,* 86:149, 1973)

21.   **E.**   The alpha receptor is associated with relaxation of the gut. All other statements are correct.
(*Am Heart J,* 86:149, 1973)

22.   **B.**   There may be as few as one neurofibroma on the skin in patients with Von Recklinghausen's disease, or there may be literally thousands. In addition, neurofibromas may be found in the bowel, stomach, bladder, kidney, or liver.
(*Hosp Med,* 7:9, 1971)

23.   **D.**   Methysergide therapy has been associated with retroperitoneal fibrosis and other fibrotic lesions involving the heart valves, lungs, pleura, great vessels, and gastrointestinal tract.
(*JAMA,* 213:1571, 1970)

24.   **B.**   Cyclic 3'5'-AMP mediates beta-adrenergic effects on effector tissue and its available level is increased by methylxanthines which pharmacologically block the action of phosphodiesterase.
(*CIBA Clin Symposia,* 27:27, 1975)

25.   **A.**   The scrotal hernia is an inguinal hernia, almost always of the indirect type, and of sufficient size to permit the hernial sac and its contents to enter the scrotum together with the contents of the spermatic cord.
(1:255)

26.   **A.**   The second heart sound results from aortic and pulmonary valve closure.
(1:162)

27.   **True.**   Care must be exercised when adding calcium to intravenous solutions with other electrolytes such as bicarbonate, since they may precipitate out as the calcium salt.
(*Ann Int Med,* 82:64, 1975)

28.   **True.**   Because the pathogenesis of heat stroke involves failure of the heat-regulating mechanism with cessation of sweating, external means of heat dissipation must be employed. The most effective measure is to immerse the patient in an ice-water bath.
(3:57)

29.   **False.**   Widened pulse pressure indicates an increase in cardiac stroke volume.
(2:103)

30.   **True.**   It has become clear that the level of blood pressure is not necessarily an indicator of effective microcirculation. More emphasis must be placed on urinary output and arterial pO_2 which reflect blood flow to very sensitive capillary beds.
(2:96)

31.   **Erythrocyte.**   Adenyl cyclase is found in all animal cells except the mature erythrocyte.
(*Curr Med Digest,* 39:1117, 1972)

32.   **Thymomas.**   Thymomas and germinal-cell neoplasms constitute most of the masses that occur in the anterior mediastinum.
(*Hosp Practice,* 8:104, 1973)

33.   **Virilism.**   Virilism is a state of masculinization in the female.
(1:40)

34.   **C.**   Both statements are true of very low-density lipoprotein (VLDL).
(*JAMA,* 233:275, 1975)

35.   **A.**   Evidence of increased erythrocyte production includes reticulocytosis, usually greater than 5% and erythroid hyperplasia of the bone marrow.
(*Res Staff Phys,* 18:35, 1972)

36.   **A.**   With the use of aspirin, tinnitus and hearing loss are dose-related and completely reversible.
(*Res Staff Phys,* 18:35, 1972)

37.   **C.**   Blood pressure is dependent upon cardiac output and peripheral vascular resistance.
(2:96)

38.   **A.**   Hyponatremic patients who are volume-contracted may have diarrhea and vomiting. Some patients on diuretic therapy, especially the overdiuresed, and patients with Addison's disease may also fit into this category.
(*Patient Care,* 9:22, 1975)

39.   **A.**   Pyelographic contrast media are rapidly eliminated by the kidneys. All other statements are correct.
(*AFP,* 3:73, 1971)

40.   **A.**   Prostaglandin E_1, prostaglandin E_2, epinephrine, isoproterenol, and theophylline are all stimulators of cyclic AMP accumulation in the cell.
(*Ann Intern Med,* 78:401, 1973)

41.   **D.**   Serum osmolality may be estimated by multiplying the serum sodium concentration by 2 and adding 10. This approximation holds true in the absence of significant hyperglycemia, azotemia, hyperlipemia or blood alcohol levels. Because of the prevalence of drinking, alcohol may be the commonest cause of hyperosmolality.
(*Med Challenge,* p. 29, Nov 1975)

42.   **E.**   Ringer's lactate solution is contraindicated in patients with hyperkalemia, hypercalcemia and

metabolic alkalosis; one should be reluctant to use it in treating hyponatremia. It more closely resembles the normal composition of extracellular fluid volume than does saline. All other statements are correct. (*Ann Intern Med,* 82:64, 1975)

43. **A.**   (*J Allergy,* 49:142, 1972)

44. **B.**   (*J Allergy,* 49:142, 1972)

Textbook References for Chapter 15

1. Judge, R.D. and Zuidema, G.D., Editors (1974): *Physical Diagnosis: A Physiologic Approach to the Clinical Examination,* Little, Brown and Company, Boston.

2. Lauler, D.P., Editor-in-Chief (1971): *Gram Negative Sepsis,* Medcom, Incorporated, Clifton, New Jersey.

3. Isselbacher, K.J., Editor (1980): *Harrison's Principles of Internal Medicine,* Ninth Edition, McGraw-Hill Book Company, New York.

CHAPTER 16

Musculoskeletal System

Directions: For each of the following multiple-choice questions, select the ONE CORRECT answer.

1. Vitamin D therapy in high doses is contraindicated in osteitis fibrosa because

    A. it has little beneficial effect on symptoms
    B. it actually increases bone resorption
    C. there is a risk of metastatic calcification
    D. all of the above
    E. none of the above

2. Thyrotoxic myopathy

    A. involves weakness and wasting especially of the proximal muscles of the limbs and the trunk muscles
    B. is associated with increased tendon reflexes
    C. should not be expected to disappear when the thyroid condition is treated
    D. all of the above
    E. none of the above

3. Muscular disorders responsible for facial paralysis include

    A. myasthenia gravis
    B. muscular dystrophy
    C. dystrophia myotonica

    D. all of the above
    E. none of the above

Directions: For each of the incomplete statements below, ONE or MORE of the completions given is correct. In each case, select
    A. if 1, 2, and 3 are correct
    B. if 1 and 3 are correct
    C. if 2 and 4 are correct
    D. if only 4 is correct
    E. if all statements are correct

4. Skeletal syndromes associated with hyperparathyroidism include

    1. bone cysts (brown tumor)
    2. chondrocalcinosis
    3. osteitis fibrosa cystica
    4. osteoporosis

5. Osteomalacia is associated with

    1. malabsorption syndrome
    2. normal or low serum calcium
    3. depressed serum phosphate
    4. normal serum alkaline phosphatase

6. Osteolytic lesions can be produced by

    1. almost any type of aggressive neoplasia
    2. tumors in the upper respiratory tract
    3. tumors in the lung
    4. tumors in the thyroid gland and breast

201

Directions: Use the key below to answer questions 7 and 8.
A. if A is greater than or more appropriate than B
B. if B is greater than or more appropriate than A
C. if A and B are equal or approximately equal

7. A vertebral body fracture is most conspicuous on

    A. lateral x-rays
    B. anteroposterior x-rays

8. Fasciculation is likely caused by a lesion of

    A. anterior horn cells
    B. anterior root

Directions: Indicate whether each of the following statements is true or false.

9. A subluxation is a partial dislocation of one bone from the articular surface of its partner.

10. Dislocation of the shoulder joint decreases the overall length of the limb.

11. In hyperthyroidism, muscle involvement may take the form of myopathy, or very rarely, myasthenia or periodic paralysis.

12. There is increased lactate accumulation in subjects with hereditary muscle phosphorylase deficiency.

13. Patients with hyperparathyroidism usually show increased bone turnover, as evidenced by a more rapid disappearance of bone-seeking isotopes after intravenous injection.

Directions: Use the key below to answer questions 14 through 17.
A. if the position described is a heel in varus
B. if the position described is a heel in valgus

14. The axis of the heel is tilted away from the midline of the body

15. The heel is tilted toward the midline of the body

16. Associated with club foot and cavus foot

17. Associated with flat feet

Directions: Use the key below to answer questions 18 and 19.
A. if the statement defines sprain
B. if the statement defines strain

18. A total tear or avulsion

19. Stretch or partial tear

Directions: For each of the incomplete statements below, ONE or MORE of the completions given is correct. In each case, select
A. if 1, 2, and 3 are correct
B. if 1 and 3 are correct
C. if 2 and 4 are correct
D. if all statements are correct
E. if all statements are incorrect
F. if another combination is correct

20. Paget's disease of the bone

    1. is estimated to involve 3% of subjects over 40 years of age
    2. may disseminate widely and produce severe skeletal deformities, neurologic deficits, deafness, and congestive heart failure
    3. has been shown to be consistently suppressed by mithramycin as reflected by changes in serum alkaline phosphatase and urinary hydroxyproline levels, and the occurrence of symptomatic relief
    4. is rarely asymptomatic

21. McArdle's disease

    1. is a rare, genetically determined, recessive disorder
    2. is associated with intermittent muscular weakness, pain, and stiffness particularly following exercise

3. following arm exercise with a cuff occluding the arterial circulation, the normal rise in blood pyruvate and lactate do not occur
4. is characterized by an excess of muscle phosphorylase

22. The principal causes of muscular hypertonia include
1. neural shock, either cerebral or spinal
2. lesions of the cerebellum
3. chorea
4. lower motor neuron lesions

23. Fasciculation
1. is seen in its most characteristic form as the result of degeneration of motor ganglion cells in motor neuron disease
2. does not occur when the cells of the motor neurons are rapidly injured or destroyed, as in the acute stage of poliomyelitis
3. is often seen in some muscles of the upper limbs in patients with cervical myelopathy due to spondylosis
4. may be observed in some cases of polymyositis and in thyrotoxic myopathy and may occur as the result of a lesion of a spinal anterior root; e.g., in a limb when the relevant root is compressed by an intervertebral disc protrusion

24. In lead neuropathy,
1. there is predilection for the motor fibers of the nerves supplying the muscles most used in an occupation
2. there is usually wrist- and finger-drop
3. deterioration of the anterior horn cells and degeneration of the corticospinal tracts may occur
4. involvement of the lower limbs is common

25. Physiologically, as is best seen in the case of a partial or progressive upper motor neuron lesion,

1. it becomes more difficult to move a segment of the limb in isolation, so that in any attempted movement the limb tends to move as a whole
2. it is the less voluntary and the less skilled movements which suffer most
3. muscular tone is characteristically increased, the tendon reflexes are exaggerated, clonus is often present, and if the upper motor neurons concerned in movement of the lower limb are involved, the corresponding plantar reflex is extensor
4. emotional movement of the face is more impaired than voluntary movement

Directions: For each of the following statements, fill in the correct answer.

26. _____ fracture is a generic term for ankle fractures in general.

27. In renal failure severe hypocalcemia, if unresponsive to a decrease in serum phosphorus, suggests _____ .

28. Conspicuous muscular wasting sometimes occurs, especially in the upper limb, as the result of a lesion of the opposite parietal lobe causing sensory loss of the cortical type. This is sometimes called " _____ wasting."

29. A swelling over the medial aspect of the metatarsophalangeal joint of the great toe is termed a _____ and may be associated with a medial deviation of more than 15 degrees when compared with the lateral four metatarsals (metatarsus primus varus), or with lateral deviation of the great toe (hallux valgus).

30. The term hereditary paramyotonia describes a hereditary disorder characterized by the occurrence of myotonia only when the sufferer is exposed to _____ .

Directions: For each of the following multiple-choice questions, select the ONE INCORRECT answer.

31. Hypercalcemia secondary to increased bone resorption occurs with

    A. hyperparathyroidism
    B. hyperthyroidism
    C. immobilization
    D. neoplasia
    E. sarcoidosis

32. In dystrophia myotonica,

    A. muscular dystrophy, myotonia, and other dystrophic disturbances, especially cataract and gonadal atrophy can be present
    B. symptoms of the fully developed form of the disorder usually first appear between the ages of 15 and 40
    C. muscular weakness or myotonia is usually the first symptom noted
    D. muscular wasting is most conspicuous in the facial muscles, the sternocleidomastoids, the muscles of the shoulder girdle, forearms and hands, the quadriceps, and the legs
    E. affected families have normal intelligence

33. Pseudohypertrophic muscular dystrophy

    A. is the commonest variety
    B. usually appears in about the middle of the first decade of life
    C. affects females more frequently than males
    D. involves some muscles which are palpably enlarged due to an excess of fat
    E. causes the proximal muscles of the limbs to be more liable to waste than the distal ones, and wasting is almost always present in the sternal part of the pectoralis major and latissimus dorsi

Directions: For each of the following questions, select
    A. if the question is associated with A only
    B. if the question is associated with B only
    C. if the question is associated with both A and B
    D. if the question is associated with neither A nor B

34. Von Graefe's sign

    A. is characterized by lag of the upper lid in following the downward movement of the eye
    B. is seen in hypothyroidism
    C. both
    D. neither

35. Administration of large amounts of vitamin D in the treatment of renal osteodystrophy may

    A. result in hypocalcemia
    B. be associated with severe metastatic calcification
    C. both
    D. neither

36. Radiographic examination of bone can make the diagnosis of hyperparathyroidism more accurate. In the phalanges, characteristic subperiosteal resorption proximally and loss of tufts distally may be demonstrated more often by special radiographic techniques. A ground-glass appearance in the skull with loss of definition of the tables and loss of lamina dura around the teeth are characteristic but less frequently seen. A combination of these lesions with bone cysts is diagnostic of

    A. primary hyperparathyroidism
    B. secondary hyperparathyroidism
    C. both
    D. neither

Directions: For each of the following statements, fill in the correct answer.

37. A fracture which might be defined as Colles' fracture, except that the distal radial fragment is tilted toward the volar rather than the dorsal side, is called a _____ fracture.

38. Subluxation of an upper vertebra on a lower one is best seen in a _____ projection of the cervical spine in a neutral or forward flexed position.

39. _____ is the name for a rotated attitude of the head brought about by clonic or tonic contraction of the cervical muscles.

Answers and Commentary

1. **D.** Vitamin D therapy in high doses is contraindicated in osteitis fibrosa due to all the reasons listed. (*Med Clin North Am*, 56:961, 1972)

2. **A.** The tendon reflexes in patients with thyrotoxic myopathy are diminished, and the disorder may be expected to disappear when the thyroid condition is treated. (1:386)

3. **D.** All the muscular disorders listed may be responsible for facial paralysis. (1:55)

4. **E.** All the skeletal syndromes listed, as well as pathologic fractures, have been associated with hyperparathyroidism. (*Med Clin North Am*, 56:941, 1972)

5. **A.** Osteomalacia is associated with elevated serum alkaline phosphatase. The other disorders listed may be associated with this condition. (*N Engl J Med*, 281:1115, 1969)

6. **E.** Osteolytic lesions can be produced by any of the disorders listed. (*N Engl J Med*, 281:1120, 1969)

7. **A.** A vertebral body fracture is usually caused by compression forces, and the consequent reduction in height of the involved vertebral body is most conspicuous on lateral x-rays. (2:327)

8. **A.** Involvement of the anterior horn cells leads to the symptoms of a lower motor neuron lesion identical with those of a lesion of an anterior spinal root, except that a progressive lesion of the anterior horn cells is more likely to cause fasciculation in the muscles innervated than an anterior root lesion. (1:309)

9. **True.** A subluxation is a partial dislocation. Contact between the articular surfaces is less than normal. (2:324)

10. **False.** Dislocation of some joints, such as the shoulder, increases the overall length of the limb. (2:324)

11. **True.** In hyperthyroidism, muscle involvement may take the form of myopathy, or very rarely, myasthenia or periodic paralysis. (*Br Med J, 2*, 5810:399, 1972)

12. **False.** Defective glycogenolysis due to hereditary muscle phosphorylase deficiency can produce muscle cramping early in brisk exercise, and can even result in muscle damage as reflected by myoglobinemia and myoglobinuria. However, if the exercise is gradually increased, oxygen and free fatty acid utilization can be accelerated, and eventually, strong exercise can be done by individuals with this rare disorder in glycogen metabolism. Obviously, there is no lactate accumulation in affected subjects. (3:504)

13. **True.** Hyperparathyroid patients usually will show increased bone turnover, as evidenced by a more rapid disappearance of bone-seeking isotopes after intravenous injection. This effect also occurs in other disorders including hyperthyroidism, osteomalacia, and Paget's disease. Bone biopsies normally show an increased number of osteoclasts, an increased resorptive surface on microradiography, and certain biochemical changes (but these changes may also occur in osteoporosis, osteomalacia, and cancer). (*N Engl J Med*, 285:1006, 1971)

14. **B.** (2:299)

15. **A.** (2:299)

16. **A.** (2:299)

17. **B.** (2:299)

18. **B.** (2:325)

19. **A.** (2:325)

20. **A.** Paget's disease of the bone is commonly asymptomatic. All other statements are correct. (*JAMA*, 213:1153, 1970)

21. **A.** The chief interest in McArdle's disease arises from the fact that the biochemical defect has actually been demonstrated and is the result of a deficiency of muscle phosphorylase which is necessary for the breakdown of glycogen. All other statements are true of this rare condition. (1:386–87)

22. **D.** All the disorders listed are principal causes of muscular hypertonia. Also included are lesions involving the sensory afferents and primary degeneration of the muscles themselves. (1:80)

23. **D.** All statements are true of fasciculation. (1:89)

24. **A.** Lead neuropathy usually affects the extensor muscles of the wrist and fingers, bilaterally, causing wrist- and finger-drop, the brachioradialis escaping. An upper arm type of paralysis involves the spinati, deltoid, biceps, brachialis, and brachioradialis muscles. Involvement of the lower limbs is rare. There is no sensory loss. All other statements are true. (1:374)

25. **B.** In upper motor neuron lesions, it is the more voluntary and the more skilled movements which suffer most, while the less voluntary and less skilled are relatively spared. Thus the voluntary movement of the face is more impaired than emotional movement, and the finer movements of the fingers than the grosser movements of the shoulder and elbow. Though disuse may lead to a little loss of volume in the affected muscles, conspicuous wasting does not occur after an upper motor neuron lesion. All other statements are true. (1:93)

26. **Pott's.** Pott's fracture is a generic term for ankle fractures in general. (2:337)

27. **Osteomalacia.** In renal failure severe hypocalcemia, if unresponsive to a decrease in serum phosphorus, suggests osteomalacia. (*Med Clin North Am*, 56:961, 1972)

28. **Parietal.** Conspicuous muscular wasting sometimes occurs, especially in the upper limb, as the result of a lesion of the opposite parietal lobe causing sensory loss of the cortical type. This is sometimes called "parietal wasting." (1:207)

29. **Bunion.** A swelling over the medial aspect of the metatarsophalangeal joint of the great toe is termed a bunion and may be associated with a medial deviation of more than 15 degrees when compared with the lateral four metatarsals (metatarsus primus varus), or with lateral deviation of the great toe (hallux valgus). (2:299)

30. **Cold.** The term hereditary paramyotonia describes a hereditary disorder characterized by the occurrence of myotonia only when the sufferer is exposed to cold. (1:384)

31. **E.** Hypercalcemia secondary to increased bone resorption may occur in hyperparathyroidism, hyperthyroidism, immobilization (particularly with Paget's disease) and in neoplastic states. (*Hosp Physician*, 10:71, 1974)

32. **E.** Low intelligence and mental subnormality are common in families affected by dystrophia myotonica. All other statements are true. (1:382–84)

33. **C.** Pseudohypertrophic muscular dystrophy may occur sporadically or affect several siblings, and males suffer very much more frequently than females. All other statements are true of this disorder. In addition, tendon reflexes are diminished and ultimately lost. (1:381–82)

34. **A.** Lag of the upper lid in following the downward movement of the eye is known as von Graefe's sign. The common cause of lid retraction is thyrotoxicosis, but it is occasionally a symptom of organic nervous disease, such as tabes or Parkinsonism. (1:37)

35. **B.** Hypercalcemia and severe metastatic calcification have been reported when large amounts of vitamin D have been used in the treatment of renal osteodystrophy. (*Lancet, 1,* 7815:1273, 1973)

36. **C.** A combination of the radiographic lesions listed, as well as bone cysts, is diagnostic of either primary or secondary hyperparathyroidism. (*N Engl J Med*, 285:1006, 1971)

37. **Smith's.** A fracture which might be defined as a Colles' fracture, except that the distal radial fragment is tilted toward the volar rather than the dorsal side, is called a Smith's fracture. (2:337)

38. **Lateral.** Subluxation of an upper vertebra on a lower one is best seen in a lateral projection of the cervical spine in a neutral or forward flexed position. (2:327)

39. **Torticollis.** Torticollis is the name of a rotated attitude of the head brought about by clonic or tonic contraction of the cervical muscles. (1:300)

Textbook References for Chapter 16

1. Bannister, Roger (1978): *Brain's Clinical Neurology*, Fifth Edition, Oxford Medical Publications, New York.

2. Judge, R.D. and Zuidema, G.D., Editors, (1974): *Physical Diagnosis: A Physiologic Approach to the Clinical Examination*, Little, Brown and Company, Boston.

3. Isselbacher, K.J., Editor (1980): *Harrison's Principles of Internal Medicine*, Ninth Edition, McGraw-Hill Book Company, New York.

CHAPTER 17

Nephrology

Directions: For each of the following multiple-choice questions, select the ONE CORRECT answer.

1. The main cause of renal failure in children as well as young and middle-aged adults is

    A. pyelonephritis
    B. glomerulonephritis
    C. polycystic disease
    D. renal vascular disease
    E. drug nephropathy

2. Glomerular filtration rate at the age of 60 is about what percentage of the normal observed in young adults?

    A. 10%
    B. 30%
    C. 50%
    D. 70%
    E. 90%

3. Associated with decreased potassium excretion is/are

    A. alkalosis
    B. decreased total body potassium content
    C. increased sodium delivery to the distal tubule
    D. mineralocorticoid excess
    E. all of the above

4. To cause shock, the magnitude of volume deficit must be in excess of what percentage of the blood volume?

    A. 2%
    B. 5%
    C. 10%
    D. 15%
    E. over 20–30%

5. About what percentage of calcium stones, usually oxalate, are formed without elevation of serum or urine calcium (idiopathic)?

    A. 10%
    B. 30%
    C. 50%
    D. 70%
    E. 90%

6. Duration of action of furosemide is

    A. 1 to 3 hours
    B. 3 to 5 hours
    C. 6 to 8 hours
    D. 9 to 12 hours
    E. 15 hours

Directions: For each of the following multiple-choice questions, select the ONE INCORRECT answer.

7. Characteristics of idiopathic hypercalciuria include

A. normal serum calcium
B. serum phosphorus sometimes depressed
C. increased intestinal absorption of calcium
D. abnormal bones
E. a tendency, when calcium intake is raised to about 800 to 1000 mg, for calcium excretion to rise more precipitously than in normal subjects

8. Conditions causing increased blood lactate and pyruvate with a normal lactate/pyruvate ratio include

   A. hypoventilation
   B. bicarbonate administration
   C. infusion of pyruvate
   D. infusion of lactate
   E. infusion of glucose

9. Neurological manifestations of uremia include

   A. respiratory asterixis
   B. myoclonic muscle spasm
   C. involuntary muscle twitching
   D. choreoathetoid movements
   E. seizures

10. Chronic interstitial nephritis due to lead toxicity is associated with

    A. glycosuria, aminoaciduria, proteinuria, and cylindruria
    B. increased excretion of lead, delta-aminolevulinic acid, coproporphyrin, and urobilinogen
    C. hypertension and hyperuricemia, rarely
    D. intranuclear inclusion bodies in tubular cells which may be seen in the urine sediment
    E. tubular degeneration, calcification, and interstitial nephritis, which are sometimes accompanied by nonspecific vascular disease, resulting in renal failure

11. Causes of glomerular proteinuria include

    A. immune complexes
    B. sarcoidosis

C. antiglomerular basement membrane antibodies
D. deposition of abnormal material as in amyloidosis or diabetes mellitus
E. pyelonephritis

12. Uremic myocardiopathy with acute, extreme dilatation of the heart

    A. may occur in association with pleurisy and pericarditis, especially in patients with accelerated hypertension
    B. can be distinguished from pericardial tamponade by radioisotope or sonar scanning techniques
    C. responds well to digitalization
    D. responds well to intensive hemodialysis
    E. responds well to ultrafiltration

13. Classical renal tubular acidosis is

    A. proximal
    B. characterized by inability to establish a hydrogen ion (pH) gradient across the epithelium of the distal nephron
    C. characterized by urine that is inappropriately alkaline (5.5) for any level of plasma pH and bicarbonate concentration
    D. primary or secondary due to hyperglobulinemia, amphotericin B toxicity, or hypercalcemia
    E. characterized by urinary bicarbonate wastage, which is minimal, and hypokalemia, which is common, and responds well to alkali therapy because daily acid accumulation is not massive

14. Hypomagnesemia and tissue magnesium depletion may occur in

    A. steatorrhea
    B. malnutrition
    C. alcoholism
    D. chronic diuretic use
    E. chronic constipation

15. In Goodpasture's syndrome,

    A. patients usually present with hemoptysis, pallor, and anemia

B. microscopic or gross hematuria may be a presenting symptom

C. kidneys are large, soft, and pale

D. basement membrane are present as is a linear pattern of deposition of immune globulin and complement on the glomerular basement membrane

E. the course is characteristically slow with a good prognosis

16. Thyrocalcitonin

A. is secreted by the parafollicular cells of the parathyroid gland

B. inhibits bone resorption when the latter is stimulated by vitamin D, parathyroid hormone or vitamin A, which lowers serum calcium and urinary hydroxyproline excretion

C. since it is stimulated by high levels of calcium and magnesium, appears to serve as a counterregulatory hormone

D. tends to normalize serum calcium and inhibit abnormal bone resorption

E. increases sodium, phosphate, calcium, and magnesium excretion

17. Cardinal clinical features of cystic disease of the renal medulla include

A. anemia

B. urinary tract infection

C. marked urinary abnormalities

D. "renal salt wasting"

E. progressive uremia

18. "Pseudoaldosteronism" is associated with

A. high blood pressure

B. low plasma renin

C. high adrenal secretory rates of aldosterone

D. normal or hyperplastic adrenal glands

E. hypertension which is cured by bilateral adrenalectomy

19. Syndrome of inappropriate secretion of antidiuretic hormone (SIADH)

A. results either from sustained, uncontrolled release of ADH from the neu-

rohypophysis or from the synthesis or secretion of ADH-like substances by neoplastic or infected tissue

B. manifests hyponatremia as the consequence of water retention due to sustained ADH activity

C. is characterized by urine that is often hypertonic to plasma; but even though its tonicity may occasionally be somewhat lower than plasma, it is still higher than is appropriate for the level of hyponatremia

D. is characterized by urine sodium concentration of less than 30 mEq/liter

E. is characterized by absence of clinical dehydration and edema

20. In diabetes mellitus with renal involvement,

A. proteinuria may be marked

B. there may be diffuse glomerulosclerosis or nodular glomerulosclerosis or both

C. there is no known therapy

D. electron microscopy shows an increase in mesangial matrix and thickening of the basement membrane

E. immunofluorescence findings are specific

21. Patients with staghorn calculi

A. are usually male

B. always have infected urine

C. have a continual loss of renal parenchyma

D. have gradually deteriorating renal function

Directions: Indicate whether each statement is true or false.

22. Patients with the syndrome of inappropriate ADH usually have decreased creatinine clearances.

23. Hypercalciuria in excess of 500 mg/24 hours is common in hyperparathyroidism.

24. Severe secondary hyperparathyroidism may lead to raised serum calcium in a minority of patients with chronic renal failure.

25. Acute acidosis stimulates tubular potassium secretion.

26. Patients in shock frequently have metabolic (lactic) acidosis which is usually reversed by volume replacement.

27. The position, shape, and size of kidneys can often be determined on the plain film of the abdomen.

28. Renal artery stenosis does not occur in normotensive patients.

29. Patients with lipoid nephrosis generally excrete more high-molecular weight proteins.

30. In anti-glomerular-basement-membrane-antibody disease, there is a completely continuous (linear) accumulation of immunoglobulins and complement along the basement membrane.

31. The protein fractional curve in tubular proteinuria differs from glomerular proteinuria in that larger quantities of low-molecular weight proteins appear in the urine along with small amounts of albumin.

32. Generally, metabolic alkalosis responds well to therapy with saline solutions.

33. In renal disease, the capacity of the kidney to lower urinary pH to less than 6.0 is lost early.

34. It is uncommon for lactic acidosis to be associated with diabetic ketoacidosis.

35. Azotemia induced by diuretics is irreversible.

36. Inhibition of amino acid absorption may account for the aminoaciduria accompanying the secondary hyperparathyroidism of vitamin D deficiency.

37. In polycystic disease of the kidney, a salt loss tendency with dehydration and hyponatremia is rarely found.

38. A pure lipoid nephrosis may occur with lymphomas, as in Hodgkin's disease, and radiation therapy of the latter may result in a dramatic response of the nephrosis.

Directions: For each of the incomplete statements below, ONE or MORE of the numbered completions is correct. In each case, select
  A. **if 1, 2, and 3 are correct**
  B. **if 1 and 3 are correct**
  C. **if 2 and 4 are correct**
  D. **if only 4 is correct**
  E. **if all statements are correct**

39. Hemodialysis
    1. restores calcium and phosphorus homeostasis to normal
    2. abolishes vitamin D resistance
    3. corrects gastrointestinal absorption of calcium
    4. alleviates uremic symptoms

40. Decreased nerve conduction velocity in uremia
    1. usually starts symmetrically in the lower extremities
    2. usually spares the autonomic nervous system
    3. is associated with "restless leg syndrome" and paresthesias of the feet, followed by sensory loss, loss of stretch reflexes, motor loss, and atrophy of distal muscles
    4. is always associated with neurologic symptoms

41. Intraluminal causes of obstructive uropathy include

    1. stone
    2. bladder and ureteral tumors
    3. papillary necrosis (diabetes)
    4. clot

42. In minimal change glomerular disease,

    1. the most common first symptom is edema which develops insidiously and often reaches mammoth proportions
    2. characteristics of the nephrotic syndrome may be present, including: heavy proteinuria (more than 5 g/day), hypoalbuminemia, and usually hypercholesterolemia
    3. the plasma urea and creatinine are usually normal
    4. when given steroids, most patients rapidly lose their proteinuria and all other signs

43. A palpable mass in the renal area may be produced by

    1. neoplasm
    2. hydronephrosis
    3. polycystic kidney
    4. perinephric abscess

44. Causes of hyperchloremic acidosis include

    1. disorders causing the Fanconi syndrome
    2. medullary cystic disease
    3. amphotericin B toxicity
    4. systemic lupus erythematosus and other hyperglobulinemias

45. Renal vein thrombosis

    1. may follow thrombosis of the aorta, renal artery, and pulmonary arteries
    2. may result in thromboembolism of the pulmonary artery
    3. can result in heavy proteinemia and a nephrotic syndrome
    4. pathological changes include thickening of the basement membrane, prominent margination of polymorphonuclear leukocytes in the capillaries, and marked interstitial edema

46. Renal failure in multiple myeloma is often preceded by

    1. dehydration
    2. renal infection
    3. nephrotic syndrome
    4. hypocalcemia

47. Viruses implicated in human immune complex nephritis include those of

    1. measles
    2. mumps
    3. hepatitis
    4. common cold

48. In chronic interstitial nephritis due to obstructive uropathy,

    1. tubular abnormalities such as impaired salt and water conservation may occur
    2. hyperchloremic acidosis may be present
    3. urea retention may be disproportionate to creatinemia
    4. it only occurs with infection

49. "Benign" hematuria with focal glomerulitis is associated with

    1. recurrent or persistent hematuria with red cell casts, minimal proteinuria, and normal renal function
    2. adults are more commonly affected than children
    3. kidneys that show minimal local, focal proliferative changes
    4. hypertension in the majority of cases

50. Causes of hypertension and hypokalemia include

    1. primary aldosteronism
    2. renal artery stenosis
    3. ACTH-secreting carcinomas
    4. adrenal hypersecretion of other mineralocorticoids (deoxycorticosterone, corticosterone)

51. Important causes of partial nephrogenic diabetes insipidus and hypertonic dehydration include

    1. hypocalcemia
    2. hypercalcemia

3. hyperkalemia
4. hypokalemia

52. Weak diuretics include

    1. spironolactone
    2. ethacrynic acid
    3. triamterene
    4. furosemide

53. In hereditary nephritis,

    1. there is neurosensory hearing impairment
    2. sex distribution is approximately equal
    3. pathologic changes may resemble chronic glomerulonephritis or chronic pyelonephritis
    4. renal failure occurs more often in females

54. Nephrotic syndrome refers to the clinical association of

    1. heavy proteinuria
    2. hypoalbuminemia
    3. generalized edema
    4. hypertension and azotemia

55. Renovascular hypertension differs from essential hypertension in that

    1. it is likely to be of shorter duration
    2. obesity is uncommon
    3. hypokalemia and bacteriuria are more common
    4. it is more frequent in the black population

56. Bartter's syndrome is associated with

    1. renal potassium wastage
    2. hypokalemic metabolic alkalosis
    3. variably elevated aldosterone secretory rates and plasma renin levels
    4. high blood pressure

57. Causes of hypercalcemia include

    1. hyperthyroidism
    2. metastatic breast cancer
    3. Paget's disease
    4. thiazide diuretics

58. Medullary sponge kidney

    1. is usually symptomatic
    2. may be discovered radiographically
    3. frequently causes renal failure
    4. may be discovered because of nephrolithiasis, hematuria, or renal infection

Directions: Use the key below to answer questions 59 to 61.
    A. if the disease is induced by sulfonamides
    B. if the disease is induced by penicillamine
    C. if the disease is induced by probenecid

59. Immune-complex glomerulonephritis

60. Allergic vasculitis

61. Minimal change disease

Directions: Indicate whether each of the following statements is true or false.

62. Hypercalcemia results in deficits of body sodium and water which, unless corrected, reduce urinary calcium excretion, exaggerate the hypercalcemia, and increase the propensity for systemic toxicity and renal damage.

63. When analgesic nephropathy is detected and the offending drugs, especially those containing phenacetin, are discontinued, the disease will usually stabilize or improve, provided renal failure is not too far advanced.

64. In the nephrotic syndrome, hypovolemia secondary to hypoalbuminemia may produce a sharp decline in renal function which is potentially reversible.

65. Repeated finding of pure cultures of organisms in properly collected urine when associated with relevant symptoms or urinary sediment abnormalities signifies infection only if greater than 10^5 organisms/ml urine are cultured.

66. The predominant factor influencing survival in malignant hypertension has been the status of renal function at the time of diagnosis.

67. In ischemic renal tubular injury, observed structural changes far exceed the functional loss.

68. A majority of patients with lipoid nephrosis develop focal glomerulosclerosis.

69. In uncomplicated cases of acute tubular necrosis in which there is no serious underlying disease and treatment is optimal, survival rates in excess of 70 to 80% are common.

70. A dilute urine with clinical dehydration suggests impairment in renal function.

71. Symptomatic bone disease during the early stages of renal insufficiency (GFR 20 to 60 ml/min/1.73 sq m) is rare except in patients with long-standing acidosis due to chronic pyelonephritis or to inherited forms of renal disease, such as the various syndromes of renal tubular insufficiency, renal tubular acidosis, and medullary cystic disease.

72. When magnesium ammonium phosphate hexahydrate (triple phosphate, struvite) occurs in kidney stones, it is the hallmark of alkaline (urea-splitting) infection.

73. In acute renal failure, the survival rate is increased by dialysis to hold the BUN to below 100 mg% and allow a higher protein intake which may enhance regeneration.

74. Acute renal failure, an abrupt loss of renal function, most often results from toxic or ischemic injury to the renal tubules, which usually show overt necrosis.

75. The minority of uric acid stones occur in pure form.

76. During the oliguric phase of ischemic renal tubular injury, increased fibrin degradation products are found in the blood, suggesting a possible role of intravascular coagulation in tubular necrosis.

77. Hyponatremia may be viewed basically as an abnormality in the renal excretion of (electrolyte-free) water.

78. Thiazide diuretics are of considerable value in patients with renal insufficiency.

79. Chronic renal failure is a likely sequel to acute pyelonephritis.

80. Triamterene depends on the presence of mineralocorticoids for its action.

81. Ionizing radiation exceeding 1000 rads may cause chronic interstitial nephritis with anemia, proteinuria, renal failure, and hypertension, which may occasionally be malignant.

82. Clinically, hypernatremia is commonly associated with sodium depletion and hypovolemia.

83. Marked elevations of serum cholesterol are more common in lupus erythematosus than in other forms of nephrotic syndrome.

84. In multiple myeloma, tubular atrophy favors urinary excretion of filterable low molecular weight proteins, kappa chains or Bence Jones proteins, while renal failure favors their accumulation in plasma.

85. The most important factor in treatment of nephrotic syndrome is the proper use of diuretics.

86. In acute renal failure, mannitol infusion has rarely restored renal function, even when administered during or immediately after a renal insult.

Directions: For each of the following incomplete statements, select
- **A.** if the answer is associated with A only
- **B.** if the answer is associated with B only
- **C.** if the answer is associated with both A and B
- **D.** if the answer is associated with neither A nor B

87. In uremia, erythrokinetic studies show

   A. abnormal iron turnover rates
   B. normal red cell utilization of iron
   C. both
   D. neither

88. Diseases in which selective proteinuria indicates a good prognosis include

   A. congenital nephrotic syndrome
   B. renal amyloidosis
   C. both
   D. neither

89. The following may manifest azotemia, anemia, impaired renal conservation of salt and water, small kidneys with medullary cysts, little urinary sediment, osteomalacia and early death in renal failure:

   A. juvenile nephrophthisis
   B. cystic disease of the renal medulla
   C. both
   D. neither

90. Dehydrocholesterol

   A. depends on renal metabolism for its action
   B. may be useful in the treatment of patients with kidney disease
   C. both
   D. neither

91. *Staphylococcus aureus*

   A. is a common cause of pyelonephritis
   B. may lead to renal abscess formation
   C. both
   D. neither

92. Acute interstitial nephritis occurs as a manifestation of

   A. some systemic infections (e.g., syphilis)
   B. hypersensitivity to drugs such as penicillins, sulfonamides, diphenylhydantoin, and colistin
   C. both
   D. neither

93. Inability to concentrate the urine maximally occurs frequently due to

   A. loss of nephrons
   B. damage to various parts of the medulla, notably the loop of Henle as in sickle cell disease, hypercalcemia, or potassium depletion
   C. both
   D. neither

94. Myeloma

   A. most often causes renal failure by the development of dense, wide, laminated casts surrounded by a ring of disintegrated tubular cells and extensive tubular atrophy
   B. renal sodium wastage, the Fanconi syndrome, and tubular acidosis may precede renal failure
   C. both
   D. neither

95. Major forms of immunologically mediated glomerular diseases recognized from experimental studies include

   A. immune-complex glomerulonephritis
   B. anti-glomerular-basement-membrane-antibody disease
   C. both
   D. neither

96. Anti-glomerular-basement-membrane-antibody diseases include

   A. glomerulonephritis associated with Goodpasture's syndrome
   B. some cases classified as rapidly progressive or chronic glomerulonephritis
   C. both
   D. neither

Answers and Commentary

1. **B.** Glomerulonephritis is the main cause of renal failure in children as well as young and middle-aged adults. (2:1352)

2. **D.** Glomerular filtration rate at the age of 60 is approximately 70% of the normal observed in young adults. (*N Engl J Med*, 290:785, 1974)

4. **E.** To cause shock, the magnitude of volume sociated with decreased potassium excretion. (*JAMA*, 231:631, 1975)

4. **D.** To cause shock, the magnitude of volume deficit must be in excess of 20 to 30% of the blood volume. (1:75)

5. **C.** About 50% of calcium stones, usually oxalate, are formed without elevation of serum or urine calcium (idiopathic). (1:86)

6. **C.** The duration of action of furosemide is 6 to 8 hours. (*Am Fam Physician*, 8:186, 1973)

7. **D.** Idiopathic hypercalciuria is characterized by normal bones. All other statements are correct. (1:86)

8. **A.** Hyperventilation may cause increased blood lactate and pyruvate with a normal lactate/pyruvate ratio. All other causes listed are correct. (1:77)

9. **A.** Neurological manifestations of uremia include metabolic asterixis, myoclonic muscle spasm, involuntary muscle twitching, choreoathetoid movements, or seizures. (1:86)

10. **C.** Hypertension and hyperuricemia are frequent manifestations of chronic interstitial nephritis due to lead toxicity. All other signs listed are correct. (1:85)

11. **B.** Sarcoidosis is not a cause of glomerular proteinuria. In addition to those listed, causes include vascular disease (e.g., hypertension and congestive heart failure), congenital renal disease (e.g., Alport's syndrome), causes of unknown etiology (e.g., lipoid nephrosis), and physiologic causes (e.g., exercise, postural changes, and fever). (*Am J Med*, 56:71, 1974)

12. **C.** Uremic myocardiopathy with acute, extreme dilatation of the heart may occur in association with pleurisy and pericarditis, especially in patients with accelerated hypertension. It can be distinguished from pericardial tamponade by radioisotope or sonar scanning techniques. The disorder is resistant to digitalization, but responds to intensive hemodialysis and ultrafiltration. (1:87)

13. **A.** Classical renal tubular acidosis is distal. All other characteristics listed are correct. (1:77)

14. **E.** Hypomagnesemia and tissue magnesium depletion may occur in a number of conditions including steatorrhea, malnutrition, alcoholism, chronic diuretic use, and hyperparathyroidism. (1:80)

15. **E.** Characteristically, the course of Goodpasture's syndrome is rapid with a poor prognosis. All other statements are true of this disorder. (1:82)

16. **A.** Thyrocalcitonin is secreted by the parafollicular cells of the thyroid gland. All other statements are true. (1:78, 79)

17. **C.** Cardinal clinical features of cystic disease of the renal medulla are as follows: anemia, urinary tract infection, scanty urinary abnormalities, "renal salt wasting," and progressive uremia. (*JAMA*, 228:1403, 1974)

18. **E.** Hypertension is not cured by bilateral adrenalectomy in patients with pseudoaldosteronism. All other statements are true. (1:78)

19. **D.** A typical patient with the syndrome of inappropriate secretion of antidiuretic hormone manifests a urine sodium concentration greater than 30 mEq/liter. All other statements are true of this syndrome. (1:72)

20. **E.** Immunofluorescence findings are nonspecific in diabetic patients with renal involvement. All other statements are true. (1:82)

21. **A.** Patients with staghorn calculi are usually female. All other statements are correct. (*Emerg Med*, 4:91, 1972)

22. **False.** Workers have measured creatinine clearances on patients they felt had the syndrome of inappropriate ADH and found them to be routinely elevated. Whereas normal clearances were approximately 110 to 120 ml/min, patients with the syndrome had elevations as high as 230 to 240 ml/min. Their experience was that creatinine clearance measurement is helpful in differentiating volume contraction from inappropriate ADH. (*Patient Care*, 9:22, 1975)

23. **False.** When renal function is normal, the occurrence of hypercalcemia usually results in an increase in the filtration of calcium and hypercalciuria. PTH facilitates renal tubular reabsorption of calcium and acts to minimize hypercalciuria in hyperparathyroidism. Hypercalciuria in excess of 500 mg/24 hours is unusual in hyperparathyroidism. Comparable levels of serum calcium in various other hypercalcemic disorders (with suppression of PTH secretion) are often associated with appreciably greater hypercalciuria. Impaired renal function diminishes hypercalciuria because the filtered load of calcium is reduced. (*Med Clin North Am*, 56:941, 1972)

24. **True.** In a minority of patients with chronic renal failure, severe secondary hyperparathyroidism can result in hypercalcemia. (*Lancet*, 1:1273, 1973)

25. **False.** Acute alkalosis stimulates and acute acidosis inhibits tubular potassium secretion. (1:78)

26. **True.** Patients in shock frequently have metabolic (lactic) acidosis which is usually reversed by volume replacement. (1:75)

27. **True.** Plain film of the abdomen is often helpful in the diagnosis of genitourinary disease. The position, shape, and size of the kidneys can often be determined on the plain film. Evidence of bony abnormalities and soft-tissue densities may be identified, as may calcification in the region of the adrenals, kidneys, ureter, bladder, and prostate. (3:252)

28. **False.** It is well known that renal artery stenosis may exist in normotensive patients, or as an incidental finding rather than an etiologic factor in hypertension. (*JAMA*, 221:368, 1972)

29. **False.** Patients with lipoid nephrosis generally excrete fewer high-molecular weight proteins. (*Am J Med*, 56:71, 1974)

30. **True.** In anti-glomerular-basement-membrane-antibody disease, there is a completely continuous (linear) accumulation of immunoglobulins and complement along the basement membrane. (*N Engl J Med*, 288:564, 1973)

31. **True.** The protein fractional curve in tubular proteinuria differs from glomerular proteinuria in that larger quantities of low-molecular weight proteins appear in the urine along with small amounts of albumin. (*Am J Med*, 56:71, 1974)

32. **True.** Generally, metabolic alkalosis responds well to therapy with saline solutions. (1:77)

33. **False.** The capacity of the kidney to lower urinary pH to less than 6.0 is retained until the very end stages of renal acidosis. (1:76)

34. **False.** It is not uncommon for lactic acidosis to be associated with diabetic ketoacidosis. When this occurs, the alteration in the "redox state" may increase the proportion of ketoacids existing as beta-hydroxybutyrate (which does not react with the commonly used nitroprusside reagent). (1:77)

35. **False.** Azotemia induced by diuretics is reversible. (*Am Fam Physician*, 8:186, 1973)

36. **True.** Inhibition of aminoacid absorption may account for the amino aciduria accompanying the secondary hyperparathyroidism of vitamin D deficiency. (1:78)

37. **False.** In polycystic disease of the kidney, a salt loss tendency with dehydration and hyponatremia is common. (*Res Staff Physician*, 20:82, 1974)

38. **True.** A pure lipoid nephrosis may occur with lymphomas, as in Hodgkin's disease, and radiation therapy of the latter may result in a dramatic response of the nephrosis. (1:82)

39. **D.** Although hemodialysis alleviates uremic symptoms, it does not restore calcium and phosphorus homeostasis to normal. Vitamin D resistance persists. Gastrointestinal absorption of calcium, though variable, usually remains defective and most studies indicate a persisting and slight negative calcium balance. Hyperphosphatemia also persists, partly because of the increased intake of phosphate with the liberalized diet and partly because of the low clearance of phosphate with conventional dialyzers, and probably to some extent, due to the increased resorption of phosphate from the bone.
(*Med Clin North Am*, 86:961, 1972)

40. **A.** Decreased nerve conduction velocity in uremia is more common in men. Relatively few patients have significant neurologic symptoms. All other statements are correct. (1:86, 87)

41. **E.** Stones, bladder tumors, papillary necrosis (diabetes), clots, and ureteral tumors are all intraluminal causes of obstructive uropathy. Intramural causes may be congenital, such as bladder neck obstruction, or acquired, such as urethral stricture. Extramural causes of obstructive uropathy include prostatic obstruction, pelvic tumor, aortic aneurysm, periureteral fibrosis, and retroperitoneal nodes. (2:1448)

42. **E.** All the statements concerning minimal change glomerular disease are true. In addition, the disease has a remarkable tendency to remit.
(2:1392)

43. **E.** A palpable mass in the renal area may be produced by neoplasm, hydronephrosis, polycystic kidney, or perinephric abscess. (3:247)

44. **E.** All the disorders listed may be causes of hyperchloremic acidosis. (1:85)

45. **E.** All the statements are true of renal vein thrombosis. In addition, hematuria is common.
(1:83)

46. **A.** Renal failure in multiple myeloma is often preceded by dehydration (as in pyelographic preparation), hypercalcemia, renal infection, or secondary amyloidosis and nephrotic syndrome.
(1:85)

47. **B.** Viruses implicated in human immune complex nephritis are those of hepatitis and measles. (1:81)

48. **A.** Chronic interstitial nephritis due to obstructive uropathy may occur without infection. All other statements are true. (1:85)

49. **B.** "Benign" hematuria with focal glomerulitis, commonly reported in pediatric literature, also occurs in adults. The clinical characteristics include recurrent or persistent hematuria with red cell casts and minimal proteinuria (less than 1 g/day), normal renal function, and the absence of hypertension. (1:83)

50. **E.** All the listed disorders may cause hypertension and hypokalemia. Excessive ingestion of licorice is also a cause. (1:78)

51. **C.** Hypercalcemia and hypokalemia continue to be important causes of partial nephrogenic diabetes insipidus and hypertonic dehydration. (1:73)

52. **B.** Spironolactone and triamterene are weak diuretics. Furosemide and ethacrynic acid are termed high ceiling or potent diuretics. (1:74)

53. **A.** In hereditary nephritis, renal failure occurs more often in males. All other statements are correct. (1:82)

54. **A.** The term nephrotic syndrome refers to the clinical association of heavy proteinuria, hypoalbuminemia, and generalized edema. By definition, hypertension and azotemia are not necessary in order to have the nephrotic syndrome. (2:1387)

55. **A.** Renovascular hypertension is less frequent in the black population. All other statements are correct. (1:75)

56. **A.** Several cases of renal potassium wastage associated with hypokalemic metabolic alkalosis, normal blood pressure, and variably elevated aldosterone secretory rates and plasma renin levels have been reported (so-called Bartter's syndrome). Hyperplasia of the renal juxtaglomerular cells has been consistently observed. (1:78)

57. **E.** All the disorders and drugs listed may cause hypercalcemia. (1:79)

58. **C.** Medullary sponge kidney is usually asymptomatic and may be discovered radiographically or because of nephrolithiasis, hematuria or renal infection; it does not cause renal failure. (1:85)

59. **B.** (2:1432)

60. **A.** (2:1427)

61. **C.** (4:1316)

62. **True.** Hypercalcemia results in deficits of body sodium and water which, unless corrected, reduce urinary calcium excretion, exaggerate the hypercalcemia, and increase the propensity for systemic toxicity and renal damage. (1:79)

63. **True.** When analgesic nephropathy is detected and the offending drugs, especially those containing phenacetin, are discontinued, the disease will usually stabilize or improve, provided renal failure is not too far advanced.
(*Internist Observer*, p3 Oct.–Nov. 1973)

64. **True.** In the nephrotic syndrome, hypovolemia secondary to hypoalbuminemia may produce a sharp decline in renal function which is potentially reversible. (*Lancet*, 2:29, 1973)

65. **False.** Most patients with urinary tract infection have greater than 10^5 organisms/ml urine when studied, but there are a significant number with fever or other relevant symptoms, or with pyuria and/or blood cell casts in their urine, who have less than 10^5 organisms/ml urine on culture, but obviously have a urinary tract infection. (1:80)

66. **True.** The predominant factor influencing survival in malignant hypertension has been the status of renal function at the time of diagnosis.
(*Ann Intern Med*, 80:754, 1974)

67. **False.** The functional loss in ischemic tubular injury far exceeds the observed structural changes. (1:83)

68. **False.** A minority of patients with lipoid nephrosis develop focal glomerulosclerosis. (1:82)

69. **True.** In uncomplicated cases of acute tubular necrosis in which there is no serious underlying disease and treatment is optimal, survival rates in excess of 70 to 80% are common. (2:1374)

70. **True.** A dilute urine with clinical dehydration suggests impairment in renal function.
(*Ann Intern Med*, 82:64, 1975)

71. **True.** Symptomatic bone disease during the early stages of renal insufficiency (GFR 20 to 60 ml/min/1.73 sq m) is rare except in patients with long-standing acidosis due to chronic pyelonephritis or to inherited forms of renal disease, such as the various syndromes of renal tubular insufficiency, renal tubular acidosis, and medullary cystic disease.
(*Med Clin North Am*, 56:961, 1972)

72. **True.** When magnesium ammonium phosphate hexahydrate (triple phosphate, struvite) occurs in kidney stones, it is the hallmark of alkaline (urea-splitting) infection. (1:85, 86)

73. **True.** In acute renal failure, the survival rate is increased by dialysis to hold the BUN to below 100 mg% and allow a higher protein intake which may enhance regeneration. (1:83)

74. **False.** Acute renal failure, an abrupt loss of renal function, most often results from toxic or ischemic injury to the renal tubules, which rarely show overt necrosis. (1:83)

75. **False.** Most uric acid stones occur in pure form (85%). (1:86)

76. **True.** During the oliguric phase of ischemic renal tubular injury, increased fibrin degradation products are found in the blood, suggesting a possible role of intravascular coagulation in tubular necrosis. (1:83)

77. **True.** Hyponatremia may be viewed basically as an abnormality in the renal excretion of (electrolyte-free) water. (1:71)

78. **False.** Thiazide diuretics are of little value in patients with renal insufficiency and may become ineffective when compensatory mechanisms, such as fall in GFR or enhanced sodium resorption at a more proximal nephron site, diminish the delivery of sodium to their site of action. (1:74)

79. **False.** Chronic renal failure is an unlikely sequel to acute pyelonephritis. (1:84)

80. **False.** Spironolactone is an antagonist of aldosterone, while triamterene does not depend on the presence of mineralocorticoids for its action. (1:74)

81. **True.** Ionizing radiation exceeding 1000 rads may cause chronic interstitial nephritis with anemia, proteinuria, renal failure, and hypertension, which may occasionally be malignant. (1:85)

82. **True.** Hypernatremia may occur at various levels of total body sodium content, although clinically it is commonly associated with sodium depletion and hypovolemia. (1:73)

83. **False.** In nephrotic syndrome, plasma cholesterol may rise to 1500 mg/100 ml, but the level of this and of the other lipids varies considerably, even in patients with the same type of nephrotic syndrome. (2:1389)

84. **True.** In multiple myeloma, tubular atrophy favors urinary excretion of filterable low molecular weight proteins, kappa chains or Bence Jones proteins, while renal failure favors their accumulation in plasma. (1:85)

85. **True.** The most important factor in treatment of nephrotic syndrome is the proper use of diuretics. Except in cases of profound hypoalbuminemia or when the syndrome is complicated by severe renal failure, edema can nearly always be controlled by diuretics alone. (2:1389)

86. **False.** Mannitol infusion has often restored renal function, when administered during or immediately after a renal insult. (1:83)

87. **D.** In uremia, erythrokinetic studies show normal iron turnover rates, but defective red cell utilization of iron. (1:87)

88. **D.** There appear to be only two exceptions to the general rule that a highly selective proteinuria indicates a good prognosis, and both are uncommon: congenital nephrotic syndrome, a rare and invariably fatal disease, and occasional cases of renal amyloidosis. (2:1389)

89. **C.** Both juvenile nephrophthisis and cystic disease of the renal medulla may manifest anemia, azotemia, impaired renal conservation of salt and water, small kidneys with medullary cysts, little urinary sediment, osteomalacia, and early death in renal failure. (1:85)

90. **B.** Dehydrocholesterol does not depend on renal metabolism for its action and may be useful in the treatment of patients with kidney disease. (1:79)

91. **B.** *Staphylococcus aureus* is a rare cause of pyelonephritis but may lead to renal abscess formation. (1:84)

92. **C.** Acute interstitial nephritis occurs as a manifestation of some systemic infections (e.g., syphilis) and of hypersensitivity to penicillins, sulfonamides, diphenylhydantoin, colistin, and other drugs. (1:84)

93. **C.** Inability to concentrate the urine maximally occurs frequently due to loss of nephrons or damage to various parts of the medulla, notably the loop of Henle as in sickle cell disease, amphotericin B toxicity, lupus erythematosus, and other hyperglobulinemias, hypercalcemia, and potassium depletion. (1:85)

94. **C.** Myeloma, a multifocal plasma cell neoplasia, most often causes renal failure by the development of dense, wide, laminated casts surrounded by a ring of disintegrated tubular cells and extensive tubular atrophy. Renal sodium wastage, the Fanconi syndrome, and tubular acidosis may precede renal failure which is often precipitated by dehydration (as in pyelographic preparation), by hypercalcemia, by renal infection, or by secondary amyloidosis and nephrotic syndrome. (1:85)

95. **C.** Both disorders listed are major forms of immunologically mediated glomerular diseases. (*N Engl J Med*, 288:564, 1973)

96. **C.** Both conditions are types of anti-glomerular-basement-membrane antibody diseases. (*N Engl J Med*, 288:564, 1973)

Textbook References for Chapter 17

1. American College of Physicians (1974): *Medical Knowledge Self-Assessment, Program III: Recent Developments in Internal Medicine,* R.G. Petersdorf, General Editor, American College of Physicians, Philadelphia.

2. Beeson, P.B. and McDermott, W. (1979): *Cecil Textbook of Medicine*, Fifteenth Edition, W.B. Saunders Company, Philadelphia.

3. Judge, R.D. and Zuidema, G.D., Editors (1974): *Physical Diagnosis: A Physiologic Approach to the Clinical Examination,* Little, Brown, and Company, Boston.

4. Isselbacher, K.J., Editor (1980): *Harrison's Principles of Internal Medicine*, Ninth edition, McGraw-Hill Book Company, New York.

CHAPTER 18

Neurology

Directions: For each of the following questions, select the ONE INCORRECT answer.

1. In jacksonian seizures,
   A. there are lesions in the sensory cortex
   B. the seizure starts with convulsive twitchings of one portion of the body, usually the distal part of one extremity
   C. if the seizure starts in the fingers, the spread is to the wrist, the forearm, arm, the face, and then to the homolateral leg
   D. if the movements spread to the opposite half of the body, consciousness is lost and the further manifestations are similar to those of a grand mal seizure
   E. the power of speech may be impaired or lost when the focal discharge arises in the dominant temporal or frontal lobe

2. With thrombosis of the superior sagittal sinus,
   A. there is increased intracranial pressure with headache, vomiting, and papilledema
   B. convulsions may occur
   C. veins of the scalp do not become congested
   D. paraplegia may occur due to infarction of the upper part of the cerebral hemisphere

3. Which of the following disorders occur within the spinal canal and are principal causes of lesions of the spinal dorsal nerve roots?
   A. meningovascular syphilis (causing spinal leptomeningitis)
   B. tabes dorsalis
   C. extramedullary tumor
   D. herpes zoster
   E. meralgia paresthetica

4. In acute "infective" polyneuropathy (Landry-Guillain-Barré syndrome),
   A. onset of symptoms is usually acute or subacute, and patients are frequently febrile
   B. in contrast to other forms of polyneuropathy, the proximal muscles of the limbs may suffer as severely as the distal ones, and the trunk muscles may also be involved
   C. sensory changes may be severe, slight, or even sometimes absent
   D. the cranial nerves often suffer, sometimes even the optic nerves with papilledema, and the eighth nerve causing deafness
   E. cerebrospinal fluid protein and pressure may be raised and there is usually an excess of cells

222

5. With cerebral embolism,

   A. onset of symptoms is more sudden than with either cerebral hemorrhage or thrombosis

   B. the most common cause is aortic stenosis

   C. in most cases, there is atrial fibrillation

   D. a clot formed on the mural endocardium after myocardial infarction may be causative

   E. a convulsion may occur at the onset and there is usually headache

6. With pontine hemorrhage,

   A. there is facial paralysis on the side of the lesion with flaccid paralysis of the limbs on the opposite side

   B. owing to paralysis of conjugate ocular deviation and of rotation of the head to the side of the lesion, the patient lies with his head and eyes turned toward the side of the paralyzed limbs

   C. extension of the hemorrhage involves the opposite side of the pons, and resulting paralysis of the face and limbs on both sides with bilateral exterior plantar reflexes

   D. pupils are usually dilated

   E. there is often a terminal hyperpyrexia

Directions: For each of the following incomplete statements, select
   A. **if the question is associated with A only**
   B. **if the question is associated with B only**
   C. **if the question is associated with both A and B**
   D. **if the question is associated with neither A nor B**

7. The posterior cerebral artery

   A. supplies the visual cortex of the occipital lobe

   B. when occluded, causes crossed homonymous hemianopia

   C. both

   D. neither

8. Intracranial lesions (infection, trauma, or tumor) may produce inappropriate secretion of ADH by

   A. partial destruction of the posterior lobe of the pituitary gland with escape of hormone

   B. virtue of an irritative focus that promotes the secretion of the hormone

   C. both

   D. neither

9. Drugs which are less effective than diphenylhydantoin (Dilantin) in patients with focal seizures include:

   A. phenobarbital

   B. primidone

   C. both

   D. neither

10. High temperature readings are invariably found in patients in coma due to

    A. drug intoxication

    B. metabolic acidosis

    C. both

    D. neither

11. Occlusion of one internal carotid artery leads to its territory being invaded

    A. by the basilar supply through the posterior communicating artery

    B. from the opposite internal carotid artery through the anterior communicating artery

    C. both

    D. neither

12. Which of the following may develop at any time in patients who had only petit mal seizures at the onset and are apt to persist in adult life in the patient who ceases to have petit mal attacks?

    A. grand mal seizures

    B. psychomotor seizures

    C. both

    D. neither

13. With spinal cord injury of C1 on C2, there may be

   A. paralysis of all respiratory muscles
   B. quick death
   C. both
   D. neither

14. Disorders which are improved by the administration of potassium include:

   A. hyperkalemic paralysis (adynamia episodica hereditaris of Gamstorp)
   B. normokalemic paralysis (paramyotonia congenita)
   C. both
   D. neither

15. Jacksonian and generalized seizures with a focal onset

   A. usually occur in patients with a structural lesion in the nervous system
   B. are more common than the other forms of seizures
   C. both
   D. neither

16. The diagnosis of myasthenia gravis can be corroborated in most instances by "double blind" pharmacologic tests using

   A. edrophonium (Tensilon)
   B. neostigmine (Prostigmin)
   C. both
   D. neither

Directions: For each of the following questions, select the ONE CORRECT answer.

17. The electroencephalographic concomitants of psychomotor-temporal lobe seizures are characterized by discharges of spikes, complexes, and sharp and slow waves localized from the involved temporal lobe in at least what percentage of instances?

   A. 10%
   B. 25%
   C. 40%
   D. 55%
   E. 75%

18. Approximately what percentage of patients with convulsions suffer with seizures of the grand mal type?

   A. 10%
   B. 30%
   C. 50%
   D. 70%
   E. 90%

19. In deep coma, the last reflexes to be lost are the

   A. corneal reflexes
   B. tendon reflexes
   C. pupillary reflexes
   D. plantar reflexes
   E. none of the above

20. Pituitary tumors account for approximately what percentage of all intracranial tumors?

   A. 1%
   B. 5%
   C. 10%
   D. 25%
   E. 50%

21. Effect of intravenous diphenhydramine hydrochloride (Benedryl) is greatest on phenothiazine-induced

   A. parkinsonian syndrome
   B. akathisia (constant restlessness)
   C. acute muscle spasms and dystonia
   D. choreoathetosis
   E. none of the above

Directions: Indicate whether each statement is true or false.

22. Weakness of both legs with increased tone, "leg jumps" (flexor spasms), and upgoing toes suggest spinal cord pathology.

23. In advancing vertebrobasilar infarcts, angiography is mandatory.

24. In lesions of the brainstem after the corticofungal fibers have crossed, the patient's

head and eyes are turned away from the side of the hemiplegia.

25. Petit mal seizures frequently have their onset after the age of twenty.

Directions: For each of the following incomplete statements, select
    A. if the question is associated with A only
    B. if the question is associated with B only
    C. if the question is associated with both A and B
    D. if the question is associated with neither A nor B

26. Akinetic seizures may occur in patients with
    A. petit mal attacks
    B. grand mal seizures
    C. both
    D. neither

27. Ptosis of the upper lid resulting from third nerve paralysis is usually associated with
    A. a dilated and fixed pupil
    B. paralysis of external ocular muscles
    C. both
    D. neither

28. In the management of transient ischemic attacks (TIAs), anticoagulants may
    A. decrease the frequency of attacks
    B. augment longevity
    C. both
    D. neither

29. Which of the following is/are effective in psychomotor seizures?
    A. diphenylhydantoin (Dilantin)
    B. primidone (Mysoline)
    C. both
    D. neither

30. Compared to L-dopa in Parkinson's disease, amantadine hydrochloride has a
    A. more pronounced effect
    B. longer duration of action
    C. both
    D. neither

31. Entrapment neuropathies include
    A. meralgia paresthetica
    B. thoracic outlet syndrome
    C. both
    D. neither

Directions: For each of the following multiple-choice questions, select the ONE CORRECT answer.

32. Intracranial hemorrhage that is almost invariably traumatic is
    A. extradural
    B. subdural
    C. subarachnoid
    D. intracerebral
    E. none of the above

33. The most common first sign or symptom of multiple sclerosis as proved by clinical study and autopsy has been found to be
    A. diplopia and impaired vision
    B. weakness
    C. tremor, ataxia, and incoordination
    D. paresthesias
    E. dizziness or vertigo

34. Primary intracerebral hemorrhage originates most commonly in the
    A. thalamus
    B. cerebellum
    C. pons
    D. putamen
    E. none of the above

35. The spinal fluid gammaglobulin is elevated in approximately what percentage of multiple sclerosis cases in exacerbation?
    A. 5%
    B. 20%
    C. 45%
    D. 60%
    E. 85%

Directions: Use the key below to answer questions 36 through 40. If the electroencephalographic configuration indicates
  A. grand mal and focal motor seizure pattern
  B. petit mal seizure
  C. psychomotor seizure pattern
  D. minor myoclonic and akinetic seizure pattern
  E. infantile myoclonic seizure pattern

36. Hypoarrhythmia

37. Polyspike-and-wave and 2/sec slow spike-and-wave

38. 3/sec spike-and-wave

39. Temporal-lobe spikes-and-sharp waves

40. Spikes, spike-and-wave and sharp waves

Directions: Indicate whether each of the following statements is true or false.

41. Babinski toe sign may be absent or equivocal even though the corticospinal tracts are involved.

42. If the number of attacks is considered, grand mal is the most common seizure.

43. In primary intracerebral hemorrhage, the mortality rate is under 50%.

44. Contrary to general opinion, no gross lesion can be demonstrated by clinical examination in many patients who develop seizures after the age of twenty.

45. When evaluating seizure patients, it should be remembered that generalized seizures are more likely to be associated with structural lesions such as brain tumors than are focal seizures.

46. A pontine lesion, usually a hemorrhage, produces very large pupils.

47. The frequency of convulsive seizures in organic diseases of the central nervous system is directly related to the severity or degree of cerebral damage.

48. There is no pathological support for the concept that many cases of diabetic mononeuropathy are caused by infarcts in the nerves.

49. The aura of migraine may occur without a subsequent vasodilatation, headache phase.

Directions: For each of the following multiple-choice questions, select the ONE CORRECT answer.

50. Intracardiac mural thrombosis develops in about 44% of patients with myocardial infarction. Approximately what percentage of these will have a cerebral embolism within the first 6 weeks following their infarction?
  A. 1%
  B. 5%
  C. 10%
  D. 22%
  E. 30%

51. Proximal bilateral weakness suggests
  A. a myopathic process
  B. spinal cord pathology
  C. polyneuropathy
  D. all of the above
  E. none of the above

52. In myasthenia gravis, thymectomy produces improvement or remission in what percentage of patients?
  A. 5 to 10%
  B. 20 to 30%
  C. 45 to 65%
  D. 75 to 90%
  E. 100%

Directions: For each of the following statements, fill in the correct answer(s).

53. The two most common types of headaches are muscle contraction and _____ .

54. The most common hereditary ataxia is _____ ataxia.

55. Wernicke-Korsakoff syndrome is characterized by a triad of signs: _____ , ataxia, and mental confusion.

56. The two principal reflexes mediated by the trigeminal nerve are the _____ reflex and the _____-jerk.

57. Transient ischemic attacks (TIAs) are usually related to _____ disease.

58. Herpes zoster of the geniculate ganglion may cause _____ paralysis, the syndrome of Ramsay _____ .

Directions: For each of the incomplete statements below, ONE or MORE of the numbered completions is correct. In each case, select
A. if 1, 2, and 3 are correct
B. if 1 and 3 are correct
C. if 2 and 4 are correct
D. if only 4 is correct
E. if all statements are correct

59. Regarding status epilepticus,
    1. it is characterized by frequent recurrence of generalized convulsions with failure to regain consciousness between exacerbations
    2. rapid withdrawal of anticonvulsants is the most common precipitating factor
    3. fever, electrolyte imbalance, hypoglycemia and structural brain damage may predispose to status epilepticus
    4. when the seizure is typically tonic and the patient apneic, emergency treatment is required

60. "Acquired non-Wilsonian chronic hepatocerebral degeneration" involves
    1. dementia
    2. dysarthria
    3. ataxia of gait
    4. tremor

61. Meniere's syndrome
    1. involves recurrent attacks of severe giddiness usually leading to vomiting and prostration and is associated with tinnitus and increasing deafness
    2. runs a protracted course with a tendency towards disappearance of the vertigo as the deafness increases
    3. has been shown to result from gross dilation of the endolymph system of the internal ear without evidence of infection or trauma, causing degenerative changes in the cochlear and vestibular sense organs
    4. during the attack, the patient usually lies on the sound side and exhibits a rotary nystagmus which is most evident at the side of affected ear

62. Disorders of the lower motor neuron tend to present with
    1. hypertonia
    2. hypertrophy
    3. increased tendon reflexes
    4. weakness

63. Ocular abnormalities in Wernicke-Korsakoff syndrome include
    1. horizontal and vertical nystagmus
    2. internal strabismus
    3. diplopia
    4. weakness or paralysis of conjugate gaze

64. Myasthenia gravis
    1. is a chronic disease with a tendency to remission and relapse
    2. involves impairment of conduction at the myoneural junction which is temporarily relieved by cholinesterase inhibitors such as physostigmine and neostigmine
    3. occurs most commonly between the ages of 20 and 50
    4. affects men more frequently than women

65. Tic douloureux

    1. usually occurs in the distribution of the second or third division of the fifth cranial nerve and, less commonly, in the first
    2. may respond to diphenylhydantoin
    3. may require neurosurgical procedures
    4. commonly occurs in the seventh, ninth, or eleventh nerve

Directions: Use the key below to answer questions 66 through 68. If the symptoms are characteristic of

A. **Alport's syndrome**
B. **Pendred's disease**
C. **Waardenburg's disease**

66. Hereditary deafness with goiter

67. Hereditary deafness with nephritis

68. Hereditary deafness with skin abnormalities such as albinism, lentigines, piebaldness, and white forelock

Directions: For each of the following multiple-choice questions, select the ONE INCORRECT answer.

69. Craniopharyngioma

    A. is a hypophysial epidermoid tumor
    B. is a tumor of Rathke's pouch
    C. is derived from an embryonic remnant of the craniopharyngeal pouch which comes to lie above the sella turcica
    D. does not undergo degeneration and calcification
    E. may produce endocrine disturbances, papilledema, and visual field defects

70. Delirium tremens

    A. is the most severe form of the withdrawal syndrome
    B. has its onset between 48 and 96 hours after withdrawal
    C. is characterized by profound confusion, intense psychomotor activity, and derangements of autonomic nervous system function (tachycardia, fever, dilated pupils, intense sweating)
    D. is a relatively frequent complication of withdrawal
    E. is a potentially lethal complication of withdrawal

71. Glioblastoma multiforme

    A. is a relatively benign tumor
    B. arises in middle-age
    C. is almost invariably found in the cerebral hemisphere
    D. is a reddish, highly vascular tumor which tends to infiltrate the brain extensively

72. In migrainous neuralgia,

    A. there is a paroxysm of severe pain usually in the frontotemporal region and the eye, occurring several times a day and lasting from one-half to two hours
    B. at the height of the attack, there may be lacrimation and nasal discharge, more marked on the same side of the headache
    C. each bout tends to last a few weeks, followed by a free interval of months or even a year or more when the same series of events is repeated
    D. there is no associated abnormality to be found, and the pathogenesis of the condition is unknown
    E. ergotamine has no specific effect

73. In hyperosmolar nonketotic coma

    A. it is mostly associated with diabetes in middle-aged or elderly patients
    B. blood glucose is usually over 600 mg/ml
    C. serum osmolality is in excess of 350 mOsm/kg
    D. cerebrospinal fluid pressure is usually elevated
    E. severe acidosis is uncommon since the small quantities of plasma insulin present inhibit lipolysis

74. "Upper motor neuron" disease

    A. is due to damage in the descending motor pathway
    B. is associated with spastic weakness
    C. is associated with overactive tendon reflexes
    D. shows no Babinski sign
    E. signs may take hours or days to appear

75. In Friedreich's ataxia,

    A. the spinal cord is unusually small
    B. the heart may be enlarged
    C. the age of onset is usually between 5 and 15 years
    D. in later stages, dysarthric speech, nystagmus, extensor plantar reflexes, and loss of tendon reflexes may occur
    E. pes cavus and scoliosis are present in the minority of cases

76. Lumbar puncture headache

    A. is characterized by a steady occipitonuchal pain and frontal pain coming on a few minutes after arising from a recumbent position
    B. is relieved within a few minutes by lying down
    C. has as its cause a persistent leakage of cerebrospinal fluid into the lumbar tissues through the needle site
    D. has low cerebrospinal fluid pressure (often 0 in the lateral decubitus position)
    E. is aggravated by the injection of sterile isotonic saline solution intrathecally

77. Peroneal muscular atrophy (Charcot-Marie-Tooth disease) is characterized by

    A. interstitial neuritis, chiefly affecting the branches of the common peroneal nerve, together with degeneration of the corticospinal tracts and the posterior columns
    B. "claw feet" and steppage gait beginning usually in the second decade
    C. wasting of hand muscles
    D. presence of fasciculation and loss of tendon jerks and plantar reflexes
    E. cutaneous sensibility unaffected

Directions: For each of the following incomplete statements, select
   A. if the question is associated with A only
   B. if the question is associated with B only
   C. if the question is associated with both A and B
   D. if the question is associated with neither A nor B

78. Primary subarachnoid hemorrhage is usually due to rupture of an

    A. intracranial aneurysm
    B. arteriovenous malformation
    C. both
    D. neither

79. The headache which usually occurs in single attacks over a period of days may be associated with

    A. subarachnoid hemorrhage
    B. bacterial meningitis
    C. both
    D. neither

80. It is generally believed that thrombus formation on ulcerated areas of atheromatous plaques is important in

    A. cerebral infarction
    B. transient cerebral ischemia
    C. both
    D. neither

81. Myasthenia gravis may be associated with

    A. hyperthyroidism, hypothyroidism, goiter, and Hashimoto's thyroiditis
    B. rheumatoid arthritis, systemic lupus erythematosus, and polymyositis
    C. both
    D. neither

82. Diabetic neuropathy is limited

    A. mainly to the lower extremities
    B. to patients with long duration of the disease
    C. both
    D. neither

Answers and Commentary

1. **A.** The focal seizures described by Jackson are associated with lesions in the motor cortex. All the other statements listed are true of jacksonian seizures. (5:852–53)

2. **C.** There is often congestion of the veins of the scalp in patients with thrombosis of the superior sagittal sinus. All other statements are correct. (2:281)

3. **E.** The principal causes of lesions of the spinal dorsal nerve roots are meningovascular syphilis causing spinal leptomeningitis, tabes dorsalis, extramedullary tumor, and herpes zoster, all of which may occur within the spinal canal. (2:428–41)

4. **E.** In acute "infective" polyneuropathy, there is no excess of cells in the cerebrospinal fluid. In most cases, the outlook is good. All other statements are true. (2:369–70)

5. **B.** Mitral stenosis is now a rarer cause of cerebral embolism. It is rarely fatal unless the embolus lodges in the internal carotid artery. All other statements are true. (2:268–69)

6. **D.** Marked contraction of the pupils—"pinpoint pupils"—the result of bilateral destruction of the ocular sympathetic fibers, is characteristic of a pontine hemorrhage. All other statements are true of pontine hemorrhage. (2:276)

7. **C.** Since the posterior cerebral artery supplies the visual cortex of the occipital lobe its occlusion causes crossed homonymous hemianopia. (2:258)

8. **C.** Intracranial lesions (infection, trauma, or tumor), independent of their ability to induce seizures, may produce inappropriate secretion of ADH by partial destruction of the posterior lobe of the pituitary gland, with escape of hormone, or by virtue of an irritative focus that promotes the secretion of the hormone.
(*Ann Intern Med*, 83:736, 1975)

9. **D.** Phenobarbital and primidone are more effective in patients with focal seizures than diphenylhydantoin.(*N Engl J Med*, 286:464, 1972)

10. **D.** Subnormal temperature readings are commonly found in patients in coma due to drug intoxication or metabolic acidosis. (4:36)

11. **C.** Occlusion of one internal carotid artery leads to its territory being invaded by the basilar supply through the posterior communicating artery, and also from the opposite internal carotid through the anterior communicating artery. (2:255)

12. **C.** Grand mal or psychomotor seizures may develop at any time in patients who had only petit mal seizures at the onset, and are apt to persist in adult life in the patient who ceases to have petit mal attacks. (5:858)

13. **C.** An odontoid fracture represents a perilous injury in view of potential instability of C1 on C2 and the limited space available to the spinal cord if displacement occurs. When cord injury does occur at this level, there may be immediate paralysis of all respiratory muscles and quick death. (4:328)

14. **D.** Hyperkalemic and normokalemic paralysis are uncommon and are worsened by the administration of potassium. (1:94)

15. **A.** Jacksonian and generalized seizures with a focal onset usually occur in patients with a structural lesion in the nervous system and are less common than the other forms of seizures. They

will be found to be more common than generally supposed, however, if the symptoms at onset of supposedly generalized attacks are carefully analyzed. (5:852)

16. **C.** The diagnosis of myasthenia gravis can be corroborated in most instances by "double blind" pharmacologic tests using edrophonium or neostigmine. (1:93)

17. **E.** The electroencephalographic concomitants of psychomotor-temporal lobe seizures are characterized by discharges of spikes, complexes, and sharp and slow waves localized from the involved temporal lobe in at least 75% of instances, and are often enhanced by sleep. Frequently, however, the abnormalities are bitemporal or more generalized and asynchronous representing transmission and diffusion of the paroxysmal discharges. This is particularly true in the electroencephalograms of children with this type of epilepsy. (5:854)

18. **E.** Approximately 90% of patients with convulsions suffer with seizures of the grand mal type. (5:851)

19. **C.** Reflex responses vary with the depth of unconsciousness. The plantar reflexes early become extensor; in deeper coma the corneal reflexes, tendon reflexes, and pupillary reflexes are lost. (2:157)

20. **C.** Pituitary tumors account for approximately 10% of all intracranial tumors. By far the most common pituitary tumor is the chromophobe adenoma which is usually nonsecretory in nature. Active pituitary tumors usually secrete only one pituitary hormone in excess. Tumors secreting GH, ACTH, MSH, TSH, and LTH have all been described, although the last three types of tumor are very rare. FSH- or LH-secreting tumors are notable by their absence. (6:1675)

21. **C.** The effect of intravenous diphenhydramine hydrochloride is greatest on phenothiazine-induced acute muscle spasms and dystonia. (1:101)

22. **True.** Weakness of both legs with increased tone, "leg jumps" (flexor spasms), and upgoing toes suggest spinal cord pathology. (1:91)

23. **False.** In advancing vertebrobasilar infarcts whose clinical pattern is so characteristic, angiography can usually be omitted.
(*Br Med J,* 1:91, 1972)

24. **False.** In lesions of the brainstem after the corticofungal fibers have crossed, the patient's head

and eyes may be turned toward the side of the hemiplegia. (*Med Clin North Am,* 57:1363, 1973)

25. **False.** Petit mal seizures are a manifestation of epilepsy in childhood and rarely have their onset after the age of twenty. They are also characteristic of so-called idiopathic epilepsy. They may occur in patients with birth injuries or developmental defects or may develop following acute febrile illnesses in childhood, but they are most commonly seen in children with no gross lesion in the nervous system and practically never appear for the first time in adult patients with cerebral tumors or abscesses, or following cerebral trauma. (5:855)

26. **C.** Akinetic seizures may occur in patients who have typical petit mal attacks, but they also occur in patients whose clinical seizures are of the grand mal type. (5:857)

27. **C.** Ptosis of the upper lid resulting from third nerve paralysis is usually associated with a dilated and fixed pupil and paralysis of external ocular muscles. (2:42)

28. **A.** In the management of transient ischemic attacks, anticoagulants may decrease the frequency of attacks, but not augment longevity.
(*JAMA,* 228:757, 1974)

29. **C.** Both diphenylhydantoin and primidone are effective in treating psychomotor seizures. (1:96)

30. **D.** Compared to L-dopa in Parkinson's disease, amantadine hydrochloride has a less pronounced effect and shorter duration of action. (1:97)

31. **C.** There are several types of entrapment neuropathies. These include meralgia paresthetica, thoracic outlet syndrome, carpal tunnel syndrome, tardy ulnar nerve palsy, acute radial nerve palsy, acute and tardy peroneal nerve palsy, and tarsal tunnel syndrome. (3:901–02)

32. **A.** Extradural hemorrhage is almost invariably traumatic. (2:269)

33. **B.** Several studies have shown that weakness is the most frequent first symptom of multiple sclerosis, and that at some time during the course of the disorder, it occurs in the majority of patients. (3:847)

34. **D.** Primary intracerebral hemorrhage usually originates in putamen (44%), thalamus (13%), cerebellum (9%), or pons (9%). (1:98)

35. **E.** The spinal fluid gammaglobulin is elevated in approximately 85% of multiple sclerosis cases in exacerbation. (1:97)

36. **E.** (*N Engl J Med*, 286:464, 1974)

37. **D.** (*N Engl J Med*, 286:464, 1974)

38. **B.** (*N Engl J Med*, 286:464, 1974)

39. **C.** (*N Engl J Med*, 286:464, 1974)

40. **A.** (*N Engl J Med*, 286:464, 1974)

41. **True.** Babinski toe sign may be absent or equivocal even though the corticospinal tracts are involved. (*Med Clin North Am*, 57:1363, 1973)

42. **False.** If the number of attacks is considered, petit mal is the most common seizure because it is not unusual for many attacks to occur daily in patients who are subject to this form. (5:851)

43. **False.** The mortality rate is over 50% in primary intracerebral hemorrhage. (1:98)

44. **True.** It is correct that no gross lesion can be demonstrated by clinical examination in many of the patients who develop seizures after the age of twenty. As a rule, the later the onset of seizures, the greater the probability that they are associated with some gross organic lesions of the brain. (5:844)

45. **False.** When evaluating seizure patients, it should be remembered that focal seizures are far more likely to be associated with structural lesions such as brain tumors than are generalized seizures. (1:95)

46. **False.** A pontine lesion, usually a hemorrhage, produces very small pupils, the result perhaps of a combination of parasympathetic irritation and sympathetic paresis. (*Med Clin North Am*, 57:1363, 1974)

47. **False.** It is of interest to note that the frequency of convulsive seizures in organic diseases of the central nervous system is not directly related to the severity or degree of cerebral damage. The incidence of convulsive seizures, although significantly greater than in the general population, is relatively low in certain diseases of the nervous system in which there is extensive cortical or subcortical damage. Examples of such conditions are uncomplicated cases of cerebral arteriosclerosis, with or without areas of encephalomalacia, and multiple sclerosis. (5:849)

48. **False.** There is pathological support for the concept that many cases of diabetic mononeuropathy are caused by infarcts in the nerves. (1:99)

49. **True.** The aura of migraine may occur without a subsequent vasodilatation, headache phase. (2:191)

50. **B.** Intracardiac mural thrombosis develops in about 44% of patients with myocardial infarction and about 5% of these will have a cerebral embolism within the first 6 weeks following their infarction. (1:98)

51. **A.** Proximal bilateral weakness suggests a myopathic process; distal weakness with or without glove-stocking hypesthesia and with decreased tendon reflexes suggests polyneuropathy; weakness of both legs with increased tone, "leg jumps" (flexor spasms) and upgoing toes suggest spinal cord pathology. (1:91)

52. **D.** In myasthenia gravis, thymectomy produces improvement or remission in 75 to 90% of patients. (1:93)

53. **Migraine.** The two most common types of headaches are muscle contraction headache and migraine. (1:98)

54. **Friedreich's.** The most common hereditary ataxia is Friedreich's ataxia. (2:452)

55. **Ophthalmoplegia.** Wernicke-Korsakoff syndrome is characterized by a triad of signs—ophthalmoplegia, ataxia, and mental confusion. (1:100)

56. **Corneal, jaw.** The two principal reflexes mediated by the trigeminal nerve are the corneal reflex and the jaw-jerk. (2:49)

57. **Atherosclerotic.** Transient ischemic attacks are usually related to atherosclerotic disease. (1:97)

58. **Facial, Hunt.** Herpes zoster of the geniculate ganglion may cause facial paralysis, the syndrome of Ramsay Hunt. (2:55)

59. **E.** All the statements are true of status epilepticus. (*N Engl J Med*, 286:464, 1972)

60. **E.** A fixed neurological syndrome consisting of dementia, dysarthria, ataxia of gait, and tremor has been described under the name "acquired non-Wilsonian chronic hepatocerebral degeneration." (1:99)

61. **E.** All statements are true of Meniere's syndrome. It is most common in middle-aged men. (2:66–69)

62. **D.** Disorders of the lower motor neuron tend to present with weakness, hypotonia, atrophy, and decreased or absent tendon reflexes. (1:92)

63. **E.** All the ocular abnormalities listed may be found in the Wernicke-Korsakoff syndrome. (1:100)

64. **A.** Women are affected by myasthenia gravis more frequently than men and the facial muscles are almost always affected, causing weakness of closure of eyes and of retraction of the angles of the mouth, with the production of a characteristic snarling appearance on smiling. Also, there is abnormal muscular fatigability most frequently observed in the ocular muscles resulting in ptosis or diplopia. All other statements are true of myasthenia gravis. (2:388)

65. **A.** Tic douloureux occurs rarely in the seventh, ninth, or eleventh nerve. The other statements are true of tic douloureux. (1:99)

66. **B.** (6:306)

67. **A.** (6:306)

68. **C.** (6:306)

69. **D.** Craniopharyngiomas are very liable to undergo cystic degeneration and calcification. All other statements are true of this type of tumor. (2:201)

70. **D.** Delirium tremens is a relatively rare but potentially lethal complication of withdrawal. All other statements are true. (1:101)

71. **A.** The glioblastoma multiforme is an extremely malignant glioma. All other statements are true. (2:197)

72. **E.** Ergotamine tartrate relieves the migrainous headaches by increasing the tone and so diminishing the stretch of the branches of the external carotid artery. All other statements are true of migranous neuralgia. (2:193)

73. **D.** Cerebrospinal fluid pressure is not usually elevated in patients with hyperosmolar nonketonic coma. All other statements are true of this disorder. (1:99)

74. **D.** The Babinski sign is present in upper motor neuron disease. All other statements are true. (1:92)

75. **E.** Pes cavus and scoliosis are present in almost all cases of Friedreich's ataxia; scoliosis is usually associated with a slight contracture of the muscles of the calf. In most cases, the disease is slowly and steadily progressive. All other statements are true of Friedreich's ataxia. (2:452–54)

76. **E.** Lumbar puncture headache (characterized by a steady occipitonuchal pain and frontal pain coming on a few minutes after arising from a recumbent position and relieved within a few minutes by lying down) has as its cause a persistent leakage of cerebrospinal fluid into the lumbar tissues through the needle site. The cerebrospinal fluid pressure is low (often 0 in the lateral decubitus position), and the injection of sterile isotonic saline solution intrathecally relieves it. (6:20)

77. **E.** In peroneal muscular atrophy, there is usually distal impairment of cutaneous, less often of postural, sensibility. The disease runs a slow course which may be arrested at any stage. All other statements are true of Charcot-Marie-Tooth disease. (2:454–55)

78. **C.** Primary subarachnoid hemorrhage is usually due to rupture of an intracranial aneurysm or an arteriovenous malformation. (1:98)

79. **C.** The headache of both bacterial meningitis and subarachnoid hemorrhage usually occur in single attacks over a period of days. (6:26)

80. **C.** It is generally believed now that thrombus formation on ulcerated areas of atheromatous plaques is important in both cerebral infarction and transient cerebral ischemia. (*Br Med J*, 1:89, 1972)

81. **C.** Myasthenia gravis is associated with all the disorders listed. (1:93)

82. **D.** Diabetic peripheral neuropathy is not limited mainly to the lower extremities and to patients with long duration of disease. In one study, the subjects with juvenile onset diabetes had impaired light-touch and two-point perception thresholds of the upper as well as the lower extremity. The abnormalities in light-touch critical flicker fusion and electric taste were present within two years of onset of clinically recognized disease. (*N Engl J Med*, 286:1233, 1972)

Textbook References for Chapter 18

1. American College of Physicians (1974): *Medical Knowledge Self-Assessment, Program III: Recent Developments in Internal Medicine,* Petersdorf, R.G., General Editor, American College of Physicians, Philadelphia.

2. Bannister, Roger (1978): *Brain's Clinical Neurology,* Fifth Edition, Oxford Medical Publications, New York.

3. Beeson, P.B. and McDermott, W. (1979): *Cecil Textbook of Medicine,* Fifteenth Edition, W.B. Saunders Company, Philadelphia.

4. Judge, R.D. and Zuidema, G.D., Editors (1974): *Physical Diagnosis: A Physiologic Approach to the Clinical Examination,* Little, Brown and Company, Boston.

5. Merritt, Houston H. (1979): *A Textbook of Neurology,* Sixth Edition, Lea and Febiger, Philadelphia.

6. Isselbacher, K.J., Editor (1980): *Harrison's Principles of Internal Medicine,* Ninth Edition, McGraw-Hill Book Company, New York.

CHAPTER 19

Pharmacology

1. Of the following sulfonylureas, the longest duration of effect occurs with

    A. tolbutamide (Orinase)
    B. acetohexamide (Dymelor)
    C. chlorpropamide (Diabinese)
    D. tolazamide (Tolinase)
    E. glyburide (Diabeta, Micronase)

Directions: Indicate whether each of the following statements is true or false.

2. The medication which most frequently alters the concentration of thyroid-binding proteins is female hormone.

3. Spironolactone (Aldactone) is contraindicated in severe congestive heart failure.

4. Digitalis is associated with toxicity in at least 15% of patients receiving it.

5. Anticonvulsant drugs may obscure insulin reactions.

6. The use of digoxin in treating sinus tachycardia secondary to significant congestive heart failure will generally evoke a therapeutic response, but if the sinus tachycardia is secondary to some other cause, no response may be seen until the dosages are in the toxic range.

7. Large amounts of propranolol may cause hyperosmolar nonketotic coma in persons with untreated diabetes by blocking lipolysis or interfering with the insulin response or both.

8. Propranolol is contraindicated for arrhythmias associated with Wolff-Parkinson-White syndrome.

9. Furosemide (Lasix) does not concentrate urine to the same degree as the thiazides and has less tendency to produce hyponatremia.

10. Long-term corticosteroid therapy is associated with a decreased incidence of arteriosclerotic vascular disease.

Directions: Answer questions 11 and 12 by using the key below:
A. if both the statement and reason are true and are related as to cause and effect
B. if both the statement and reason are true, but are not related as to cause and effect
C. if the statement is true, but the reason is false
D. if the statement is false, but the reason is true
E. if both the statement and reason are false.

11. Demeclocycline may be the treatment of choice in the chronic form of the syndrome of inappropriate ADH secretion because the response to the drug is instantaneous.

12. Since nearly all normal subjects treated with lithium acquire a diabetes insipidus syndrome, there is considerable reason to suspect that lithium would be effective in the management of all cases of the syndrome of inappropriate secretion of antidiuretic hormone.

Directions: For each of the following incomplete statements, select
A. if the question is associated with A only
B. if the question is associated with B only
C. if the question is associated with both A and B
D. if the question is associated with neither A nor B

13. Phenobarbital
    A. has been used in all seizure states including grand mal, petit mal, psychomotor and other focal seizures
    B. is most useful in limited dosage in combination with other drugs such as diphenylhydantoin (Dilantin)
    C. both
    D. neither

14. Cromolyn sodium (disodium cromoglycate)
    A. has a steroid-sparing effect
    B. is essentially a therapeutic agent
    C. both
    D. neither

15. Side effects of testosterone therapy include
    A. acne
    B. priapism
    C. both
    D. neither

16. May lead to the development of hypochloremic alkalosis, which does not interfere with its diuretic properties:
    A. furosemide
    B. ethacrynic acid
    C. both
    D. neither

17. Acetazolamide (Diamox)
    A. has been used as an adjuvant in all types of seizures, especially those in females related to menstrual cycles
    B. toxic effects include anorexia, acidosis, drowsiness, numbness of extremities, and, rarely, blood dyscrasias
    C. both
    D. neither

Directions: For the following multiple-choice question, select the INCORRECT ANSWER or ANSWERS.

18. The combination of trimethoprim (80 mg) and sulfamethoxazole (400 mg)
    A. results in a true demonstrable synergism at the ratio at which the two agents are present
    B. results in concentrations of either drug that alone would be only mildly bacteriostatic but are bacteriocidal when they are combined
    C. interferes with two consecutive steps in the normal bacterial metabolism of folic acid
    D. is effective *in vitro* against a wide variety of gram-positive and gram-negative organisms including staphylococci, streptococci, *Escherichia coli, Haemophilus influenzae, Proteus mirabilis,* and both salmonella and shigella species

E. has no antiprotozoal and antifungal activity

F. *Bacteroides* species are sensitive to the combination

G. probably should not be considered as primary medication for acute and chronic urinary tract infections

H. results in *Klebsiella-Enterobacter* sensitivity *in vitro*, despite the fact that many are completely resistant to sulfamethoxazole alone

I. may be used for bacterial infections of the upper respiratory tract, including infections of the nose, throat, and ear, when a patient's condition has failed to respond to other antibacterial therapy

Directions: For each of the incomplete statements below, ONE or MORE of the numbered completions is correct. In each case, select
A. **if 1, 2, and 3 are correct**
B. **if 1 and 3 are correct**
C. **if 2 and 4 are correct**
D. **if only 4 is correct**
E. **if all statements are correct**

19. Carbonic anhydrase inhibitors as diuretic agents

1. are associated with hyperchloremic acidosis and hypokalemia
2. have the principal site of action on the distal tubule
3. result in increased excretion of sodium, potassium, and bicarbonate, and a decrease in hydrogen excretion in urine
4. result in inhibition of enzymes involved in alkalinization of the urine

20. Amphetamines

1. possess anticonvulsant properties
2. control sleep seizures in children better than in adults
3. diminish or alleviate anticonvulsant, drug-induced drowsiness
4. control late nocturnal seizures better than early nocturnal seizures

21. Drugs which may induce pancreatitis include

1. glucocorticoids
2. chlorothiazide
3. isoniazid
4. salicylates

22. Drugs which may induce the malabsorption syndrome include

1. cholestyramine
2. colchicine
3. irritant laxatives
4. neomycin

23. Diphenylhydantoin (Dilantin)

1. may inhibit insulin release *in vitro*
2. may inhibit insulin response to an intensive and sustained glucose stimulation
3. should be used with caution in patients who have a risk factor for diabetes
4. should be used with caution in patients who are receiving other diabetogenic drugs

24. Usually effective in hypercalcemia, regardless of the cause is/are

1. calcitonin
2. mithramycin
3. phosphate
4. glucocorticoids

25. Intravenous colchicine

1. can produce a severe neutropenia since the usual warning of toxicity, gastrointestinal symptoms, does not occur
2. should be given in doses of no more than 4 mg during any acute gouty attack
3. in most patients an initial dose of 1 to 2 mg is followed in 6 hours by an additional 1 mg if necessary
4. decreases serum uric acid levels

Directions: For each of the following statements, fill in the correct answer(s).

26. The most serious toxic manifestation of gentamicin is loss of _____ function.

27. Lithium carbonate, which has been used in the treatment of inappropriate ADH secretion, carries the potential for severe toxicity if the patient becomes _____ depleted.

Directions: For each of the following multiple-choice questions, select the ONE INCORRECT answer.

28. Chlorpropamide administration has been associated with

    A. hyponatremia and serum hypo-osmolality
    B. continued sodium excretion despite hyponatremia
    C. an impaired ability to dilute urine maximally
    D. an impaired ability to excrete a water load
    E. an irreversible form of the syndrome of inappropriate APH secretion

29. Treatment of hyperthyroidism with carbimazole may

    A. provide satisfactory control in pregnancy
    B. hasten attainment of a euthyroid state after radio-iodine
    C. produce a euthyroid state in patients designated for surgery
    D. be used in patients with severe exophthalmos, in whom it is desirable to produce a euthyroid state as soon as possible
    E. commonly induce agranulocytosis

Directions: For each of the incomplete statements below, ONE or MORE of the numbered completions is correct. In each case, select
    A. if 1, 2, and 3 are correct
    B. if 1 and 3 are correct
    C. if 2 and 4 are correct
    D. if all statements are correct
    E. if all statements are incorrect
    F. if another combination is correct

30. Cromolyn sodium

    1. appears to have inhibitory effects on the vasoactive amines which are strikingly similar to the beta-adrenergic sympathomimetics
    2. inhibits specifically the release of allergic vasoactive amines (histamine serotonin and SRS-A), following the antigen-antibody reaction
    3. is most effective when administered to the extrinsic, atopic asthmatic
    4. acts as a bronchodilator and an antiinflammatory agent

31. Free T₄ index may be affected by

    1. estrogens
    2. androgens
    3. Dilantin
    4. high-dose salicylates

Directions: For each of the following incomplete statements, select
    A. if the answer is associated with A only
    B. if the answer is associated with B only
    C. if the answer is associated with both A and B
    D. if the answer is associated with neither A nor B

32. Chlorpropamide may produce the syndrome of inappropriate ADH

    A. by potentiating the action of circulating ADH on the kidney
    B. possibly by a central action on ADH secretion
    C. both
    D. neither

33. Intravenous mithramycin

    A. reduces calcium levels in hypercalcemia secondary to malignancy
    B. inhibits bone resorption in small doses
    C. both
    D. neither

34. Which of the following increases cardiac work in patients with coronary artery disease?

    A. morphine
    B. pentazocine (Talwin)
    C. both
    D. neither

35. Digitalis has a potent cholinergic effect on the
    A. sinoatrial (SA) node
    B. AV junction
    C. both
    D. neither

36. Propranolol
    A. has a direct membrane stabilizing effect on myocardial cells
    B. increases automaticity of ectopic pacemakers within the atria and ventricles
    C. both
    D. neither

37. Elevation of low-density lipoprotein (LDL) cholesterol may be treated with
    A. cholestyramine resin
    B. niacin
    C. both
    D. neither

38. Patients with metastatic islet cell carcinomas have been treated with
    A. streptozotocin
    B. diazoxide
    C. both
    D. neither

Directions: Answer questions 39 through 42 by using the key given below.
    A. if choice A is greater than or more appropriate than B
    B. if choice B is greater than or more appropriate than A
    C. if A and B are equal or approximately equal

39. Gastrointestinal absorption:
    A. digoxin
    B. digitoxin

40. A patient with a heart rate of 96 with normal beats followed by PVCs in a bigeminal pattern should be treated with
    A. atropine
    B. lidocaine

41. Protein-binding:
    A. digitoxin
    B. digoxin

42. Will increase the circulating levels of corticosteroids:
    A. liver disease
    B. kidney disease

Directions: Use the key given below for questions 43 through 45. If the statement describes
    A. **sulfonamides**
    B. **nalidixic acid**
    C. **novobiocin**

43. Inhibit(s) synthesis of DNA and RNA

44. Inhibit(s) synthesis of DNA precursors

45. Inhibit(s) DNA synthesis

Directions: Indicate whether each of the following statements is true or false.

46. Demeclocycline (7-chloro-6-demethyltetracycline), a relatively nontoxic antibiotic, can produce a reversible nephrogenic diabetes insipidus in normal persons.

47. Thiazide diuretics may decrease urinary calcium excretion and raise serum calcium concentration in any patient, but sustained high-serum calcium concentrations usually develop only in primary or secondary hyperparathyroidism.

48. The uricosuric action of probenecid is not suppressed by salicylates in man.

49. Dexamethasone possesses practically pure glucocorticoid activity and may be profitably employed when salt retention is a major problem.

50. Aminophylline is contraindicated in patients with Cheyne-Stokes breathing.

51. In healthy subjects, a 48- to 72-hour fast is usually required before ethanol will precipitate hypoglycemia.

Directions: For each of the following incomplete statements, ONE or MORE of the numbered completions is correct. In each case, select
A. if 1, 2, and 3 are correct
B. if 1 and 3 are correct
C. if 2 and 4 are correct
D. if all statements are correct
E. if all statements are incorrect
F. if another combination is correct

52. Colchicine may produce

1. alopecia
2. leukopenia
3. abdominal pain
4. thrombocytopenia and anemia

53. Probenecid

1. plasma half-life is dose-dependent but ranges from 6 to 12 hours
2. maintenance dose ranges from 500 mg to 3 g/day given in three or four divided doses
3. initiation of uricosuric therapy leads to a transient increase in uric acid excretion
4. is poorly bound to plasma protein and has both analgesic and antiinflammatory properties

54. Phenylbutazone administration

1. may be associated with the appearance of rash, sore throat, fever, melena, or fluid retention
2. may potentiate action of sulfonylureas
3. has been found helpful in primary fibrositis
4. may decrease the effect of warfarin (Coumadin)

55. Gentamicin has been found to be effective against

1. *Escherichia coli*
2. pseudomonas
3. proteus
4. klebsiella

56. Salbutamol

1. is a beta-2 agonist
2. is effective when administered as an aerosol
3. exerts a minimal effect upon the cardiovascular system
4. is less potent than isoprenaline in promoting relaxation of bronchial smooth muscle

Directions: For each of the following incomplete statements, ONE or MORE of the numbered completions is correct. In each case, select
A. if 1, 2, and 3 are correct
B. if 1 and 3 are correct
C. if 2 and 4 are correct
D. if only 4 is correct
E. if all statements are correct

57. Potential complications associated with mithramycin administration include

1. lethargy
2. nausea and vomiting
3. bone-marrow depression
4. liver and renal damage

58. Allopurinol may lead to the development of

1. gastrointestinal intolerance
2. skin rashes, sometimes with fever
3. leukopenia and thrombocytopenia
4. hepatitis and vasculitis

59. By decreasing vitamin D-mediated calcium absorption from the intestine, prednisone (40 mg daily for 7 to 10 days) will correct the hypercalcemia in most cases of

1. sarcoidosis
2. multiple myeloma
3. vitamin D intoxication
4. osseous malignancy with extensive bone invasion

60. With the use of diazepam (Valium),

1. withdrawal symptoms similar to those noted with barbiturates and alcohol have followed abrupt discontinuation of the drug

2. characteristic symptoms of withdrawal may include convulsions, tremor, abdominal and muscle cramps, and vomiting and sweating

3. addiction-prone persons have been inclined to use the drug for treatment of insomnia despite the fact that one reported adverse reaction to the drug is insomnia itself

4. overdosage generally manifests itself with symptoms of somnolence, confusion, diminished reflexes and coma

Directions: For each of the following incomplete statements, select
A. **if the question is associated with A only**
B. **if the question is associated with B only**
C. **if the question is associated with both A and B**
D. **if the question is associated with neither A nor B**

61. Perchlorate

    A. is an effective antithyroid drug
    B. may cause fatal aplastic anemia and, therefore, should not be used for treatment of hyperthyroidism
    C. both
    D. neither

62. Iodide is

    A. used in thyroid crisis and congenital thyrotoxicosis when a rapid but short-term effect is required
    B. has been used in the immediate preoperative preparation of patients for thyroidectomy
    C. both
    D. neither

63. The blood level of carbenicillin, after a continuous intravenous infusion, is about twice as high as that of ampicillin; this occurs because

    A. the rate of renal clearance is much lower for carbenicillin than for other penicillins
    B. carbenicillin has a longer half-life because it is inactivated by nonrenal mechanisms at a much slower rate than either ampicillin or penicillin G
    C. both
    D. neither

64. Vasopressors may

    A. sustain life in severe shock by preserving coronary and cerebral flow
    B. improve cardiac output by diverting blood from the vascular beds of the kidney, gut, liver, and extremities
    C. both
    D. neither

Directions: Indicate whether the following statement is true or false.

65. Bacterial isolates which have been obtained before the introduction of antibiotics do not show resistance to antibiotics.

Directions: For each of the following incomplete statements, ONE or MORE of the numbered completions is correct. In each case, select
A. **if 1, 2, and 3 are correct**
B. **if 1 and 3 are correct**
C. **if 2 and 4 are correct**
D. **if only 4 is correct**
E. **if all statements are correct**

66. Which of the following interfere(s) with the synthesis of thyroid hormone by blocking the binding of iodine?

    1. carbimazole
    2. methimazole
    3. propylthiouracil
    4. methylthiouracil

67. Antimicrobial agents which interfere with the functions of the polyribosome system include

    1. tetracyclines
    2. chloramphenicol
    3. erythromycin
    4. aminoglycosides

68. Carbenicillin

    1. is a semisynthetic penicillin whose antimicrobial spectrum resembles but is broader than that of ampicillin
    2. is also effective against pseudomonas and indole-positive proteus infections
    3. is virtually nontoxic
    4. since it has a tendency to produce drug resistance, should be given with another chemotherapeutic agent, such as an aminoglycoside, which will delay the emergence of resistance

Answers and Commentary

1. **C.** The duration of tolbutamide's effect is usually 6 to 12 hours. The duration of action of acetohexamide, tolazamide, and glyburide is 12 to 24 hours. Chlorpropamide's effect may last 24 to 48 hours. (1:1986)

2. **True.** The medication which most frequently alters the concentration of thyroid-binding proteins is female hormone.
   (*Am Fam Physician*, 3:73, 1971)

3. **False.** Spironolactone, 75 to 100 mg/day, is commonly used as a potassium-sparing diuretic. In refractory heart failure, doses of 100 to 600 mg/day have proved helpful. (1:1103)

4. **True.** Digitalis is associated with toxicity in at least 15% of patients receiving it.
   (*Internist Observer*, p. 5, Oct–Nov 1975)

5. **True.** Anticonvulsant drugs may obscure insulin reactions. (*JAMA*, 214:1119, 1970)

6. **True.** The use of digoxin in treating sinus tachycardia secondary to significant congestive heart failure will generally evoke a therapeutic response, but if the sinus tachycardia is secondary to some other cause, no response may be seen until the dosages are in the toxic range.
   (*Internist Observer*, p. 5, Oct–Nov 1975)

7. **True.** Large amounts of propranolol may cause hyperosmolar nonketotic coma in persons with untreated diabetes by blocking lipolysis or interfering with the insulin response or both.
   (*Metabolism*, 22:685, 1973)

8. **False.** Propranolol may be used for Wolff-Parkinson-White syndrome, provided the patient is not in failure and there is time to wait for a therapeutic effect. Propranolol acts quickly and it is relatively safe.
   (*Emerg Med*, 5:157, Oct, 1973)

9. **True.** Furosemide does not concentrate urine to the same degree as the thiazides and has less tendency to produce hyponatremia.
   (*Am Fam Physician*, 8:186, 1973)

10. **False.** Long-term corticosteroid therapy is associated with an increased incidence of arteriosclerotic vascular disease.
    (*Ann Rheum Dis*, 31:196, 1972)

11. **C.** The response to demeclocycline in patients with inappropriate secretion of ADH is, as in normal subjects, delayed for several days, and does not appear useful to achieve the prompt remission of an acute water intoxication, but may be the treatment of choice in the chronic form of the syndrome. (*N Engl J Med*, 293:915, 1975)

12. **E.** Since only 12% of normal subjects treated with lithium acquire a diabetes insipidus syndrome, there is little reason to suspect that lithium would be effective in the management of all cases of the syndrome of inappropriate secretion of antidiuretic hormone. Although lithium carbonate has been used in the syndrome of inappropriate secretion of ADH, several side effects of lithium should be seriously considered when long-term administration is needed. Even at low doses, gastrointestinal irritation and central nervous system dysfunction are frequently seen in lithium therapy, especially when a sodium depletion factor is present. Moreover, lithium has been occasionally associated with increased myocardial irritability, even without evidence of previous cardiac disease, and with thyroid dysfunction.
    (*N Engl J Med*, 293:915, 1975)

13. **C.** Both statements are true of phenobarbital. Its toxic effects include drowsiness, dulling, rash, fever, irritability and hyperactivity in some children.   (1:859)

14. **A.** Cromolyn sodium is essentially a prophylactic agent.
(*Curr Med Digest*, 39:1117, 1972)

15. **C.** Acne and priapism are both side effects of testosterone therapy.
(*Ann Intern Med*, 78:527, 1973)

16. **C.** Furosemide and ethacrynic acid may lead to the development of hypochloremic alkalosis which does not interfere with their diuretic properties. (*Am Fam Physician*, 8:186, 1973)

17. **C.** Both these statements are true of the use of acetazolamide (Diamox) in seizures.   (1:859)

18. **E,F,G.** The combination of trimethoprim and sulfamethoxazole has antiprotozoal and antifungal activity. Bacteroid species are not sensitive to this combination. The mixture should be considered as primary medication for acute and chronic urinary tract infections. All other statements are correct.   (*JAMA*, 231:635, 1975)

19. **B.** The principal site of action of carbonic anhydrase inhibitors is on the proximal tubule. They result in inhibition of enzymes involved in acidification of urine. They are not very potent diuretics, and lose effectiveness in a few days. As mentioned, they result in increased excretion of sodium, potassium, and bicarbonate and a decrease in hydrogen in urine. Blood studies may reveal hyperchloremic acidosis and hypokalemia.
(1:1103)

20. **B.** For reasons that at present remain obscure, adults rather than infants or very young children, and patients with early rather than late nocturnal seizures respond better to amphetamine therapy. All other statements are correct.
(*JAMA*, 233:278, 1975)

21. **E.** All the drugs listed may induce pancreatitis. In addition, pancreatitis may be induced by oral contraceptives, especially in women who have Type 4 as well as Type 5 lipid patterns before therapy, and by indomethacin.   (1:1551)

22. **E.** All the drugs listed, as well as *p*-amino salicylic acid, may result in drug-induced malabsorption syndrome.   (1:1526)

23. **E.** All statements are true of Dilantin.
(*N Engl J Med*, 286:339, 1972)

24. **A.** Calcitonin, mithramycin, and phosphate are usually effective in hypercalcemia regardless of the cause. Calcitonin may not have a sustained effect, and mithramycin, though safe in a single dose, may be toxic in multiple doses. Phosphorus should be given by mouth in moderate doses (1 to 3 g/day) since excessive phosphate loading can produce soft tissue calcification and worsening of renal function. Any of these measures, if effective, will allow the physician time to do further diagnostic studies. Glucocorticoids are particularly effective in vitamin D intoxication and sarcoidosis, may be effective in many neoplasms including peptide-secreting tumors, are less effective when there is extensive bone invasion, and are only occasionally effective in hyperparathyroidism.
(*N Engl J Med*, 286:339, 1972)

25. **A.** Intravenous colchicine does not decrease serum uric acid levels. All other statements are true.   (*Semin Drug Treat*, 1:119, 1971)

26. **Vestibular.** The most serious toxic manifestation of gentamicin is loss of vestibular function.
(2:65)

27. **Sodium.** The treatment of symptomatic chronic hyponatremia due to the syndrome of inappropriate antidiuretic hormone (ADH) secretion (for example, associated with tumors) usually requires severe water restriction and meets with limited patient acceptance. Lithium carbonate has also been used in this syndrome, but it carries the potential for severe toxicity if the patient becomes sodium depleted. (*Ann Intern Med*, 83:654, 1975)

28. **E.** Chlorpropamide has been associated with a reversible form of the syndrome of inappropriate activity of ADH. The syndrome has been found in 4% of patients receiving chlorpropamide in a clinic population. The antidiuretic action of chlorpropamide has been recognized and used in the therapy of diabetes insipidus.
(*N Engl J Med*, 284:65, 1971)

29. **E.** In the treatment of hyperthyroidism with carbimazole, rashes may occur, but agranulocytosis is extremely rare. All other statements are correct.   (*Br Med J*, 2:337, 1972)

30. **A.** Cromolyn sodium is neither a bronchodilator nor an antiinflammatory agent. All other statements are correct.
(*Curr Med Digest*, 39:1117, 1972)

31. **D.** The free T_4 index may be affected by estrogens, androgens, Dilantin, or high-dose salicylates.   (*Am Fam Physician*, 3:73, 1971)

32. **C.** Chlorpropamide may produce the syndrome of inappropriate ADH by potentiating the action of circulating ADH on the kidney or possibly by a central action on ADH secretion.
(*Mod Med*, 41:39, 1973)

33. **C.** In a study by Slayton and others, an intravenous bolus injection of mithramycin (25 µg/kg) was given to patients with malignancy-related hypercalcemia persisting after hydration. In most circumstances, a gradual but steady fall in the serum calcium occurred within the next 48 hours, accompanied by a fall in serum inorganic phosphate and 24-hour urinary calcium excretion. Aside from transient nausea and vomiting, side effects were minimal. Small doses of mithramycin inhibit bone resorption. The hypercalcemia following administration of these agents may be an expression of their antivitamin D action.
(*JAMA*, 218:2000, 1971)

34. **B.** Pentazocine increases cardiac work in patients with coronary artery disease. It is decreased by morphine.
(*N Engl J Med*, 287:623, 1972)

35. **C.** Digitalis has a potent cholinergic effect on both the sinoatrial node and AV junction.
(*Am Fam Physician*, 9:178, 1974)

36. **A.** Propranolol has a direct membrane stabilizing effect on myocardial cells and decreases automaticity of ectopic pacemakers within the atria and ventricles. (*Am Fam Physician*, 9:178, 1974)

37. **C.** Elevation of low-density lipoprotein cholesterol may be treated with either of the medications listed. (*JAMA*, 233:275, 1975)

38. **C.** Diazoxide has proved to be an effective agent in many patients with metastatic islet cell carcinomas. To counteract the sodium-retaining effect of diazoxide administered in a dose of 600 to 1000 mg/day, a natriuretic thiazide should be used. Patients may also be treated with streptozotocin. Several patients with metastatic islet cell carcinoma who were treated with streptozotocin have had complete relief from hypoglycemia and regression of tumor mass for months or years.
(*Mod Med*, 41:24, 1973)

39. **B.** Seventy-five to ninety percent of digoxin may be absorbed from the gastrointestinal tract, whereas 90 to 100% of digitoxin is absorbed.
(1:1096)

40. **A.** A patient with a rate of 96 with normal beats followed by PVCs in a bigeminal pattern should be treated with atropine.
(*Emerg Med*, 5:157, Oct, 1973)

41. **A.** Twenty-three percent of digoxin is protein-bound, as compared to 97% of digitoxin. (1:1096)

42. **A.** Liver disease will increase circulating levels of corticosteroids. (*Ration Drug Ther*, 6:1, 1972)

43. **C.** (2:35)

44. **A.** (2:35)

45. **B.** (2:35)

46. **True.** It has been shown that demeclocycline (900 mg/day) can at least partially inhibit the action of ADH in the setting of tumor-induced ADH secretion with the production of a reversible, partial nephrogenic diabetes insipidus, and with few or no side effects. Demeclocycline may be useful in the treatment of chronic inappropriate ADH secretion.
(*Ann Intern Med*, 83:654, 1975)

47. **True.** Thiazide diuretics may decrease urinary calcium excretion and raise serum calcium concentration in any patient, but sustained high-serum calcium concentrations usually develop only in primary or secondary hyperparathyroidism. Thiazide diuretics may simply increase calcium bound to serum albumin, but could also stimulate bone resorption or PTH secretion.
(*N Engl J Med*, 285:1006, 1971)

48. **False.** The uricosuric action of probenecid is suppressed by salicylates in man.
(*Semin Drug Treat*, 1:119, 1971)

49. **True.** Dexamethasone possesses practically pure glucocorticoid activity and may be profitably employed when salt retention is a major problem.
(*Ration Drug Ther*, 6:1, 1972)

50. **False.** Aminophylline is often helpful in controlling Cheyne-Stokes breathing. For cardiac patients who have a Cheyne-Stokes respiration or moderate orthopnea, a rectal suppository of aminophylline, 0.5 g given at bedtime, will frequently relieve the respiratory distress and promote sleep. (3:121)

51. **True.** In healthy subjects, a 48 to 72 hour fast is usually required before ethanol will precipitate hypoglycemia. (*Mod Med*, 41:24, 1973)

52. **D.** Colchicine may produce any of the disorders listed. In addition, it may produce ascending paralysis, respiratory failure, malabsorption, and diarrhea. (*Semin Drug Treat*, 1:119, 1971)

53. **A.** Probenecid is readily bound to plasma proteins (89 to 94%) and has no analgesic or anti-inflammatory properties. All other statements are true of probenecid.
(*Semin Drug Treat*, 1:119, 1971)

54. **A.** Phenylbutazone administration may increase the effect of warfarin. All other statements are correct. (*Johns Hopkins Med J*, 130:300, 1972)

55. **D.** Gentamicin has been found to be effective against *Escherichia coli,* pseudomonas, proteus, klebsiella, and enterobacter. (2:61)

56. **A.** Salbutamol is more potent than isoprenaline in promoting bronchial smooth muscle relaxation, and its duration of action (approx. 6 hours) is longer than that of isoprenaline.
(*Curr Med Digest*, 39:1117, 1972)

57. **E.** All of the complications listed may occur with mithramycin administration. In addition, hemorrhage has been reported. Administration of this drug is more hazardous if renal function is impaired. (*Geriatrics*, 27:104, 1972)

58. **E.** Allopurinol may lead to the development of any of the disorders listed.
(*Semin Drug Treat*, 1:119, 1971)

59. **A.** Prednisone in the stated dosage will correct the hypercalcemia in about half the cases of non-osseous malignancy including peptide-secreting tumors. It is less effective when there is extensive bone invasion and is only rarely effective in hyperparathyroidism. All other disorders listed can be effectively treated with this drug.
(*Ann Intern Med*, 82:64, 1975)

60. **E.** All statements listed are true of the use of diazepam. In addition, adverse paradoxical reactions have been observed, including acute hyper-excited states, anxiety, hallucinations, muscle spasticity, and rage.
(*N Engl J Med*, 290:807, 1974)

61. **C.** Both statements are true of perchlorate.
(*Br Med J*, 2:337, 1972)

62. **C.** Both statements are true of iodide.
(*Br Med J*, 2:337, 1972)

63. **C.** Both factors cause the blood level of carbenicillin (after a continuous intravenous infusion) to be twice as high as that of ampicillin.
(2:66)

64. **C.** Both statements are true of vasopressors.
(2:96)

65. **False.** Bacterial isolates which had been obtained before the introduction of antibiotics still show resistance to antibiotics. (2:27)

66. **E.** Carbimazole, methimazole, propylthiouracil and methylthiouracil all interfere with the synthesis of thyroid hormone by blocking the binding of iodine. (*Br Med J*, 2:337, 1972)

67. **E.** All the antimicrobial agents listed interfere with the functions of the polyribosome system.
(2:36)

68. **E.** All the statements are true of carbenicillin.
(2:61, 65, 66)

Textbook References for Chapter 19

1. Beeson, P.B. and McDermott, W. (1979): *Cecil Textbook of Medicine*, Fifteenth Edition, W.B. Saunders Company, Philadelphia.

2. Lauler, D.P. et al (1971): *Gram Negative Sepsis,* MedCom, Clifton, N.J.

3. Isselbacher, K.J., Editor (1980): *Harrison's Principles of Internal Medicine*, Ninth Edition, McGraw-Hill Book Company, New York.

CHAPTER 20

Physical Examination and History-Taking

Directions: For each of the following questions, fill in the ONE CORRECT answer.

1. Intra-abdominal inflammation which secondarily involves the iliopsoas muscle may be detected by the _____ test: the patient is asked to flex his thigh against the examiner's hand and if inflammation is present in this location, the contraction of the psoas muscle will be accompanied by pain.

2. _____ is a blind or partially blind area in the visual field.

3. The _____ reflex is tested by quickly extending or flexing the last joint of the middle finger; while suspending the limp hand by its middle finger, quickly flip the tip of the finger upward or downward.

4. _____ is edema of the optic disc ("choked disc"), usually due to increased intracranial pressure.

5. _____ is a technique which calls for lightly thrusting the fingers into the abdomen in the region of a suspected mass; the thrust will tend to displace the fluid, permitting the mass to bound upward, producing a characteristic tapping sensation against the palpating fingers.

6. There is a V-shaped row of _____ papillae at the junction of the anterior two-thirds and the posterior one-third of the tongue.

7. The tympanic membrane is usually found on a slanted plane with the anterior inferior quadrant farthest away from the examiner. This accounts for the triangle of light reflecting anteroinferiorly from the _____ .

8. The parotid duct orifice is found in the posterior mucosal surface of the cheek opposite the maxillary _____ molar.

9. When the secondary component of an apparently split first sound is louder at the base of the heart than at the apex, and is of sharp quality, the additional sound is probably a(n) _____ sound.

10. The _____ gland can be palpated directly under the ramus of the mandible about halfway between the chin and the angle of the jaw.

Directions: Indicate whether each of the following statements is true or false.

11. In healthy adults, the muscles are normally somewhat hypertonic.

12. The liver edge may normally be felt during palpation, especially in men.

13. A reflex is considered truly absent if it cannot be elicited by a direct, smart strike to the tendon or bone with a reflex hammer.

14. Since the left kidney normally is somewhat lower than the right, it is usually palpable.

15. The spleen must be two or three times normal size before it becomes palpable.

16. Tricuspid regurgitation causes a murmur similar to that of mitral insufficiency which is best heard over the tricuspid area; it can also be distinguished by the fact that it may become softer with inspiration.

17. With intestinal obstruction, peristaltic waves may be particularly visible passing across the abdomen.

18. When delineating the upper and lower borders of the liver during a physical examination, the borders should be more than 10 cm apart.

19. Splitting of the first heart sound is common normally, particularly in the tricuspid area.

20. Sinusitis usually causes generalized headache.

21. Applying the cuff too loosely will give falsely depressed blood pressure values.

22. Light pressure over the jugular bulb causes the neck veins to collapse.

23. The pulmonary component of the second heart sound is softer than the aortic component and is normally heard only at and around the second left interspace (pulmonic area).

24. Because the pulmonic and tricuspid valves are located near the chest, their sounds are transmitted to nearby auscultatory areas.

25. The systolic pressure in the lower extremities is usually about 10 mm Hg below that in the upper extremities.

26. A gross estimate of the diastolic pressure is possible at times by palpation.

27. When trying to detect low-pitched sounds and murmurs, the stethoscope bell should be applied as forcefully as possible.

28. Generalized hyperresonance not due to full-held inspiration is found when the lung contains more air than normal, as in obstructive emphysema.

29. Although rhonchi and some loud, interrupted crackling rales are sometimes misleadingly called "dry," all of these sounds indicate the presence of fluid somewhere within the respiratory tract.

Directions: For each of the following incomplete statements, ONE or MORE of the numbered completions is correct. In each case, select
  A. if 1, 2, and 3 are correct
  B. if 1 and 3 are correct
  C. if 2 and 4 are correct
  D. if only 4 is correct
  E. if all statements are correct

30. Normally, the pupils
  1. are equal in size
  2. are about 2 to 3 mm in diameter
  3. react to light directly
  4. do not react to light consensually, or to convergence

31. Giant "a" waves
  1. result from very forceful right atrial contraction
  2. are seen with tricuspid stenosis
  3. more commonly result from loss of diastolic compliance accompanying right ventricular hypertrophy, as in pulmonary stenosis and pulmonary hypertension
  4. do not disappear following onset of atrial fibrillation

32. Common causes of a weak pulse include

    1. mitral stenosis
    2. acute myocardial infarction
    3. shock
    4. constrictive pericarditis

33. In arterial occlusion, examination of the affected extremity may show

    1. diminished or absent pulses, and audible systolic bruits extending into early diastole heard over major arteries (femoral or subclavian)
    2. reduced or absent hair peripherally (over the digits and dorsum of the hands or feet)
    3. atrophy of muscles and soft tissues
    4. thickened nails with rough transverse ridges and longitudinal curving

34. Venous pulse

    1. is diffuse and undulant
    2. disappears in the sitting position
    3. is obliterated by light pressure over the jugular bulb
    4. increases with inspiration

35. Venous hum is

    1. a phasic roaring heard in about 25% of normal adults
    2. heard at the lower border of the sterno-cleidomastoid muscle in the recumbent position
    3. immediately interrupted by compression over the jugular bulb and the Valsalva maneuver
    4. a serious finding

36. Vesicular breath sounds

    1. are breezy or swishy in character
    2. are high-pitched, and the inspiratory phase predominates
    3. expiration is heard only as a short, fainter, lower pitched puff less than one-fourth as long as inspiration
    4. when occurring over most of the lungs, they are an abnormal finding

37. The specialized mucosa of the dorsum of the tongue presents papillations of

    1. filiform types
    2. fungiform types
    3. circumvallate types
    4. foliate types

38. Carotid pulse

    1. is localized and swift
    2. is affected by position
    3. does not change with respiration
    4. is changed by light pressure over the jugular bulb

Directions: Use the key below to answer questions 39 through 42. If the procedure is used in testing the

    A. Babinski reflex
    B. Chaddock reflex
    C. Oppenheim reflex
    D. Gordon reflex

39. Stroking the lateral edge of the foot from the heel to the toes just above the sole

40. Firmly pressing down on the skin with the knuckles from the knee to the ankle

41. Stroking the sole of the foot with a pointed instrument from the heel, along the lateral edge of the foot, and then across the ball of the foot medially

42. Squeezing the calf firmly

Directions: For each of the following multiple-choice questions, select the ONE INCORRECT answer.

43. Cremasteric reflex

    A. is unrelated to the abdominal reflexes
    B. appropriate stimulus is a light scratch along the inner aspect of the upper part of the thigh and the response is a contraction of the cremasteric muscles, with elevation of the testicle
    C. arc runs through the first lumbar spinal segment

D. is diminished or abolished by a lesion of the corticospinal tract

E. is usually diminished or absent in a patient with varicocele and is usually extremely brisk in children

44. Vitamin B₁₂ neuropathy

A. equally affects the sexes in contrast to the female preponderance in pernicious anemia

B. has glove-and-stockings distribution of superficial sensory loss

C. is usually associated with moderate muscular wasting, especially in the peripheral muscles of the limbs

D. is less closely related to glossitis than is the anemia

E. does not occur without severe anemia or obvious changes in the blood film or bone marrow

45. In Rinne's test,

A. a vibrating tuning fork is applied to mastoid process, the ear being closed by examiner's finger

B. when the patient ceases to hear the sound, the tuning fork is placed at the external acoustic meatus

C. in middle-ear deafness, sound cannot be heard by air conduction after bone conduction has ceased to transmit it

D. in nerve deafness, sound cannot be heard by air conduction after bone conduction has ceased to transmit it

Directions: Use the key below to answer questions 46 through 49. If the statement is characteristic of the
A. **Trendelenburg gait**
B. **antalgic gait**

46. Marked by a fall of the pelvis, rather than the normal rise, on the side opposite the involved hip when it is weight-bearing

47. "Antipain" gait; the patient attempts to minimize the force bearing through the hip by leaning over the involved hip as weight bears through it

48. The body's center of gravity is moved toward the hip joint, decreasing the force exerted on the hip

49. Weakness of the abductor muscles due to intrinsic muscle disease, lack of normal innervation of the muscle, or an unstable hip joint

Directions: For the following multiple-choice questions, select the ONE CORRECT answer.

50. The most common variation in hard-palate structure is seen in a midline hard swelling or exostosis (torus palatinus) which occurs in what percentage of the adult population?
A. 5%
B. 10%
C. 20%
D. 50%
E. 75%

51. The blood vessels of the retina emerge from and enter the disc in how many main pairs?
A. 2
B. 4
C. 8
D. 16
E. 20

52. The corneal reflex
A. can be tested by carefully placing a fine, elongated wisp of cotton on the cornea while the patient is looking away from the approaching cotton
B. both eyes should blink quickly with stimulation
C. each eye should be tested separately
D. all of the above
E. none of the above

53. Hoffmann's reflex is
A. physiologically identical with the flexor finger jerk, which is elicited by tapping the palmar surface of the slightly flexed fingers

B. a positive response consisting of a sharp twitch of adduction and flexion of the thumb and flexion of the fingers

C. an index of muscular hypertonia rather than of an upper motor neuron lesion as such

D. all of the above

E. none of the above

54. The reaction of accommodation

A. is part of the near reflex

B. consists of convergence, accommodation of the eyes, and miosis

C. is impaired with midbrain lesions

D. all of the above

E. none of the above

55. Major source(s) of inaccurate observation include

A. oversight

B. forgetting

C. bias

D. all of the above

E. none of the above

56. Palpable parathyroid adenomas occur in what percentage of cases of primary hyperparathyroidism?

A. less than 2%

B. 5%

C. 10%

D. 24%

E. 50%

57. In obstructive emphysema,

A. there is barrel-shaped deformity of the chest

B. the ribs are more horizontal

C. the subcostal angle is less than 65 degrees with variation during respiration

D. B and C

E. A and B

Directions: Use the key below to answer questions 58 through 61. If the statement defines

A. dyschezia

B. tympanites

C. obstipation

D. tenesmus

58. Painful defecation

59. Persistent failure to pass any stool

60. The sensation of the need to evacuate the bowels, but without result

61. Distention of the abdomen due to presence of gas or air in the intestine or peritoneal cavity

Directions: Indicate whether each of the following statements is true or false.

62. Intensity of fremitus and the breath sounds are influenced in the same direction.

63. Dullness is elicited with pulmonary infiltration of almost any cause, regardless of the state of patency of the supplying bronchus, whenever the air content of the lung is partially or completely replaced by fluids or solids.

64. Dullness to percussion occurs when the air content of the underlying tissue is decreased and its solidity is increased.

65. Large, bulky tumors, pleural effusion, and pneumothorax usually draw the mediastinum toward the same side as the disorder.

66. Auscultation of the abdomen is probably one of the most rewarding aspects of the physical examination of a patient with abdominal pain.

67. The neutral question should be avoided whenever possible when interviewing patients.

68. The normal thyroid gland is visible.

69. Subnormal temperature is common in many individuals.

70. During a history-taking interview, an attempt should be made to record the complete history in final form.

71. Localized increased fremitus occurs when the transmission of sound from the trachea through the vibrating lung to the examining finger is interfered with by any cause.

72. Helpful in the diagnosis of intrathoracic disease is a change in the normally obtuse angle the skin makes with the base of the nail; in clubbing, the nail is raised and this angle lost and flattened.

73. Even with careful percussion, the extent and equality of diaphragmatic excursion will be poorly evaluated in most patients.

74. The retinal arterioles are somewhat darker than the veins and are about one-third wider.

75. The diastolic murmur of tricuspid stenosis is similar in timing and quality to the mitral murmur but is frequently higher-pitched and localized near the tricuspid area or along the left sternal border; inspiration usually makes it louder.

76. A thyroid bruit is almost pathognomonic of hyperthyroidism.

77. The simple direct question is always open because it requires simply a yes or no answer.

78. The patient will almost universally respond in a nonbiased manner to a question which conveys the possibility of serious consequences.

79. The single most useful physical finding in patients with chronic obstructive pulmonary disease is diminished intensity of breath sounds which is probably produced by decrease in airflow combined with hyperinflation.

80. A major reason for overtreatment of hypertension is the failure to get blood pressures in both the supine and upright positions.

Directions: Use the key below to answer questions 81 through 83. Select
 A. if the statement defines ectropion
 B. if the statement defines exophthalmos
 C. if the statement defines entropion

81. Inversion of the lid border

82. Eversion of the lid border

83. Protrusion of the eyeball

Directions: Use the key below to answer questions 84 and 85. If the statement is characteristic of
 A. women
 B. men

84. Tend to breathe largely with costal cage, and thoracic expansion is easily noted

85. Respiration is largely diaphragmatic and bulging of the abdomen with inspiration is seen

Answers and Commentary

1. **Iliopsoas.** Intra-abdominal inflammation which secondarily involves the iliopsoas muscle may be detected by the iliopsoas test. The patient is asked to flex his thigh against the resistance of the examiner's hand. If inflammation is present in this location, the contraction of the psoas muscle will be accompanied by pain. (2:224)

2. **Scotoma.** Scotoma is a blind or partially blind area in the visual field. (2:342)

3. **Hoffmann.** The Hoffmann reflex is tested by quickly extending or flexing the last joint of the middle finger. While suspending the limp hand by its middle finger, quickly flip the tip of the finger upward or downward. Normally there is very little if any response to this maneuver, but a flexion response of the thumb and fingers is not an unequivocal sign of pyramidal tract disease. It is significant only when markedly exaggerated or unilaterally present. (2:349)

4. **Papilledema.** Papilledema is edema of the optic disc ("choked disc"), usually due to increased intracranial pressure. (2:341)

5. **Ballottement.** Ballottement is a technique which calls for lightly thrusting the fingers into the abdomen in the region of the suspected mass. The thrust will tend to displace the fluid, permitting the mass to bound upward, producing a characteristic tapping sensation against palpating fingers. (2:212)

6. **Circumvallate.** There is a V-shaped row of circumvallate papillae at the junction of the anterior two-thirds and the posterior one-third of the tongue. These papillae receive taste fibers from the ninth glossopharyngeal nerve and have a more important taste function than the taste fibers from the lingual nerve (chorda tympani) which innervates the taste buds on the anterior two-thirds of the tongue. (2:98)

7. **Umbo.** The tympanic membrane is usually found on a slanted plane with the anterior inferior quadrant farthest away from the examiner. This accounts for the triangle of light reflecting anteroinferiorly from the umbo. (2:95)

8. **Second.** The parotid duct orifice is found in the posterior mucosal surface of the cheek opposite the maxillary second molar. (2:85)

9. **Ejection.** When the secondary component of an apparently split first sound is louder at the base of the heart than at the apex, and is of sharp quality, the additional sound is probably an ejection sound. (*JAMA*, 224:1133, 1973)

10. **Submaxillary.** The submaxillary gland can be palpated directly under the ramus of the mandible and about halfway between the chin and the angle of the jaw. It has a firm, irregular consistency. This gland can be more accurately palpated bimanually. Place the index finger of one hand in the floor of the mouth, between the lateral aspect of the tongue and the teeth. The other hand palpates the gland externally. The submaxillary glands descend and become more prominent with advancing age; this is frequently misinterpreted as an enlargement of the glands. (2:97)

11. **False.** In healthy adults, the muscles are normally somewhat hypotonic. (2:348)

12. **False.** The liver edge may normally be felt during palpation, particularly in women and children. (2:206)

13. **False.** In normal young adults, the reflexes may be minimal or apparently absent and may be elicited only by asking the patient to "reinforce" by pulling with one hand against the other at the time the tendon is tapped. A reflex is not considered truly absent until it has been proved that it cannot be elicited by this maneuver. (2:349)

14. **False.** Since the right kidney normally is somewhat lower than the left, it is occasionally palpable, particularly in asthenic patients. (2:242)

15. **True.** The spleen must be two or three times normal size before it becomes palpable. (2:234)

16. **False.** Tricuspid regurgitation may become louder with inspiration. (2:187)

17. **True.** With intestinal obstruction, peristaltic waves may be visible passing across the abdomen. (2:210)

18. **False.** When delineating the upper and lower borders of the liver in the midclavicular line, they should be no more than 10 cm apart. However, liver dullness along the lower border may be partially obliterated by gas in the overlying bowel, making the overall dimension less than 10 cm. (2:205)

19. **True.** The mitral valve closes from 0.02 to 0.03 seconds before the tricuspid. Splitting of the first heart sound is therefore common normally, particularly in the tricuspid area. Since tricuspid closure is usually not well heard at the apex, a single-component first sound due entirely to the mitral valve is usually heard. (2:162)

20. **False.** Sinusitis rarely causes generalized headache. More frequently, there is pain and tenderness over the involved sinus. (2:100)

21. **False.** Applying the cuff too loosely will give a falsely elevated blood pressure value. (2:153)

22. **False.** Light pressure over the jugular bulb causes the neck veins to distend, and release is followed by collapse to the previous level. (2:158)

23. **True.** The aortic component of the second heart sound is widely transmitted to the neck and over the precordium. It is as a rule entirely responsible for the second sound at the apex. The pulmonary component is softer and is normally heard only at and around the second left interspace (pulmonic area). Splitting of the second sound is therefore audible only in this region. (2:162)

24. **True.** There are four reference points used for localization of sounds on the surface of the chest:

Pulmonary, aortic, tricuspid, and mitral. Because the pulmonic and tricuspid valves are located near the chest, their sounds are transmitted to nearby auscultatory areas. The aortic and mitral valves, however, are situated deep in the chest, and their sounds are transmitted in the direction of blood flow to points closer to the chest wall. The mitral sounds are referred to the apex; the aortic sounds follow the ascending aorta as it curves forward and are heard in the second right interspace, where the aorta most closely approximates the anterior chest wall. (2:150)

25. **False.** The systolic pressure in the lower extremities is usually about 10 mm Hg above that in the upper extremities. (2:153)

26. **True.** A gross estimate of the diastolic pressure is possible at times by palpation. With further deflation of the cuff, the brachial pulse assumes a bounding quality and then abruptly becomes normal. This point of change, when evident, roughly approximates the diastolic pressure. (2:143)

27. **False.** With the stethoscope bell, the skin becomes the diaphragm and the natural frequency varies depending on the amount of pressure exerted, much as the tympani player varies the pitch of his instrument. It probably ranges from 40 cps with light pressure to 150 to 200 cps with firm pressure. When trying to detect low-pitched sounds and murmurs, therefore, the bell should be applied as lightly as possible. A rubber nipple cut to size and fitted to the end of the bell may promote a better seal with lighter pressure. (2:149)

28. **True.** The normal percussion note is resonant over all of the lungs, except at the right apex where occasionally slight dullness is detected. Generalized hyperresonance not due to full-held inspiration is found when the lung contains more air than normal, as in obstructive emphysema. Localized areas of hyperresonance are noted when pneumothorax is present, and occasionally over solitary bullae. Impaired resonance is difficult to evaluate but may be noted adjacent to areas of greater pathology and over lungs partially consolidated, as in diffuse bronchopneumonia. (2:130)

29. **True.** Although rhonchi and some loud, interrupted crackling rales are sometimes misleadingly called "dry," all of these sounds indicate the presence of fluid somewhere within the respiratory tract. (2:131–32)

30. **A.** Normally, the pupils react quickly to light consensually and to convergence. All other statements are true. (2:344)

31. **A.** Giant "a" waves disappear following onset of atrial fibrillation. All other statements are true. (2:174)

32. **E.** Weak pulse (pulsus parvus) has a normal contour but a low amplitude. It feels weak and "thready." The pulse pressure is narrowed by a low stroke volume and associated peripheral vasoconstriction. It is present with low-output failures of all types. Common causes include mitral stenosis, acute myocardial infarction, shock, and constrictive pericarditis. (2:172)

33. **E.** Examination of the affected extremity with arterial occlusion may show any of the listed findings. In addition, there may be mild brawny edema or coolness on palpation. The skin is thin, shiny, and taut. Intense grayish pallor may appear on elevation of the extremity. Dependency after a minute or two of elevation produces a dusky, plum-colored rubor which develops very gradually (30 seconds to 1 minute). The superficial veins are flat and collapsed. There is delayed venous filling time. (2:169–70)

34. **A.** The venous pulse decreases with inspiration. All other statements are correct. (2:156–158)

35. **B.** The venous hum is heard at the lower border of the sternocleidomastoid muscle in the sitting position. This is an innocent finding of no consequence. (2:163)

36. **A.** Vesicular breath sounds are normal over most of the lungs. All other statements are true. (2:124)

37. **A.** The specialized mucosa of the dorsum of the tongue presents papillations of filiform, fungiform, and circumvallate types, while at the posterolateral borders of the tongue, ridges of foliate papillae are noted. (2:86)

38. **B.** The carotid pulse is localized and swift, is unaffected by position, does not change with respiration and is unchanged by pressure over the bulb. (2:158)

39. **B.** (2:349)

40. **C.** (2:349)

41. **A.** (2:349)

42. **D.** (2:349)

43. **A.** The cremasteric reflex is closely related to the abdominal reflexes. All other statements are correct. (1:100)

44. **E.** When vitamin B12 neuropathy is a symptom of Addisonian anemia, gastric achlorhydria is constantly present, and the blood and bone marrow show the changes characteristic of the anemia, though the actual degree of anemia may be slight. All other statements are correct. (1:449–50)

45. **D.** In Rinne's test, a vibrating tuning fork is applied to the patient's mastoid process, the ear being closed by the observer's finger. The patient is asked to say when he ceases to hear the sound, and the fork is then placed at the external acoustic meatus. In middle-ear deafness, the sound cannot be heard by air conduction after bone conduction has ceased to transmit it. In nerve deafness, as in normal individuals, the reverse is true. (1:61)

46. **A.** (2:296)

47. **B.** (2:296)

48. **B.** (2:296)

49. **A.** (2:296)

50. **C.** The most common variation in hard-palate structure is seen as a midline swelling or exostosis (torus palatinus). It occurs in 20% of the adult population. Such bony growths are benign and are significant only when the surface mucosa becomes ulcerated or dental prosthetic requirements necessitate their removal. (2:85)

51. **B.** The blood vessels of the retina emerge from and enter the disc in four main pairs. Examine the superior nasal vessels first, following them out as far as possible without having the patient turn his eye. This is followed in order by the inferior nasal, inferior temporal, and superior temporal pairs. The retina adjoining each of these pairs is inspected at the same time. Then ask the patient to look up, up and in, directly toward the nose, down and in, straight down, down and out, directly outward, and then up and out. This covers eight successive overlapping zones of the retinal areas seen along with inspection of the vessels. The central retina and macular area are visualized last, the patient being asked to look directly at the light if necessary. The foveal pit is seen as a small, bright dot produced by light reflection from the indention. (2:69–70)

52. **D.** All statements are true of the corneal reflex. (2:345)

53. **D.** All statements are true of Hoffmann's reflex. (1:99)

54. **D.** All statements are true of the reaction of accommodation.
(*Med Clin North Am,* 57:1363, 1973)

55. **D.** The three major sources of inaccurate observation are oversight, forgetting, and bias. Oversights are minimized by habituation to method and by fractionating observations into logical, sequential small units. Forgetting is minimized by jotting down immediate notes and reminders, and by transferring the information to the permanent record as promptly as possible. Bias is a lifelong challenge. It may be lessened by an understanding of how it distorts. By repeated self-analysis, by being on guard, you may minimize the tendency. (2:33)

56. **A.** Palpable parathyroid adenomas occur in fewer than 2% of cases of primary hyperparathyroidism. (*JAMA,* 233:907, 1975)

57. **E.** Barrel-shaped deformity of the chest is common in older patients with obstructive emphysema. The ribs are more horizontal, and the subcostal angle is greater than 90 degrees without variation during respiration. (2:127)

58. **A.** (2:201)

59. **C.** (2:201)

60. **D.** (2:202)

61. **B.** (2:202)

62. **True.** Intensity of fremitus and the breath sounds are influenced in the same direction. (2:130)

63. **True.** Dullness is elicited with pulmonary infiltration of almost any cause, regardless of the state of patency of the supplying bronchus, whenever the air content of the lung is partially or completely replaced by fluids or solids. When correlated with the character of the breath sounds on auscultation and fremitus during palpation, the status of the underlying parenchyma in a dull area can be reliably predicted. Dullness also is noted when the pleurae and pleural cavity are thickened or filled with anything except air. (Rarely, air under great tension will give a dull rather than a hyperresonant note.) Extreme dullness or flatness is noted when no air at all underlies the pleximeter, as occurs, for practical purposes, only with pleural effusion. Tympany is rare over the lungs themselves. It occasionally occurs over a large pneumothorax. (2:130)

64. **True.** The normal percussion note varies with the thickness of the chest wall and the force applied by the examiner. The clear, long, low-pitched sound elicited over the normal lung is termed resonance. Dullness occurs when the air content of the underlying tissue is decreased and its solidity increased. The sound is short, high-pitched, soft, and thudding, and lacks the vibratory quality of a resonant sound. It is heard normally over the heart and is accompanied by an increased sense of resistance (of minor importance) in the pleximeter finger. (2:121–22)

65. **False.** Conditions such as large, bulky tumors or pleural effusion and pneumothorax which increase the volume of one hemithorax usually cause a shift of the entire mediastinum to the opposite side, as evidenced by shift of the trachea and the apex beat. (2:129)

66. **False.** Much attention has been paid to the presence or absence of peristaltic sounds, their quality, and their frequency. Auscultation of the abdomen is probably one of the least rewarding aspects of the physical examination of a patient with abdominal pain. Severe catastrophes such as strangulating small intestinal obstruction or perforated appendicitis may occur in the presence of normal peristalsis. Conversely, when the proximal part of the intestine above an obstruction becomes markedly distended and edematous, peristaltic sounds may lose the characteristics of borborygmi and become weak or absent even when peritonitis is not present. It is usually the severe chemical peritonitis of sudden onset which is associated with the truly silent abdomen. (3:37)

67. **False.** The neutral question should be used whenever possible. It is structured so that it does not suggest any particular response as being more acceptable to the physician or more beneficial to the patient. A neutral question can be open or closed. The open neutral question simply establishes a topic: "Tell me more about your headaches." The closed neutral question incorporates several alternative answers in the question: "Are your headaches more likely to occur in the morning, afternoon, or evening?" (2:10)

68. **False.** Usually the normal thyroid gland is not visible. An enlargement may be evident as a subtle fullness which glides upward transiently upon deglutition. (2:43)

69. **True.** Subnormal temperature is common in many individuals. (2:36)

70. **False.** During the interview, no attempt should be made to record the complete history in final form. There are several good reasons for this. In the first place, it is literally impossible; it distracts the patient and disrupts the procedure. Jotting

down reminders, dates, ages, and numbers is not only acceptable but indispensable. Second, the medical record is not meant to be a repository for raw data. The information must be suitably condensed, logically sequenced, and converted as far as possible into crisp, pertinent medical terminology before recording it. This requires time and thought. (2:13)

71. **False.** Localized diminution of fremitus occurs when the transmission of sound from the trachea through the vibrating lung to the examining finger is interfered with by any cause. It is therefore absent in patients with a tracheostomy or an obstructed bronchus, when air or fluid in the pleural space is interposed, or when the chest wall is considerably thickened or edematous. Generalized diminution in fremitus occurs with diffuse bronchial obstruction. (2:130)

72. **True.** Inspection for respiratory disease requires inspection of more than the thorax. Clubbing, cyanosis, use of accessory respiratory distress, and marked sweating are important extrathoracic signs of intrathoracic disease. Clubbing of the fingers is especially important. The ends of the fingers and toes are swollen, at times grotesquely so. The nails are curved convexly from base to tip and from side to side. The tissue at the base of the nail is spongy and the nail itself loosely attached; its free edge may be palpable. Helpful in diagnosis is a change in the normally obtuse angle the skin makes with the base of the nail; in clubbing, the nail is raised and this angle lost and flattened. If the syndrome of pulmonary osteoarthropathy accompanies the clubbing, the periosteum over the ends of the long bones of the forearm and leg are palpably tender. (2:126–27)

73. **False.** The extent and equality of diaphragmatic excursion are well evaluated in most patients by percussion. Fluoroscopy is more reliable though less available. Tell the patient to inhale deeply and hold his breath. Note the line of change in the percussion note between the resonant lung and the abdominal viscera posteriorly. Then ask the patient to exhale completely and hold his breath. The lower level of pulmonary resonance has now moved upward. The distance between these two points represents the extent of diaphragmatic excursion. Complementary to this is the actual measurement of costal expansion, which requires a flexible tape measure placed around the chest at the nipple level. (2:21)

74. **False.** The retinal veins are somewhat darker than the arterioles, and are about one-third wider. (2:70)

75. **True.** The diastolic murmur of tricuspid stenosis is similar in timing and quality to the mitral murmur but is frequently higher-pitched and localized near the tricuspid area or along the left sternal border. Inspiration usually makes it louder. (2:189)

76. **True.** A thyroid bruit is almost pathognomonic of hyperthyroidism. (*Br Med J, 2,* 5810:399, 1972)

77. **False.** A simple direct question is always closed because it requires simply a yes or no answer: "Do your headaches upset your stomach?" Direct questions may or may not be neutral, depending on such factors as voice inflection, context, and previous questions. Although direct questions will speed the interview, too many of them tend to overwhelm the patient and put words in his mouth. They are indispensable but require moderation. (2:10–11)

78. **False.** The patient will almost universally respond in a biased manner to a question which conveys the possibility of serious consequences. This is not necessarily due to conscious falsification of information. The response is simply affected by his subconscious fears. After you have created an atmosphere in which the patient feels safe to communicate fully without fear of being judged, you can further motivate him by involving him more deeply in the topic at hand. As the patient forgets himself and focuses on the problem, more delicate areas can be explored without fear of his withdrawal. (2:9)

79. **True.** The single most useful physical finding in patients with chronic obstructive pulmonary disease is diminished intensity of the breath sounds, which is probably produced by decrease in airflow combined with hyperinflation.
(*Mod Med,* 41:32, 1973)

80. **True.** A major reason for overtreatment of hypertension is the failure to get blood pressures in both the supine and upright positions.
(*Internist Observer,* p. 5, Oct–Nov 1975)

81. **C.** (2:61)

82. **A.** (2:61)

83. **B.** (2:61)

84. **A.** (2:119)

85. **B.** (2:119)

Textbook References for Chapter 20

1. Bannister, Roger (1978): *Brain's Clinical Neurology*, Fifth Edition, Oxford Medical Publications, New York.

2. Judge, R.D. and Zuidema, G.D., Editors (1974): *Physical Diagnosis: A Physiologic Approach to the Clinical Examination*, Little, Brown and Company, Boston.

3. Isselbacher, K.J., Editor (1980): *Harrison's Principles of Internal Medicine*, Ninth Edition, McGraw-Hill Book Company, New York.

CHAPTER 21

Pulmonary Diseases

Directions: For each of the following multiple-choice questions, select the ONE CORRECT answer.

1. The arterial blood gases in patients with cardiogenic pulmonary edema usually show

    A. metabolic acidosis
    B. metabolic alkalosis
    C. respiratory acidosis
    D. respiratory alkalosis
    E. none of the above

2. With normal arterial pCO_2 and pH, low arterial pO_2 is not a good ventilatory stimulant until arterial pO_2 approximates

    A. 20 mm Hg
    B. 40 mm Hg
    C. 60 mm Hg
    D. 80 mm Hg
    E. 90 mm Hg

3. The overall frequency of hypercalcemia in patients with untreated bronchogenic carcinoma is approximately

    A. 0.1%
    B. 1.2%
    C. 12.5%
    D. 32%
    E. 50%

4. Under basal conditions oxygen transport is approximately how many ml per kg body weight per minute?

    A. 1
    B. 2
    C. 4
    D. 8
    E. 12

5. Aspirin sensitivity occurs in about what percentage of asthmatics?

    A. 1%
    B. 3%
    C. 5%
    D. 10%
    E. 20%

6. In primary lung cancers, slowest growth rate occurs with

    A. squamous cell carcinomas
    B. undifferentiated carcinomas
    C. adenocarcinomas
    D. all rates are approximately the same

7. In pulmonary embolism the triad of increased LDH, normal SGOT, and increased bilirubin has been found in about what percentage of proven cases?

    A. 2%
    B. 12%

C. 32%
D. 52%
E. 72%

8. Tracheal intubation and ventilator support is required in about what percentage of patients hospitalized with refractory asthma?

A. 1%
B. 5%
C. 10%
D. 25%
E. 50%

Directions: For the following multiple-choice questions, select the ONE INCORRECT answer.

9. In atypical mycobacteria infection,

A. it should be suspected if a patient has far advanced cavitary disease with few signs or symptoms
B. infection often occurs in white persons of middle-class background
C. over half the infections are pulmonary, but atypical strains may infect the pleura, kidneys, joints, meninges, nodes or skin
D. differential skin tests distinguish typical and atypical infections in adults
E. in a child with a positive skin test from myobacterial infection, species-specific atypical antigen usually introduces an even larger tuberculin reaction

10. Centrilobular emphysema

A. lesions are selectively localized in the respiratory bronchioles and predominantly in the central portion of the secondary lobules
B. is more frequent in females
C. is very rare in nonsmokers
D. is often associated with chronic bronchitis

Directions: For each of the following incomplete statements, ONE or MORE of the numbered completions is correct. In each case, select

A. if 1, 2, and 3 are correct
B. if 1 and 3 are correct
C. if 2 and 4 are correct
D. if only 4 is correct
E. if all statements are correct

11. Carbon dioxide production

1. varies with metabolic activity, increasing approximately 7% for each centigrade degree oi fever
2. is increased with hypothyroidism
3. is reduced with hypothermia
4. is reduced by drugs which increase cellular metabolism

12. Blood from a low ventilation/perfusion region of the lung will reflect

1. low pO_2
2. high pO_2
3. high pCO_2
4. low pCO_2

13. Ventilatory lung scan

1. is easy to perform
2. aids in the diagnosis of pulmonary embolism
3. helps assess the course of disease or the efficacy of treatment
4. is associated with high radiation exposure

14. In endurance athletes, probably as much as a 20-fold increase in total oxygen transport may be mediated by

1. an increase in arteriovenous oxygen extraction to about three times normal (150 cc/liter vs. 50 cc/liter)
2. selective deflection of blood flow away from high flow, low utilization organs such as the skin, the kidneys and the gut
3. doubling the heart rate
4. doubling the stroke volume

15. Exudate in the respiratory tract may result from

    1. infection
    2. inflammation
    3. aspiration
    4. edema

16. Implicated in interstitial pulmonary fibrosis is/are

    1. methysergide
    2. hexamethonium
    3. busulfan
    4. nitrofurantoin

17. High-altitude pulmonary edema is associated with

    1. normal or decreased pulmonary arteriolar wedge pressure
    2. excessive arterial desaturation, not corrected by 100% oxygen
    3. normal or decreased cardiac output
    4. decreased pulmonary artery pressure

18. In emphysema, maximum voluntary ventilation may be reduced due to

    1. loss of lung elasticity
    2. bronchospasm
    3. chest deformity
    4. poor movement of the diaphragm

19. Anti-lung antibodies have been found in patients with

    1. chronic bronchitis
    2. bronchial asthma
    3. emphysema
    4. pulmonary tuberculosis

20. According to modern concepts, in sensitized persons with extrinsic asthma there is a correlation between the asthma and

    1. history of exposure to allergen
    2. positive immediate scratch, prick, or intradermal tests to the allergen
    3. an immediate decrease in vital capacity after inhalation of an aerosolized extract of the antigen
    4. evidence of bronchial obstruction

21. Disodium cromoglycate

    1. appears to be useful in some patients with atopic asthma
    2. appears to be useful in some patients with adult onset asthma
    3. its greatest value appears to be as "steroid sparer"
    4. cannot be administered by aerosol

22. In a severe, acute attack of asthma, which of the following may occur?

    1. pneumomediastinum
    2. evidence of mucoid impaction of bronchi
    3. peripheral cyanosis with a commensurate reduction in PaO_2
    4. transient electrocardiographic manifestations of acute right ventricular strain

23. Patients with aspirin intolerance and asthma usually have

    1. nasal polyps
    2. eosinophilia
    3. sinusitis
    4. intolerance to sodium salicylate

24. Malignant neoplasm can cause pleural effusions by

    1. direct pleural involvement
    2. postobstructive pneumonia
    3. hypoproteinemia
    4. lymphatic obstruction and complete obstruction of a bronchus

25. Maximum mid-expiratory flow

    1. correlates better than any other ventilatory parameter with such tests as frequency dependence of compliance, closing volume determination, and flow volume curves
    2. is more sensitive than any other ventilatory test
    3. may better reflect the course of obstructive lung disease and the response to bronchodilators
    4. reflects the effort-dependent portion of forced expiration

26. Precise calculation of left to right shunts requires the measurement of mixed venous oxygen content from a sample of blood obtained

1. from the pulmonary artery
2. in the right ventricle
3. by a Swan-Ganz catheter
4. by a central venous catheter

27. In the treatment of adult respiratory distress syndrome, P E E P

1. is not useful
2. decreases the functional residual capacity
3. increases the amount of anatomic-like shunting
4. permits the maintenance of adequate levels of oxygenation at a lower concentration of oxygen in the inspired air

28. In asthma,

1. xanthines act by increasing the production of intracellular mediators of bronchodilation, probably cyclic AMP
2. beta-adrenergic agents probably act by inhibiting or retarding intracellular metabolic degradation of bronchodilator mediators by phosphodiesterase
3. the administration of steroids may decrease the arrhythmogenic potential of beta-adrenergic agents, particularly the concentrated nebulizer preparations
4. beta-adrenergic agents and xanthines appear to be synergistic in activity

Directions: For each of the following multiple-choice questions, select the ONE INCORRECT answer.

29. In interstitial pulmonary fibrosis,

A. adrenocorticosteroid therapy may be beneficial
B. immunosuppressive therapy may be beneficial
C. familial aggregation suggests a genetic component
D. high titers of rheumatoid factor and antinuclear antibodies may be found
E. articular symptoms do not occur

30. Anaerobic pleuropulmonary infections are characteristically subacute or chronic indolent illnesses accompanied by

A. pulmonary necrosis, foul-smelling sputum, and/or empyema fluid
B. failure to isolate a pathogen by conventional aerobic culture techniques
C. necrotizing pneumonitis, pulmonary abscess, and empyema as the most common x-ray findings
D. a marked tendency for exacerbation or recurrence
E. organisms which rarely originate in the mouth

31. In aspergillus infection,

A. the organism is rarely cultured from the sputum
B. positive immediate skin reactions are often demonstrable
C. positive delayed skin reactions are often demonstrable
D. serum precipitin reactions to the antigen of the fungus are usually readily demonstrable
E. systemic and topical antifungal therapy is of little value

Directions: For each of the following incomplete statements, ONE or MORE of the numbered completions is correct. In each case, select
A. if 1, 2, and 3 are correct
B. if 1 and 3 are correct
C. if 2 and 4 are correct
D. if only 4 is correct
E. if all the statements are correct

32. Alpha-1-antitrypsin deficiency is characterized by

1. absence of a history of chronic bronchitis prior to exertional dyspnea in almost half the patients
2. lower than normal proportion of female patients
3. lesions localized primarily in the lower lobes
4. onset of symptoms at a relatively late age

33. The presence of an increased concentration of deoxyhemoglobin stimulates the red cell production of 2, 3 DPG in patients
    1. residing at high altitude
    2. with congenital cyanotic heart disease
    3. who are hypoxic due to underlying lung disease
    4. with low-output congestive heart failure

Directions: Use the key below to answer questions 34 through 36.
    A. if asthma is characteristic of the type of chronic obstructive pulmonary disease listed
    B. if emphysema is characteristic of the type of chronic obstructive pulmonary disease listed
    C. if chronic bronchitis is characteristic of the type of chronic obstructive pulmonary disease listed

34. Type A

35. Type B

36. Type C

Directions: Use the key below to answer questions 37 through 42. If the feature is associated with
    A. extrinsic asthma
    B. intrinsic asthma

37. Age of onset at middle age

38. Positive family history of allergies

39. Raised IgE levels

40. Significant association with aspirin sensitivity

41. Nasal polyps

42. Positive skin tests

Directions: Indicate whether each of the following statements is true or false.

43. In extrinsic asthma, there is a hereditary predisposition to sensitization by allergens.

44. The presence of wheezing and of sputum eosinophils, and an improvement of pulmonary function tests after bronchodilator therapy have been considered useful in selecting patients with chronic obstructive pulmonary disease who might benefit from steroid therapy.

45. When hypoxemia is due to interstitial fibrosis, the use of positive-end expiratory pressure is frequently of little value.

46. The diagnostic yield of scalene node biopsy exceeds that of mediastinoscopy even if no supraclavicular nodes are palpable.

47. When hyperventilation is accompanied by faintness, the pattern of symptoms can be reproduced readily by having the subject breathe rapidly and deeply for 2 to 3 minutes.

48. Asthma is more severe in whites than in blacks.

49. Hypoxemia without associated hypercapnia is commonly observed in asthma.

50. Respiratory infection is the most frequent precipitating cause of respiratory failure in patients with chronic obstructive pulmonary disease.

51. In obstructive disease of the smaller airways, the magnitude of the ventilation-perfusion defect is aggravated by hyperpnea as proportionately more air at high flow rates is deflected away from partially obstructed airways.

52. Ventilation is low in relation to perfusion in the upper zones of the lung.

53. When small-airway collapse occurs in or above the range of tidal breathing (i.e., when closing volume is greater than functional residual capacity), hypoxemia develops.

54. The observation that arterial oxygenation after myocardial infarction can be improved with diuretics strongly supports the hypothesis that after acute myocardial infarction, there is fluid retention in the lung.

55. Operative treatment is seldom beneficial in patients with lung cancer if mediastinoscopy discloses lymph node metastases.

56. Bronchography is of considerable value in studying small peripheral coin lesions.

57. Arteriovenous malformation often presents as a solitary nodule and pulmonary sequestration may present as mass lesions.

58. Benign intracranial hypertension may occur secondary to pulmonary encephalopathy.

59. Metastases from bronchogenic carcinoma are most frequently found in the opposite lung, regional lymph nodes, the adrenal glands, bone, brain, kidney, and liver.

60. In a healthy subject, the time required for maximal forced expiration after maximal inspiration (forced vital capacity) is about 6 seconds.

61. The three most common causes of chronic obstructive pulmonary disease are emphysema, chronic bronchitis, and asthma.

62. Disodium cromoglycate has not been shown to exert a significant inhibitory effect on exercise-induced bronchospasm.

63. Serial radioisotope lung scan studies indicate that the natural course of pulmonary embolism is toward rapid and complete resolution.

64. A normal PaO_2 and lung scan essentially exclude acute pulmonary embolism.

65. EKG patterns of right heart strain are seen in more than 25% of proven cases of pulmonary embolism.

66. Radioactive lung scans during acute asthmatic attacks frequently show grossly nonuniform pulmonary perfusion which may simulate the large perfusion defects characteristic of pulmonary embolism.

67. A barrel deformity of the chest is diagnostic of obstructive pulmonary disease.

68. Benign tumors of the lung and tracheobronchial tree are common.

69. In the adult respiratory distress syndrome following a wide variety of conditions, the final common pathway may be an abnormality of pulmonary capillary permeability (a pulmonary capillary leak syndrome).

70. Arterial hypoxemia is rarely seen in patients with acute myocardial infarction in the absence of congestive heart failure or cardiogenic shock.

71. The pathogenesis of heroin-induced pulmonary edema is probably cardiac in origin.

72. In the presence of severe respiratory acidosis complicating cardiogenic pulmonary edema, tracheal intubation and ventilatory assistance are frequently required.

73. In response to an increased volume load, pulmonary vascular resistance normally rises.

74. Interstitial pulmonary edema produces no clinical manifestations on physical examination.

75. The carbon monoxide uptake appears to provide the best readily available correlation with the presence and extent of emphysematous changes found at necropsy.

76. A negative intermediate tuberculin reaction excludes active tuberculosis.

77. With the notable exception of *Bacteroides fragilis*, most anaerobic pathogens are sensitive to penicillin as well as to erythromycin and tetracycline.

78. In acute asthmatic attacks, a paradoxical pulse may reflect increased respiratory muscle work with resultant generation of high intrathoracic pressures.

79. As in other forms of acidosis, gastric dilatation may be a serious complication of the ventilatory failure of status asthmaticus.

80. The primary site of normal airway resistance is in the smaller airways.

81. The pressure in the pulmonary circuit is so low that apical portions of the lung receive relatively little blood flow in the upright position.

82. A large percentage of patients with chronic obstructive pulmonary disease and acute ventilatory failure require or benefit from tracheal intubation and ventilator therapy.

83. When pulmonary embolism is suspected, lung scans should be done early and should be repeated periodically.

84. Continuous inhalation of a gas mixture containing more than 70% oxygen for 24 hours or less does not cause symptoms of tracheobronchial and pulmonary irritation.

85. In Wegener's granulomatosis, pulmonary lesions are always associated with systemic involvement.

86. Collapsible airways in the dependent portions of the lung close during exhalation at levels of lung inflation well above the residual volume.

87. An elevated closing volume (early airway closure before and tidal volume during exhalation) may be responsible for arterial hypoxemia in many clinical disorders.

88. Voluntary hyperventilation associated with reduction in arterial pCO_2 to levels of less than 20 to 30 mm Hg has not been shown to produce significant bronchospasm in normal man.

Directions: For each of the following incomplete statements, select
   A. if the question is associated with A only
   B. if the question is associated with B only
   C. if the question is associated with both A and B
   D. if the question is associated with neither A nor B

89. Small-cell carcinoma is the most common cell type of bronchogenic carcinoma associated with

   A. ectopic ACTH production
   B. antidiuretic hormone production
   C. both
   D. neither

90. In status asthmaticus, steroids

   A. are not beneficial until a latent period of 4 to 6 hours
   B. appear to act by potentiating or restoring responsiveness to beta-adrenergic but not methylxanthine bronchodilators
   C. both
   D. neither

91. *Bacteroides fragilis* is sensitive to

   A. clindamycin
   B. chloramphenicol
   C. both
   D. neither

92. In an asthmatic requiring mechanical ventilation, narcotics such as intravenous meperidine are contraindicated

   A. before intubation
   B. after intubation

C. both
D. neither

93. The physical properties of the lung, and not patient or subject effort, influence all of the air flow rate during expiration except the

    A. first 10%
    B. last 5%
    C. both
    D. neither

94. Most parenchymal lung disease as well as obstructive airway disease disturb

    A. perfusion
    B. ventilation
    C. both
    D. neither

95. The asthmatic's airway resistance

    A. is greatest at night and least in the morning
    B. apparently responds to a circadian rhythm of the parasympathetic nervous system

C. both
D. neither

96. "Atopic" asthma is referred to as

    A. extrinsic
    B. intrinsic
    C. both
    D. neither

97. The delivery of air under pressure to the airways, as with IPPB treatment, can

    A. increase airway resistance
    B. act as an irritant, especially in individuals with asthma
    C. both
    D. neither

98. Alveolar-cell carcinoma and adenocarcinoma of the lung

    A. are thought to have an etiologic relation to smoking
    B. can cause persistent pulmonary infiltrates without bronchial obstruction
    C. both
    D. neither

Answers and Commentary

1. **D.** The arterial blood gases in patients with cardiogenic pulmonary edema usually show respiratory alkalosis. (1:112)

2. **C.** With normal arterial pCO_2 and pH, low arterial pO_2 is not good ventilatory stimulant until arterial pO_2 approximates 60 mm Hg.
(*Ann Intern Med*, 78:401, 1973)

3. **C.** The relation of hypercalcemia, histologic cell type, and osseous neoplastic involvement was studied in 200 consecutive patients with untreated bronchogenic carcinoma. The overall frequency of hypercalcemia was 12.5%. Twenty-three percent of patients with epidermoid carcinoma, 12.7% with large-cell anaplastic carcinoma, 2.5% with adenocarcinoma, and none with small-cell carcinoma presented with or developed hypercalcemia. Fourteen of 25 patients (56%) with elevated calcium did not have osseous metastases. Osseous involvement was most frequently observed in patients with small-cell carcinoma (66%) and adenocarcinoma (50%).
(*Ann Intern Med*, 80:205, 1974)

4. **C.** Under basal conditions, oxygen transport is approximately 4 ml per kg body weight per minute. (1:115)

5. **C.** Aspirin sensitivity occurs in about 5% of asthmatics. (1:108)

6. **C.** Generally, squamous cell and undifferentiated carcinomas tend to grow rapidly, while the growth rate of adenocarcinomas is slower. (1:113)

7. **B.** In pulmonary embolism the triad of increased LDH, normal SGOT, and increased

bilirubin has been found in about 12% of proven cases. (1:111)

8. **D.** Tracheal intubation and ventilator support is required in about 25% of patients hospitalized with refractory asthma. (1:107)

9. **D.** Differential skin testing does not distinguish typical and atypical mycobacteria infections in adults. All other statements are true.
(*Res-Int Consult*, 2:22, 1973)

10. **B.** Centrilobular emphysema is more frequent in males. All other statements are true of this disorder. (*Phys World*, 1:41, 1973)

11. **B.** Carbon dioxide production is reduced with hypothyroidism and by drugs which reduce cellular metabolism. (1:114)

12. **B.** Blood from a low ventilation/perfusion region of the lung will reflect low pO_2 and high pCO_2. (*Ann Intern Med*, 78:401, 1973)

13. **A.** Ventilatory lung scan is not associated with high radiation exposure; all other statements are true of this procedure.
(*N Engl J Med*, 282:1334, 1970)

14. **E.** An increase in total oxygen transport in endurance athletes may be mediated by any of the actions listed. (1:115)

15. **E.** All the items listed, as well as retained secretions, may cause exudate in the respiratory tract. Spasm of the bronchial musculature and edema of the bronchial wall may exaggerate rhonchal sounds caused by exudate within the lumen.
(3:132)

16. **E.** All the drugs listed have been implicated in interstitial pulmonary fibrosis. (1:111)

17. **A.** High-altitude pulmonary edema is associated with elevated pulmonary artery pressure. All other statements are correct. (1:112)

18. **E.** In emphysema, maximum voluntary ventilation may be reduced due to any of the factors listed. (*Hosp Med*, 9:8, 1973)

19. **E.** Anti-lung antibodies have been found in patients with all the disorders listed, as well as in pneumoconiosis and diffuse fibrosing alveolitis (interstitial fibrosis). (*N Engl J Med*, 286:1166, 1972)

20. **E.** According to modern concepts, in sensitized persons with extrinsic asthma there is a correlation between the asthma and all the items listed. (*N Engl J Med*, 286:1166, 1972)

21. **A.** Disodium cromoglycate is effective only if administered as a finely dispersed powder by aerosol, a somewhat cumbersome, inconvenient, and sometimes irritating means of administration. (1:108)

22. **E.** All the disorders listed may occur in a severe acute attack of asthma. Pneumothorax may also occur under these circumstances. (1:107)

23. **A.** Patients with aspirin intolerance and asthma usually have a tolerance to sodium salicylate. All other statements are true. (1:108)

24. **E.** Malignant neoplasm can cause pleural effusions by any of the factors listed. (*Arch Intern Med*, 132:854, 1973)

25. **E.** All the statements are true of maximum mid-expiratory flow. (1:118)

26. **A.** Precise calculation of left to right shunts requires the measurement of mixed venous oxygen content from a sample of blood obtained in either the pulmonary artery or the right ventricle. Such a sample can be obtained through the Swan-Ganz catheter. (1:121)

27. **D.** In the treatment of adult respiratory distress syndrome, positive end-expiratory pressure is particularly useful. It results in raising the functional residual capacity, thereby decreasing the amount of anatomic-like shunting. (1:121)

28. **D.** Xanthines probably act by inhibiting or retarding intracellular metabolic degradation of bronchodilator mediators by phosphodiesterase.

Beta-adrenergic agents, such as isoproterenol, act by increasing the production of intracellular mediators of bronchodilation, probably cyclic AMP. There is considerable experimental evidence that the administration of steroids greatly increases the arrhythmogenic potential of beta-adrenergic agents, particularly the concentrated nebulizer preparations. (1:107)

29. **E.** Most patients with idiopathic interstitial pulmonary fibrosis have articular symptoms. All other statements are true. (1:105)

30. **E.** The organisms of anaerobic pleuropulmonary infections most often originate in the mouth, perhaps in a periodontal infection, and are aspirated into the tracheobronchial tree. All other statements are correct. (1:105)

31. **A.** The aspergillus organism is readily cultured from the sputum. All other statements are correct. (1:110)

32. **B.** Alpha-1-antitrypsin deficiency is characterized by a higher than normal proportion of female patients with onset of symptoms at a relatively early age (60% of patients in one study were under 40 and 90% under 50). All other statements are correct. (*Phys World*, 1:41, 1973)

33. **E.** All of the factors listed, as well as anemia, can result in the presence of an increased concentration of deoxyhemoglobin stimulating the red cell production of 2, 3 DPG. (1:116)

34. **B.** (*Curr Med Digest*, 39:1117, 1972)

35. **C.** (*Curr Med Digest*, 39:1117, 1972)

36. **A.** (*Curr Med Digest*, 39:1117, 1972)

37. **B.** (2:956)

38. **A.** (2:956)

39. **A.** (2:956)

40. **B.** (2:956)

41. **B.** (2:956)

42. **A.** (2:956)

43. **True.** In extrinsic asthma, there is a hereditary predisposition to sensitization by allergens, possibly because of defects in the respiratory mucosa, leading to the production of specific tissue-sensitizing antibodies of the IgE class that

attach themselves to mast cells in the respiratory mucosa. (*N Engl J Med*, 286:1166, 1972)

44. **True.** The presence of wheezing and of sputum eosinophils, and an improvement of pulmonary function tests after bronchodilator therapy, have been considered useful in selecting patients with chronic obstructive pulmonary disease who might benefit from steroid therapy.
(*Mod Med*, 41:32, 1973)

45. **True.** When hypoxemia is due to interstitial fibrosis, the use of positive-end expiratory pressure is frequently of little value. (1:121)

46. **False.** The diagnostic yield of mediastinoscopy exceeds that of scalene node biopsy if no supraclavicular nodes are palpable. (1:119)

47. **True.** When hyperventilation is accompanied by faintness, the pattern of symptoms can be reproduced readily by having the subject breathe rapidly and deeply for 2 to 3 minutes. This test is often of therapeutic value also because the underlying anxiety tends to be lessened when the patient learns that he can produce and alleviate the symptoms at will simply by controlling his breathing. (4:82)

48. **False.** Asthma is more severe in blacks than in whites. (*Ann Allergy*, 30:623, 1972)

49. **True.** Hypoxemia without associated hypercapnia is commonly observed in asthma.
(*Ann Intern Med*, 78:401, 1973)

50. **True.** Respiratory infection is the most frequent precipitating cause of respiratory failure in patients with chronic obstructive pulmonary disease, and is often the inciting factor in patients with acute asthmatic exacerbations. (1:115)

51. **True.** In obstructive disease of the smaller airways, the magnitudes of the ventilation-perfusion defect are aggravated by hyperpnea as proportionately more air at high flow rates is deflected away from partially obstructed airways. (1:117)

52. **False.** Ventilation is high in relation to perfusion in the upper zones and low in relation to perfusion in the lower lung zones. (1:114)

53. **True.** When small-airway collapse occurs in or above the range of tidal breathing (i.e., when closing volume is greater than functional residual capacity), hypoxemia develops. (2:841)

54. **True.** The observation that arterial oxygenation after myocardial infarction can be improved with

diuretics strongly supports the hypothesis that after acute myocardial infarction there is fluid retention in the lung.
(*N Engl J Med*, 290:761, 1974)

55. **True.** Operative treatment is seldom beneficial in patients with lung cancer if mediastinoscopy discloses lymph node metastases.
(*Scand J Thorac Cardiovasc Surg*, 6:293, 1972)

56. **False.** Bronchography is of little value in studying small peripheral coin lesions.
(*New Phys*, 23:35, 1974)

57. **True.** Arteriovenous malformation often presents as a solitary nodule and pulmonary sequestration may present as mass lesions.
(*New Phys*, 23:35, 1974)

58. **True.** Benign intracranial hypertension may occur secondary to pulmonary encephalopathy. This pulmonary encephalopathy may result from paralytic hypoventilation and emphysema, as well as the Pickwickian syndrome. (2:871)

59. **True.** Metastases from bronchogenic carcinoma are most frequently found in the opposite lung, regional lymph nodes, the adrenal glands, bone, brain, kidney, and liver.
(*N Engl J Med*, 262:505, 1970)

60. **False.** In a healthy subject, the time required for maximal forced expiration after maximal inspiration (forced vital capacity) is never greater than 4 seconds. (*Mod Med*, 41:32, 1973)

61. **True.** The three most common causes of chronic obstructive pulmonary disease are emphysema, chronic bronchitis, and asthma.
(*Mod Med*, 41:32, 1973)

62. **False.** Disodium cromoglycate has been shown to exert a significant inhibitory effect on exercise-induced bronchospasm.
(*Ann Intern Med*, 78:401, 1973)

63. **True.** Serial radioisotope lung scan studies indicate that the natural course of pulmonary embolism is toward rapid and complete resolution. (1:111)

64. **True.** While a normal PaO_2 and lung scan essentially exclude acute pulmonary embolism, a low systemic arterial oxygen tension and an abnormal lung scan pattern are not specifically diagnostic of pulmonary embolism. (1:111)

65. **False.** Electrocardiogram changes in patients with pulmonary embolism, if present, are usually

nonspecific. Patterns of right heart strain are seen in less than 10% of proven cases. (1:111)

66. **True.** Radioactive lung scans during acute asthmatic attacks frequently show grossly nonuniform pulmonary perfusion which may simulate the large perfusion defects characteristic of pulmonary embolism. (1:108)

67. **False.** A barrel deformity of the chest is not diagnostic of obstructive pulmonary disease. In fact, the anteroposterior diameter of the chest was not abnormal nor increased in a group of patients with obstructive pulmonary disease recently studied and reported. The authors of this investigation concluded that the body habitus of their patients with small anteroposterior abdominal dimension gave a spurious impression of increased anteroposterior chest diameter. (1:109)

68. **False.** Benign tumors of the lung and tracheobronchial tree are uncommon, or exceedingly rare. (1:113)

69. **True.** In the adult respiratory distress syndrome following a wide variety of conditions, the final common pathway may be an abnormality of pulmonary capillary permeability (a pulmonary capillary leak syndrome). (1:113)

70. **False.** Arterial hypoxemia is frequently seen in patients with acute myocardial infarction even in the absence of congestive heart failure or cardiogenic shock. (1:112)

71. **False.** The pathogenesis of heroin-induced pulmonary edema is unclear, but it is probably noncardiac in origin. (1:112)

72. **True.** In the presence of severe respiratory acidosis complicating cardiogenic edema, tracheal intubation and ventilatory assistance are frequently required. (1:112)

73. **False.** In response to an increased volume load, pulmonary vascular resistance normally falls. (1:112)

74. **True.** Interstitial pulmonary edema produces no clinical manifestations on physical examination. The chest roentgenogram, however, usually shows evidence of congestion. (1:112)

75. **True.** The carbon monoxide uptake appears to provide the best readily available correlation with the presence and extent of emphysematous changes found at necropsy. (1:109)

76. **False.** A negative intermediate tuberculin reaction does not exclude active tuberculosis. (1:105)

77. **True.** With the notable exception of *Bacteroides fragilis*, most anaerobic pathogens are sensitive to penicillin as well as to erythromycin and tetracycline. (1:106)

78. **True.** In acute asthmatic attacks, a paradoxical pulse may reflect increased respiratory muscle work with resultant generation of high intrathoracic pressures. (1:107)

79. **True.** As in other forms of acidosis, gastric dilatation may be a serious complication of the ventilatory failure of status asthmaticus. (1:107)

80. **False.** The primary site of normal airway resistance is in the larger airways. The smaller airways constitute very little of the work of respiration because the cross-sectional area of the tracheobronchial tree is so much larger at the smaller airway level than it is higher up. (1:117)

81. **True.** The pressure in the pulmonary circuit is so low that apical portions of the lung receive relatively little blood flow in the upright position, compared to the dependent parts of the lung which receive most of the blood. (1:114)

82. **False.** Only a small percentage of patients with chronic obstructive pulmonary disease and acute ventilatory failure require or benefit from tracheal intubation and ventilator therapy. (1:110)

83. **True.** When pulmonary embolism is suspected, lung scans should be done early and should be repeated periodically. (1:111)

84. **False.** In man, continuous inhalation for 24 hours or less, of a gas mixture containing more than 70% oxygen causes symptoms of tracheobronchial and pulmonary irritation. (1:110)

85. **False.** Recently, a less malignant form of Wegener's granulomatosis has been described which is characterized by pulmonary lesions without associated systemic involvement. (1:110)

86. **True.** Collapsible airways in the dependent portions of the lung close during exhalation at levels of lung inflation well above the residual volume. (1:114)

87. **True.** An elevated closing volume (early airway closure before and tidal volume during exhalation) may be responsible for arterial hypoxemia in many clinical disorders. (1:114)

88. **False.** Voluntary hyperventilation associated with reduction in arterial pCO₂ to levels of less than 20 to 30 mm Hg has been shown to produce

significant bronchospasm in normal man.
(*Ann Intern Med*, 78:401, 1973)

89. **C.** Small-cell carcinoma is the most common cell type of bronchogenic carcinoma associated with other paraneoplastic syndromes, especially ectopic ACTH and antidiuretic hormone production. Paradoxically, in contrast to some other types of bronchogenic carcinomas such as epidermoid and large-cell anaplastic carcinomas, it is uncommonly associated with hypercalcemia, although it is frequently associated with osseous metastases. (*Ann Intern Med*, 80:205, 1974)

90. **A.** In status asthmaticus, steroids appear to act by potentiating or restoring responsiveness to both the beta-adrenergic and methylxanthine bronchodilators. (1:107)

91. **C.** *Bacteroides fragilis* is sensitive to both clindamycin and chloramphenicol. (1:106)

92. **A.** Narcotics such as intravenous meperidine (Demerol), which are contraindicated before intubation, are very helpful in the intubated patient on a ventilator. (1:107)

93. **C.** The flow rate during exhalation of all but the first 10% and the last 5% of exhalation is not influenced by patient or subject effort but depends upon the physical properties of the lungs. (1:108)

94. **C.** Most parenchymal lung diseases, as well as obstructive airway disease, disturb both perfusion and ventilation. (1:120)

95. **C.** Both statements are true of the asthmatic's airway resistance. (*Ann Intern Med*, 78:401, 1973)

96. **A.** "Atopic" asthma is often referred to as extrinsic. (*N Engl J Med*, 286:1166, 1972)

97. **C.** Both statements are true of the delivery of air under pressure to the airways.
(*J Allergy Clin Immunol*, 49:137, 1972)

98. **B.** Alveolar-cell carcinoma and adenocarcinoma of the lung can cause persistent pulmonary infiltrates without bronchial obstruction, but are thought to have no etiologic relation to smoking.
(*N Engl J Med*, 282:968, 1970)

Textbook References for Chapter 21

1. American College of Physicians (1974): *Medical Knowledge Self-Assessment, Program III: Recent Developments in Internal Medicine*, R.G. Petersdorf, General Editor, American College of Physicians, Philadelphia.

2. Beeson, P.B. and McDermott, W. (1979): *Cecil Textbook of Medicine*, Fifteenth Edition, W.B. Saunders Company, Philadelphia.

3. Judge, R.D. and Zuidema, G.D., Editors (1974): *Physical Diagnosis: A Physiologic Approach to the Clinical Examination*, Little, Brown and Company, Boston.

4. Isselbacher, K.J., Editor (1980): *Harrison's Principles of Internal Medicine*, Ninth Edition, McGraw-Hill Book Company, New York.

CHAPTER 22

Rheumatology

Directions: For each of the following multiple-choice questions, select the ONE CORRECT answer.

1. In classic polyarteritis nodosa, the lowest incidence of necrotizing angiitis occurs in the

   A. heart
   B. liver
   C. lungs (pulmonary arteries)
   D. spleen
   E. kidneys

2. Next to arthralgia and arthritis, the most frequent clinical manifestation in systemic lupus erythematosus is

   A. weight loss
   B. skin lesions
   C. renal dysfunction
   D. fever
   E. cardiac involvement

3. In patients with primary hyperuricemia, the incidence of gouty arthritis was found to be approximately what percentage when the serum urate concentration was over 9 mg/100 ml in a small group of patients over a long period of follow-up?

   A. 10%
   B. 30%
   C. 50%
   D. 70%
   E. 90%

4. When using aspirin in the therapy of rheumatoid arthritis, a positive guaiac test

   A. is an indication to stop aspirin
   B. is both dangerous and significant
   C. may suggest a need for supplemental iron
   D. all of the above
   E. none of the above

5. Two surveys in Sweden and New York gave a prevalence of systemic lupus erythematosus in the population of about 1 per

   A. 1000
   B. 3000
   C. 5000
   D. 10,000
   E. 20,000

6. In patients with rheumatoid arthritis and leukopenia, treatment with gold salts has resulted in

   A. improvement in arthritis
   B. a rise in white-cell count
   C. a fall in the erythrocyte sedimentation rate
   D. all of the above
   E. none of the above

7. All of the following are true of spasmodic torticollis *except*

   A. an intermittent or continuous spasm of sternomastoid, trapezius, and other neck muscles, usually more pronounced on one side, with turning or tipping of the head

B. it is involuntary and cannot be inhibited and thereby differs from habit spasm or tic

C. should be considered a form of dystonia

D. worse when the patient sits, stands, or walks, and usually contactual stimulation of the chin or of the back of the head partially alleviates the muscle imbalance

E. psychiatric treatment is effective

8. In ankylosing spondylitis,

A. an elevated sedimentation rate occurs in about one-half of patients with active disease

B. tests for rheumatoid factor and other antibodies are consistently negative

C. x-ray examination of the sacroiliac joints can confirm or rule out the diagnosis

D. abnormalities on x-ray examination of the spine occur too late in the disease to be helpful in early diagnosis

E. gold, chloroquine, steroids, and local radiation are recommended adjuncts to treatment

9. Regarding allopurinol,

A. the doses required to reduce elevated serum urate levels to normal values range from 200 to 300 mg/day for patients with mild disease to 400 to 600 mg/day for those with moderately severe tophaceous disease

B. one dose per day is frequently adequate because of the relatively prolonged half-life of oxipurinol

C. the concomitant administration of uricosuric agents usually results in an appreciable increase of urinary uric acid excretion and a further decline in serum urate level

D. colchicine is contraindicated during the first months of therapy of gout with allopurinol

E. substantial resolution can be expected in most patients in 6 to 12 months

10. Paget's disease

A. is usually found incidentally on x-ray examination

B. may occur in approximately 3.5% of patients older than 45

C. alkaline phosphatase serum level correlates poorly with the disease's extent and activity

D. is characterized by accelerated bone resorption and disordered bone formation

E. prognosis is usually excellent but depends on the disease's extent, and complications include skeletal deformities, neurological abnormalities, deafness, hypercalcemia, renal stones, and (rarely) osteogenic sarcoma

11. In ankylosing spondylitis, physical findings include

A. flattening of the normal lumbar lordotic curve when the patient stands erect

B. limited ability to hyperextend the back

C. failure to round the lower back when flexing forward trying to touch the toes with the fingers

D. increased chest expansion

Directions: For each of the following incomplete statements, ONE or MORE of the numbered completions is correct. In each case, select

A. **if 1, 2, and 3 are correct**
B. **if 1 and 3 are correct**
C. **if 2 and 4 are correct**
D. **if only 4 is correct**
E. **if all statements are correct**

12. Autoantibodies in systemic lupus erythematosus include

1. antinuclear
2. anticytoplasmic
3. anti-RNA
4. anti-cell

13. Polyarthritis of unknown etiology includes
    1. rheumatoid arthritis
    2. juvenile rheumatoid arthritis
    3. ankylosing spondylitis
    4. psoriatic arthritis

14. The pathologic changes that have been described in polymyositis include
    1. necrosis, vacuolar, or granular change of muscle fibers, or a combination of these
    2. variation in size of muscle fibers, with central migration of sarcolemmal nuclei
    3. variable perivascular or interstitial infiltration with inflammatory cells, or both
    4. muscle regeneration

15. Familial Mediterranean fever
    1. is a familial disease prevalent among Arabs, Syrians, Turks, Sephardic Jews and their descendants, and other people whose origin is near the Mediterranean basin
    2. is characterized by bouts of fever, abdominal pain, chest pain, arthralgia, and joint pains
    3. attacks subside spontaneously and the patients are asymptomatic between them
    4. is invariably associated with renal amyloidosis

16. Secondary or acquired metabolic gout may occur in
    1. sarcoidosis
    2. chronic leukemia
    3. myeloid metaplasia
    4. polycythemia vera

17. In rheumatoid arthritis, the purpose of exercise is to
    1. preserve normal range of motion of the joint
    2. regain joint motion that has been lost
    3. maintain the strength and endurance of muscles supporting the joint
    4. improve the performance of the activities of daily living necessary for self-sufficiency

18. Necrotizing angiitis associated with drug abuse
    1. may be indistinguishable from periarteritis nodosa
    2. may be due to methamphetamine
    3. clinical presentation may vary from a complete lack of symptoms to pleomorphic systemic signs and symptoms with renal failure, hypertension, pulmonary edema and pancreatitis
    4. may result in vascular changes, including arterial aneurysms and sacculations which have been noted in the kidney, liver, pancreas, and small bowel at selective angiography

19. The incidence of gout is probably not as high in secondary hyperuricemia as it is in primary hyperuricemia except possibly in patients with
    1. polycythemia vera
    2. myeloid metaplasia
    3. glycogen storage disease due to a deficiency of glucose-6-phosphatase
    4. chronic lead poisoning

Directions: Use the key below to answer questions 20 through 26. If the statement is characteristic of
  A. **systemic lupus erythematosus**
  B. **procainamide-induced systemic lupus erythematosus**

20. Higher frequency of complete remission

21. Considerably higher female/male ratio

22. Less common in the black population

23. More commonly involves the pulmonary parenchyma

24. Higher frequency of antibody to native DNA

25. $C'H_{50}$ often depressed

26. Renal disease infrequent

Directions: Indicate whether each of the following statements is true or false.

27. In many patients with gout, the development of renal insufficiency is related to nephrosclerosis, hypertension, and other factors known to be associated with hyperuricemia.

28. Renal arteriography defines the subacute renal lesions of polyarteritis nodosa and shows regression of lesions after steroid treatment.

29. One may observe acute attacks of gouty arthritis in the back, hips, shoulders, or cervical spine, but these joints are affected only after the diagnosis has been well established for years and after many attacks in the toes, ankles, knees, hands, or elbows.

30. Arthritis of the first costovertebral joint is one cause of the symptoms of thoracic outlet syndrome.

31. Although rheumatoid vasculitis may be pathologically indistinguishable from periarteritis nodosa, renal involvement by rheumatoid vasculitis is more common.

32. If a patient with gout is already receiving hypouricemic therapy and develops an acute attack of gouty arthritis, the crystal-induced synovitis is usually treated by changing the hypouricemic therapy.

33. Muscle biopsy is the most useful diagnostic procedure in polymyositis.

34. A positive LE cell test is most common with systemic lupus erythematous but has a 6% frequency with rheumatoid arthritis and a lower frequency with scleroderma.

35. A very low carbon monoxide diffusion capacity (less than 15% of the predicted value) would be an unlikely finding of sclerodermatous involvement of the lung.

36. Approximately one-third of patients with systemic lupus erythematosus are free of renal disease.

37. The most common pulmonary manifestation of lupus is pleuritis, with some interstitial pneumonitis.

38. The distal interphalangeal (DIP) joints are rarely involved in rheumatoid arthritis.

39. The uricosuric effect of most agents studied has been attributed to inhibition of the tubular reabsorption of filtered urate.

40. Gold has no effect in osteoarthritis.

41. If a patient has constipation on high-dose aspirin therapy, giving aspirin which contains magnesium (such as Ascriptin) can cause looser stools.

42. Podagra is a usual finding in pyrophosphate arthropathy.

43. Radiographic changes are sensitive indicators for diagnosis of gout.

44. Rapid reduction in serum urate prevents exacerbation of gouty arthritis.

45. There is no evidence that aspirin may slow the progress of early osteoarthritis.

46. In ankylosing spondylitis, steroid therapy is rarely justified unless iritis is present.

47. Treatment with uricosurics leads to a transient increase in uric acid excretion whereas allopurinol consistently decreases uric acid excretion.

48. The administration of allopurinol in man is followed by a prompt decrease in the serum and urinary uric acid within 24 to 48 hours, reaching a maximum decrease in 4 days to 2 weeks, and remaining relatively constant over prolonged periods of time.

49. The development of ANA in high titer can be expected in 1 in 5 patients treated with procainamide, regardless of the dose given.

50. A majority of patients found to have polyarteritis at autopsy have positive muscle biopsy before death.

51. Sympathectomy may be of value in the treatment of severe Raynaud's phenomenon.

52. In a study of polymyositis, it was found that the erythrocyte sedimentation rate was a good indicator of disease activity.

Directions: For each of the following incomplete statements, select
   A. **if the question is associated with A only**
   B. **if the question is associated with B only**
   C. **if the question is associated with both A and B**
   D. **if the question is associated with neither A nor B**

53. In contrast to secondary Raynaud's phenomenon, primary Raynaud's disease

   A. has a poor prognosis
   B. requires the routine use of vasodilating drugs
   C. both
   D. neither

54. Colchicine

   A. alters serum concentration and renal excretion of uric acid
   B. has a significant effect upon the miscible pool of uric acid and the rate of its turnover
   C. both
   D. neither

55. Decreased renal excretion of uric acid is associated with

   A. phenylbutazone
   B. dicumarol
   C. both
   D. neither

56. Joint involvement is now a well recognized complication of systemic infections produced by

   A. RNA viruses (e.g., rubella or mumps)
   B. DNA viruses (e.g., variola)
   C. both
   D. neither

57. The presence of necrotizing arteritis

   A. is consistent with polyarteritis nodosa
   B. may be associated with rheumatoid arthritis or systemic lupus erythematosus
   C. both
   D. neither

58. Diffuse tenderness over the calcaneus is often associated with

   A. early rheumatoid arthritis
   B. Reiter's syndrome
   C. both
   D. neither

59. In acute gouty arthritis, intravenous injection of 2 to 3 mg colchicine results in a

   A. more rapid response than from oral administration
   B. higher incidence of gastrointestinal side effects than with oral administration
   C. both
   D. neither

60. Tenderness lateral or anterior to the radial head may

   A. indicate lateral epicondylitis (tennis elbow)
   B. be accentuated as the patient pronates the forearm and extends the wrist against resistance
   C. both
   D. neither

61. Vascular lesions are usually all in the same stage of activity in

   A. hypersensitivity angiitis
   B. polyarteritis nodosa
   C. both
   D. neither

62. In systemic lupus erythematosus,

    A. platelet antibody was found in the minority of patients
    B. a compensated thrombocytolytic state has been postulated
    C. both
    D. neither

63. Cervical spondylosis is

    A. one of the commonest causes of paraplegia of slow onset
    B. always associated with abnormal physical signs in the upper limbs
    C. both
    D. neither

64. Lesions of the intervertebral discs are

    A. by far the commonest cause of radiculopathy
    B. situated chiefly in the cervical and lumbar regions of the spine, though they occur occasionally in the thoracic region
    C. both
    D. neither

65. Arthralgia is a common prodromal symptom in

    A. hepatitis A
    B. hepatitis B
    C. both
    D. neither

66. Rheumatoid nodules and granulomas in adults are not unique to rheumatoid arthritis and may be

    A. an early manifestation of classic systemic lupus erythematosus
    B. a late manifestation of classic systemic lupus erythematosus
    C. both
    D. neither

67. When aspirating joint fluid,

    A. the syringe should be coated with sterile heparin to prevent clotting prior to analysis
    B. isotonic saline, not glacial acetic acid, should be used to dilute joint fluid for a white-cell count; otherwise, the fluid may coagulate resulting in a spuriously low cell count
    C. both
    D. neither

68. In drug abusers, a syndrome of necrotizing angiitis has been described which

    A. is strikingly similar to periarteritis nodosa, with severe renal, gastrointestinal, cardiac, and neurologic involvement
    B. may result in pancreatitis, renal failure, hypertension, pulmonary edema and neuropathy
    C. both
    D. neither

Directions: Use the key below to answer questions 69 and 70.
    A. if both the statement and reason are true and are related as to cause and effect
    B. if both the statement and reason are true, but are not related as to cause and effect
    C. if the statement is true, but the reason is false
    D. if the statement is false, but the reason is true
    E. if both the statement and reason are false

69. A search for occult muscle disease has been recommended in patients with pulmonary fibrosis **because** the latter has been associated with polymyositis and may be responsive to high-dose steroid therapy.

70. Juveniles, as well as some adult patients with rheumatoid arthritis, may be "seronegative" for rheumatoid factor **because** such sera may contain rheumatoid factors mainly of small molecular types (IgG and IgA) but little of the IgM rheumatoid factor particularly responsible for the agglutination reaction.

Directions: Use the key below to answer questions 71 through 78.
   A. if A is greater than or more appropriate than B
   B. if B is greater than or more appropriate than A
   C. if A and B are approximately equal

71. Likelihood of having ischemic ulcerations of fingers is greater in patients with
   A. Raynaud's phenomenon secondary to scleroderma
   B. Raynaud's disease

72. In gout, the incidence of treatment failures appears to be higher with
   A. uricosuric agents
   B. allopurinol

73. Muscular atrophy and weakness associated with
   A. rheumatoid arthritis
   B. osteoarthritis

74. Incidence in sarcoidosis
   A. hyperglobulinemia
   B. hypercalcemia

75. Erythema nodosum
   A. sarcoidosis
   B. tuberculosis

76. Contractures and ankylosis associated with
   A. rheumatoid arthritis
   B. osteoarthritis

77. As a cause of neuropathic foot deformities:
   A. diabetes
   B. tabes dorsalis

78. Poor mucin clot:
   A. neuropathic joint disease
   B. inflammatory arthritis (infectious, rheumatoid, or gouty)

Directions: For each of the following statements, fill in the correct answer(s).

79. Antinucleolar antibodies are encountered more often in _____ _____ _____ than in any other connective tissue disease.

80. Tenderness over the long head of the biceps tendon as it lies in the bicipital groove between the greater and lesser tuberosities of the humerus suggests _____ of the biceps tendon.

81. A torn meniscus is suggested by a positive _____ sign.

82. Interstitial pulmonary fibrosis occurs with connective-tissue diseases, classically with _____ , but less commonly and usually in a milder form with systemic lupus erythematosus or rheumatoid arthritis.

83. Tenderness over the lateral aspect of the distal radius suggests inflammation of the tendon sheaths of the extensor pollicis brevis and the abductor pollicis longus, known as _____ disease.

84. _____ disease must be strongly suspected in the presence of a consistently positive ANA test (other than weak homogeneous) if drug reaction, connective tissue disease, or family history of connective tissue disease are ruled out, and if no medications that can cause positive ANA tests have been taken.

85. Both allopurinol and its major metabolic product, _____ , are potent inhibitors of xanthine oxidase.

86. _____ was specifically developed for use as a uricosuric agent and is the most potent one known.

87. When mononeuritis multiplex occurs in an obscure systemic illness, it is highly suggestive of systemic necrotizing _____ .

88. Many patients with Raynaud's phenomenon ultimately develop a collagen disease, most commonly _____ .

Directions: Indicate the proper answer by using the key given below.
  A. if both the statement and reason are true and are related as to cause and effect
  B. if both the statement and reason are true, but are not related as to cause and effect
  C. if the statement is true, but the reason is false
  D. if the statement is false, but the reason is true
  E. if both the statement and reason are false

89. X-ray examination should not be carried out in all cases of sciatica, **since** virtually all causes of sciatic pain are not associated with bony changes visible on x-ray.

Directions: For each of the following questions, select the ONE CORRECT answer.

90. Sjögren's syndrome
  A. is characterized by dry eyes and mouth, salivary and lacrimal gland involvement, vasculitis, and autoantibody production
  B. is frequently associated with rheumatoid arthritis
  C. occurs with scleroderma, polyarteritis, discoid lupus, systemic lupus erythematosus, and thrombotic thrombocytopenic purpura
  D. all of the above
  E. none of the above

91. It has been found that most patients who developed ANA after procainamide did so within
  A. 1 to 2 months
  B. 3 to 6 months
  C. 8 to 12 months
  D. 24 to 28 months
  E. 30 to 40 months

92. In de Quervain's disease,
  A. onset is often but not invariably associated with unaccustomed use of the hand
  B. correctly administered hydrocortisone provides comparable if not better results than those of surgery
  C. there is stenosing vaginitis of the common synovial sheath of the extensor pollicis brevis and abductor pollicis longus
  D. all of the above
  E. none of the above

93. The antinuclear antibody is
  A. almost invariably positive in patients with systemic lupus erythematosus
  B. positive in 30% of patients with rheumatoid arthritis
  C. positive in 50 to 60% of patients with scleroderma
  D. all of the above
  E. none of the above

Directions: For each of the following statements, ONE or MORE of the numbered completions is correct. In each case, select
  A. if 1, 2, and 3 are correct
  B. if 1 and 3 are correct
  C. if 2 and 4 are correct
  D. if all statements are correct
  E. if all statements are incorrect
  F. if another combination is correct

94. Which of the following may occur with systemic lupus erythematosus?
  1. pulmonary infiltrates
  2. pleurisy with effusion
  3. progressive glomerulonephritis
  4. vasculitis and weight loss

95. The acute gouty attack may be treated with
  1. colchicine
  2. phenylbutazone
  3. oxyphenbutazone
  4. indomethacin

96. Indications for allopurinol include
  1. tophaceous gout
  2. gout complicated by renal insufficiency
  3. uric acid excretion greater than 1000 mg/day
  4. history of uric acid calculi

97. In the carpal tunnel syndrome,
  1. spontaneous compression of the median nerve occurs principally in middle-aged men
  2. early symptoms are pain and tingling felt in the thumb, index, and radial side of the ring finger
  3. the spontaneous variety is rarely bilateral
  4. weakness and wasting of abductor pollicis brevis and opponens pollicis cause conspicuous hollowing of the outer half of the thenar eminence

98. Systemic steroid therapy is indicated in
  1. systemic sclerosis
  2. osteoarthritis
  3. Reiter's syndrome
  4. ankylosing spondylitis

Answers and Commentary

1. **C.** Rose and Spencer studied 54 cases of polyarteritis nodosa and 30 with the diagnosis of allergic angiitis and granulomatosis. No involvement of the pulmonary arteries in classic polyarteritis nodosa was found. Conversely, 47% involvement of the lungs (pulmonary arteries) was found in allergic angiitis and granulomatosis ("polyarteritis with pulmonary involvement"). These workers found that the heart was involved in 35% of cases of classic polyarteritis nodosa; kidneys (glomerulitis, 30%; renal polyarteritis, 65%); stomach and intestines, 30%; liver 54%; pancreas 39%; spleen, 35%; brain, 4%; periadrenal connective tissue, 41%; and voluntary muscle, 20%. (1:37)

2. **D.** Several studies have shown that next to arthralgia and arthritis, which occur in 90% of patients with systemic lupus erythematosus, fever occurring during the course of the disease affects 83% of patients. (3:176)

3. **E.** In patients with primary hyperuricemia, the incidence of gouty arthritis was found to be approximately 90% when the serum urate concentration was over 9 mg/100 ml in a small group of patients over a long period of follow-up.
(*Semin Drug Treat*, 1:119, 1971)

4. **C.** Salicylate preparations can cause some gastrointestinal bleeding; not enough to blacken the stool but detectable with guaiac testing. This is usually not dangerous nor significant. Iron loss can be replaced with diet or supplemental iron and does not usually constitute an indication to stop aspirin. (*Res-Staff Phys*, 18:35, 1972)

5. **D.** Two surveys in Sweden and New York gave a prevalence of systemic lupus erythematosus in the population of about 1 in 10,000.
(*Am Heart J*, 84:228, 1972)

6. **D.** In patients with rheumatoid arthritis and leukopenia, treatment with gold salts has resulted in improvement in arthritis, a rise in the white-cell count, and a fall in the erythrocyte sedimentation rate. (*N Engl J Med*, 288:1007, 1973)

7. **E.** Spasmodic torticollis is an intermittent or continuous spasm of sternomastoid, trapezius, and other neck muscles, usually more pronounced on one side, with turning or tipping of the head. It is involuntary and cannot be inhibited and thereby differs from habit spasm or tic. This condition should be considered as a form of dystonia. It is worse when the patient sits, stands, or walks and usually contactual stimulation of the chin or of the back of the head partially alleviates the muscle imbalance. Psychiatric treatment is ineffectual. In severe cases, muscle sectioning, neurectomy, or section of the anterior cervical roots has given favorable results. (5:96)

8. **E.** Gold and chloroquine (used in rheumatoid arthritis) are not effective in ankylosing spondylitis. Corticosteroids are not recommended because they are less helpful than phenylbutazone and indomethacin and because toxicity is inevitable when used in higher doses for the prolonged periods necessary in this disease. Local radiation is no longer used because it is no more effective than phenylbutazone or indomethacin, does not halt progression of ankylosis, and carries a late risk of inducing leukemia.
(*Res-Intern Consult*, 1:32, 1972)

9. **D.** It is recommended that daily colchicine be given during the first months of therapy of gout with allopurinol. All other statements are true.
(*Semin Drug Treat*, 1:119, 1971)

10. **C.** In Paget's disease, the alkaline phosphatase serum level correlates well with the disease's extent and activity. All other statements are true. (*Res-Intern Consult*, 1:3, 1972)

11. **D.** Decreased chest expansion is a physical finding in ankylosing spondylitis. All other findings listed are correct. (*Res-Intern Consult*, 1:32, 1972)

12. **E.** All of the autoantibodies listed may occur in systemic lupus erythematous. In addition, there may be anti-clotting factors, antithyroid antibodies, rheumatoid factor, as well as a biologic false-positive test for syphilis. (*JAMA*, 224, Suppl.: 661, 1973)

13. **E.** Polyarthritis of unknown etiology includes all of the disorders listed as well as Reiter's syndrome. (*JAMA*, 224, Suppl.: 661, 1973)

14. **E.** All the pathologic changes listed have been described in polymyositis. (*Lahey Clin Foun Bull*, 16:247, 1967)

15. **A.** In familial Mediterranean fever, some patients develop renal amyloidosis, but this is unlikely in patients who developed the disease in the United States. (*JAMA*, 220:1253, 1972)

16. **E.** Secondary or acquired metabolic gout may occur in any of the disorders listed. (*Res Staff Phys*, p. 82, May 1974)

17. **E.** All the reasons listed are exercise goals of patients with rheumatoid arthritis. (*Bull Rheum Dis*, 21:609, 1970)

18. **E.** All the statements are true of necrotizing angiitis associated with drug abuse. (*N Engl J Med*, 238:1003, 1970)

19. **E.** The incidence of gout is probably not as high in secondary hyperuricemia as it is in primary hyperuricemia except possibly in patients with any of the disorders listed. (*Semin Drug Treat*, 1:119, 1971)

20. **B.** (*Bull Rheum Dis*, 20:604, 1970)

21. **A.** (*Bull Rheum Dis*, 20:604, 1970)

22. **B.** (*Bull Rheum Dis*, 20:604, 1970)

23. **B.** (*Bull Rheum Dis*, 20:604, 1970)

24. **A.** (*Bull Rheum Dis*, 20:604, 1970)

25. **A.** (*Bull Rheum Dis*, 20:604, 1970)

26. **B.** (*Bull Rheum Dis*, 20:604, 1970)

27. **True.** In many patients with gout, the development of renal insufficiency is related to nephrosclerosis, hypertension, and other factors known to be associated with hyperuricemia. (*Semin Drug Treat*, 1:119, 1971)

28. **True.** Renal arteriography defines the subacute renal lesions of polyarteritis nodosa and shows regression of lesions after steroid treatment. (*J Pediatr*, 80:1035, 1972)

29. **True.** One may observe acute attacks of gouty arthritis in the back, hips, shoulders, or cervical spine, but these joints are affected only after the diagnosis has been well established for years and after many attacks in the toes, ankles, knees, hands, or elbows. (*Hosp Tribune*, p. 5, Dec. 11, 1972)

30. **True.** Arthritis of the first costovertebral joint is one cause of the symptoms of thoracic outlet syndrome. (*Clin Orthop*, 86:159, 1972)

31. **False.** Although rheumatoid vasculitis may be pathologically indistinguishable from periarteritis nodosa, renal involvement by rheumatoid vasculitis is distinctly unusual. (*N Engl J Med*, 285:1250, 1971)

32. **False.** If a patient with gout is already receiving hypouricemic therapy and develops an acute attack of gouty arthritis, the crystal-induced synovitis is usually treated without changing the hypouricemic therapy. (*Semin Drug Treat*, 1:119, 1971)

33. **True.** Muscle biopsy is the most useful diagnostic procedure in polymyositis. (*Lahey Clin Foun Bull*, 16:247, 1967)

34. **True.** A positive LE cell test is most common with systemic lupus erythematosus but has a 6% frequency with rheumatoid arthritis and a lower frequency with scleroderma. (*N Engl J Med*, 288:204, 1973)

35. **False.** A very low carbon monoxide diffusion capacity (less than 15% of the predicted value) is a hallmark of sclerodermatous involvement of the lung. (*N Engl J Med*, 288:204, 1973)

36. **True.** Approximately one-third of patients with systemic lupus erythematosus are free of renal disease. (*N Engl J Med*, 288:204, 1973)

37. **True.** The most common pulmonary manifestation of lupus is pleuritis, with some interstitial pneumonitis. (*N Engl J Med*, 288:204, 1973)

38. **False.** The distal interphalangeal joints (DIP) are frequently involved in rheumatoid arthritis. (*JAMA*, 220:1252, 1972)

39. **True.** The uricosuric effect of most agents studied has been attributed to inhibition of the tubular reabsorption of filtered urate.
(*Semin Drug Treat*, 1:119, 1971)

40. **True.** Gold has no effect in osteoarthritis.
(*Hosp Phys*, 8:36, July 1972)

41. **True.** If a patient has constipation on high-dose aspirin therapy, giving aspirin which contains magnesium can cause looser stools.
(*Hosp Phys*, p. 36, July 1972)

42. **False.** Podagra is unusual in pyrophosphate arthropathy. (*Br Med J*, 4:1, 1972)

43. **False.** Radiographic changes are not sensitive indicators for diagnosis for gout.
(*Br Med J*, 4:1, 1972)

44. **False.** Rapid reduction in serum urate may provoke an exacerbation of gouty arthritis. (1:132)

45. **False.** There is some evidence that aspirin—long a mainstay in management—may slow the progression of early osteoarthritis. (1:133)

46. **True.** In ankylosing spondylitis, steroid therapy is rarely justified unless iritis is present. (1:128)

47. **True.** Treatment with uricosurics leads to a transient increase in uric acid excretion whereas allopurinol consistently decreases uric acid excretion. (*Semin Drug Treat*, 1:119, 1971)

48. **True.** ,The administration of allopurinol in man is followed by a prompt decrease in the serum and urinary uric acid, within 24 to 48 hours, reaching a maximum decrease in four days to two weeks, and remaining relatively constant over prolonged periods of time. (*Semin Drug Treat*, 1:119, 1971)

49. **True.** The development of ANA in high titer can be expected in 1 in 5 patients treated with procainamide, regardless of the dose given.
(*Am Heart J*, 84:228, 1972)

50. **False.** Only about 30% of patients found to have polyarteritis at autopsy have positive muscle biopsy before death.
(*Lahey Clin Found Bull*, 20:33, 1971)

51. **True.** Sympathectomy may be of value in the treatment of severe Raynaud's phenomenon.
(*Arch Surg*, 105:313, 1972)

52. **False.** In a study of polymyositis, it was found that the erythrocyte sedimentation rate was a poor indicator of disease activity. Eleven of 18 patients had elevated values on initial survey, and there was no correlation between the level of the sedimentation rate and the clinical or histologic severity of the disease.
(*Lahey Clin Found Bull*, 16:247, 1967)

53. **D.** In contrast to secondary Raynaud's phenomenon, primary Raynaud's disease has an excellent prognosis, and the use of vasodilating drugs is not routinely necessary.
(*N Engl J Med*, 285:290, 1971)

54. **D.** Colchicine does not alter serum concentration or renal excretion of uric acid nor does it have any significant effect upon the miscible pool of uric acid or the rate of its turnover.
(*Semin Drug Treat*, 1:119, 1971)

55. **D.** Both phenylbutazone and dicumarol enhance renal excretion of uric acid.
(*Semin Drug Treat*, 1:119, 1971)

56. **C.** Joint involvement is now a well recognized complication of systemic infections produced by both RNA and DNA viruses.
(*Lahey Clin Found Bull*, 20:33, 1971)

57. **C.** The presence of necrotizing arteritis is consistent with polyarteritis nodosa and may be associated with rheumatoid arthritis or systemic lupus erythematosus.
(*Lahey Clin Found Bull*, 20:33, 1971)

58. **C.** Diffuse tenderness over the calcaneus is often associated with early rheumatoid arthritis or with Reiter's syndrome. (4:300)

59. **A.** In acute gouty arthritis, intravenous injection of 2 to 3 mg of colchicine results in a much lower incidence of gastrointestinal side effects than with oral administration, and a more rapid response.
(1:131)

60. **C.** Tenderness lateral or anterior to the radial head may indicate lateral epicondylitis (tennis elbow) and may be accentuated as the patient pronates the forearm and extends the wrist against resistance. (4:294)

61. **A.** Vascular lesions are usually all in the same stage of activity in hypersensitivity angiitis.
(*Lahey Clin Found Bull*, 20:33, 1971)

62. **B.** In systemic lupus erythematosus, platelet antibody was found in 85% of patients and a compensated thrombocytolytic state has been postulated. (*N Engl J Med*, 284:11, 1971)

63. **A.** Cervical spondylosis is one of the commonest causes of paraplegia of slow onset, but is not always associated with any abnormal physical signs in the upper limbs. (2:329)

64. **C.** Both statements are true of lesions of the intervertebral discs. (2:341)

65. **C.** Arthralgia is a common prodromal symptom in both hepatitis A and hepatitis B.
(*Lahey Clin Found Bull*, 20:33, 1971)

66. **C.** Rheumatoid nodules and granulomas in adults may be either an early or a late manifestation of classic systemic lupus erythematosus.
(*JAMA*, 220:515, 1972)

67. **C.** Both procedures listed are correct when aspirating joint fluid.
(*Am Fam Physician*, 7:90, 1973)

68. **C.** Both statements are true of the syndrome of necrotizing angiitis in drug abusers.
(*N Engl J Med*, 283:1003, 1970)

69. **A.** A search for occult muscle disease has been recommended in patients with pulmonary fibrosis because the latter has been associated with polymyositis and may be responsive to high-dose steroid therapy. (*JAMA*, 222:1146, 1972)

70. **A.** Both the statement and reason are correct and positively related. (1:126)

71. **A.** Patients with Raynaud's phenomenon secondary to scleroderma are more likely to have ischemic ulcerations in their fingers than patients with Raynaud's disease.
(*N Engl J Med*, 285:290, 1971)

72. **A.** In gout, the incidence of treatment failures appears to be higher with uricosuric agents than with allopurinol. (*Semin Drug Treat*, 1:119, 1971)

73. **A.** Muscular atrophy and weakness are not associated with osteoarthritis.
(*Hosp Phys*, 8:36, 1972)

74. **A.** Several studies have indicated a higher incidence of hyperglobulinemia than hypercalcemia in patients with sarcoidosis. (3:213)

75. **A.** Whereas erythema nodosum is common in sarcoidosis, it is uncommon in tuberculosis.
(3:170)

76. **A.** Osteoarthritis is not associated with contractures and ankylosis. (*Hosp Phys*, 8:36, July 1972)

77. **A.** Neuropathic joint disease occurs most frequently in the knees of patients with tabes dorsalis, in the shoulders and elbows of those with syringomyelia, and in the feet of diabetics.
(*Am Fam Physician*, 7:90, 1973)

78. **B.** While the mucin clot of neuropathic joint disease is usually good, that of inflammatory arthritis (infectious, rheumatoid, or gouty) is usually poor. (*Am Fam Physician*, 7:90, 1973)

79. **Progressive systemic sclerosis.** Approximately one-third of patients with progressive systemic sclerosis have positive tests for rheumatoid factor and 60% or more have serum antinucleolar antibodies. Antinucleolar antibodies have been found in 10 to 50% of cases and are encountered more often in progressive systemic sclerosis than in any other connective tissue disease. (1:129)

80. **Tendonitis.** Tenderness over the long head of the biceps tendon as it lies in the bicipital groove between the greater and lesser tuberosities of the humerus suggests tendonitis of the biceps tendon.
(4:294)

81. **McMurray.** A torn meniscus is suggested by a positive McMurray sign. To perform the McMurray maneuver, flex the knee fully with the patient recumbent, steadying the knee with one hand, and slowly extend the knee while holding the tibia in internal rotation. A palpable or audible snap associated with momentary discomfort as the knee is extended suggests a tear in that portion of the lateral meniscus which was between the femoral condyle and the tibial plateau when the snap occurred. This test is repeated with the tibia held in external rotation which tests the posterior aspect of the medial meniscus. This test is generally not positive when the tear involves the anterior one-third of either meniscus. (4:298)

82. **Scleroderma.** Interstitial pulmonary fibrosis occurs with connective-tissue diseases, classically with scleroderma, but less commonly and usually in a milder form with systemic lupus erythematosus or rheumatoid arthritis.
(*N Engl J Med*, 288:204, 1973)

83. **de Quervain's.** Tenderness over the lateral aspect of the distal radius suggests inflammation of the tendon sheaths of the extensor pollicis brevis and the abductor pollicis longus—de Quervain's disease. (4:295)

84. **Malignant.** Malignant disease must be strongly suspected in the presence of a consistently positive ANA test, other than weak homogeneous, if drug reaction, connective-tissue disease or family history of connective-tissue disease are ruled out, and if no medications that can cause positive ANA tests have been taken.
(*Lancet*, 2:436, 1972)

85. **Oxipurinol.** Both allopurinol and its major metabolic product, oxipurinol, are potent inhibitors of xanthine oxidase.
(*Semin Drug Treat*, 1:119, 1971)

86. **Sulfinpyrazone.** Sulfinpyrazone was specifically developed for use as a uricosuric agent and is the most potent one known.
(*Semin Drug Treat*, 1:119, 1971)

87. **Arteritis.** When mononeuritis multiplex occurs in an obscure systemic illness, it is highly suggestive of systemic necrotizing arteritis.
(*Lahey Clin Found Bull,* 20:33, 1971)

88. **Scleroderma.** Many patients with Raynaud's phenomenon ultimately develop a collagen disease, most commonly scleroderma.
(*Arch Surg,* 105:313, 1972)

89. **E.** X-ray examination should be carried out in all cases of sciatica, since many causes of sciatic pain are associated with bony changes visible in radiographs. (2:346)

90. **D.** All statements are true of Sjögren's syndrome. (*JAMA,* 215:757, 1971)

91. **B.** It has been found that most patients who developed antinuclear antibodies after procainamide did so within 3 to 6 months.
(*Am Heart J,* 84:228, 1972)

92. **D.** All statements are true of de Quervain's disease. (*Br Med J,* 4:659, 1972)

93. **D.** All statements are true of the antinuclear antibody. (*N Engl J Med,* 288:204, 1973)

94. **D.** Any of the disorders listed may occur with systemic lupus erythematosus.
(*N Engl J Med,* 291:195, 1974)

95. **D.** The acute gouty attack may be treated with any of the drugs listed, as well as ACTH and newer nonsteroidal anti-inflammatory drugs.
(*Semin Drug Treat,* 1:119, 1971)

96. **D.** All the disorders listed are indications for allopurinol. It may also be used in the treatment of HG-PRT deficiency, and secondary hyperuricemia with overproduction of uric acid, when allergy to uricosurics is present and when uricosurics are ineffective or poorly tolerated.
(*Semin Drug Treat,* 1:119, 1971)

97. **C.** In the carpal tunnel syndrome, spontaneous compression of the median nerve occurs principally in middle-aged women. The spontaneous variety is frequently bilateral, but often begins in one hand some months or more before it starts in the other. The sensory changes are limited to the digits, the palmar skin escaping because the palmar branch of the nerve lies superficial to the retinaculum. (2:357–58)

98. **E.** Systemic steroid therapy is not indicated in any of the disorders listed.
(*Ration Drug Treat,* 6:1, 1972)

Textbook References for Chapter 22

1. American College of Physicians (1974): *Medical Knowledge Self-Assessment, Program III: Recent Developments in Internal Medicine,* R.G. Petersdorf, General Editor, American College of Physicians, Philadelphia.

2. Bannister, Roger (1978): *Brain's Clinical Neurology,* Fifth Edition, Oxford Medical Publications, New York.

3. Beeson, P.B. and McDermott, W. (1979): *Cecil Textbook of Medicine,* Fifteenth Edition, W.B. Saunders Company, Philadelphia.

4. Judge, R.D. and Zuidema, G.D., Editors (1974): *Physical Diagnosis: A Physiologic Approach to the Clinical Examination,* Little, Brown and Company, Boston.

5. Isselbacher, K.J., Editor (1980): *Harrison's Principles of Internal Medicine,* Ninth Edition, McGraw-Hill Book Company, New York.

CHAPTER 23

Signs and Symptoms

Directions: Indicate whether each of the following statements is true or false.

1. Nocturnal dyspnea is not characteristic of asthma.

2. If a drowsy patient responds to visual threat by blinking, but the response is asymmetric, this will rule out a homonymous field defect.

3. The physical signs of hemothorax are those of pleural effusion; these are diminished breath sounds at the base posteriorly on the involved side with dullness to percussion.

4. The commonest cause of vertigo is a disturbance of function of the labyrinth.

5. When nystagmus is due to disease of the labyrinth, it is usually not associated with paroxysmal vertigo and deafness.

6. In situations in which diabetic ketoacidosis is accompanied by lactic acidosis, a weakly positive nitroprusside reaction may not reflect the magnitude of ketonemia since the altered redox state favors conversion of acetoacetate to beta-hydroxybutyrate.

7. A classic attack of migraine begins with a visual disturbance which occurs within one pair of homonymous half-fields.

8. Certain wheezes due to extrabronchial compression or intrabronchial polypoid lesions appear only with change in position.

9. A strong clue to the likelihood of analgesic nephropathy is renal papillary necrosis with its usual symptoms of renal colic due to sloughed papilla passed down the ureter.

10. A low glucose concentration in pleural fluid tends to rule out the presence of malignancy.

11. Minor precordial movements can be amplified by observing during expiratory apnea.

12. A serum chloride below the level of 102 mEq/liter, in the absence of vomiting or respiratory acidosis, is evidence against the presence of a parathyroid adenoma.

13. Nystagmus is usually absent in cerebellar disease.

14. Eye signs may occur in the absence of active thyrotoxicosis (ophthalmic Graves' disease), so that their presence and severity are not necessarily related to the thyroid state of the patient.

15. Increased tendon reflexes normally occur in hypercalcemic states.

16. As far as motor, sensory, and speech functions are concerned, symptoms of occlusion of the middle cerebral artery are indistinguishable from those of occlusion of the internal carotid artery.

17. The early symptoms of senile cataract may include visual blurring, especially involving distance.

18. Small, contracted pupils which do not respond may be associated with midbrain damage.

19. In patients with the syndrome of inappropriate ADH, the urine must be hypertonic in order to make the diagnosis.

20. The presence of a normal or low normal serum phosphorus level in a patient with mild hypercalcemia in the presence of azotemia virtually rules out the diagnosis of hyperparathyroidism.

21. In appendicitis or other conditions secondarily affecting the psoas muscle, there is flexion of the thigh due to contraction of the psoas muscle.

22. The disappearance of the vein on both sides of the retinal blood column representing the artery is a measure of thickening of the arteriolar wall.

23. The patient with a trochlear palsy will complain of difficulty with vision in the lower field, as in reading, and if he has been able to maintain single binocular vision, his head will be tilted toward the shoulder opposite the side of the paralysis.

24. Reduction in GFR alone is insufficient to account for the modest elevations of plasma amylase activity that may sometimes be encountered in renal failure.

Directions: Use the key below to answer questions 25 through 31. If the signs and symptoms are characteristic of
A. pulmonary hypertension
B. tricuspid stenosis
C. tricuspid regurgitation
D. myocardial infarction
E. atrial septal defect
F. ventricular septal defect
G. pericarditis

25. Jugular v wave; elevated venous pressure; right ventricular parasternal lift; systolic thrill at tricuspid area; presence of regurgitant systolic murmur louder with inspiration; atrial fibrillation; early diastolic extra sound (over right ventricle)

26. Tachycardia; friction rub; diminished heart sounds and enlarged heart to percussion (with effusion); paradoxical pulse; neck vein distention; narrow pulse pressure (with tamponade)

27. Small pulse; giant "a" wave in jugular pulse; elevated jugular pressure; tricuspid opening snap (usually associated with mitral valve disease)

28. Cyanosis (at times); small pulse; narrow pulse pressure; cold extremities; atrial fibrillation (late); giant jugular "a" wave; parasternal lift; systolic lift in the pulmonic area; accentuated P-2, slightly split; presystolic extra sound at tricuspid area; pulmonary ejection click; pulmonic diastolic murmur (Graham Steell); systolic ejection murmur in pulmonic area

29. Small pulse; normal jugular pulse; parasternal lift and left ventricular apical lift; systolic thrill and loud systolic regurgitant murmur in third and fourth interspaces along left sternal border; apical diastolic rumble; slight persistent split of P-2 (variable)

30. Tachycardia; pallor; slightly elevated jugular pressure; small arterial pulse; narrow pulse pressure; soft heart sounds; presystolic

or early diastolic extra sound; pericardial friction rub; any of the arrhythmias

31. Normal pulse; sustained parasternal lift; lift over pulmonary artery; normal jugular pulse; systolic ejection murmur in pulmonic area; low-pitched diastolic rumble over tricuspid area (at times); persistent wide splitting of P-2

Directions: For each of the following statements, fill in the correct answer(s).

32. In chronic obstructive pulmonary disease, the two most reliable signs of hyperinflation (best seen on a lateral film) are the flatness of the _____ and the depth of the _____ air space.

33. There are two basic pathologic reflexes, the Babinski and its variants, and the _____ and its variants.

34. Partial damage to a peripheral nerve may be followed by a characteristic type of pain termed _____ .

35. When a hernia can no longer be reduced and the contents of the hernial sac cannot be returned to the peritoneal cavity, it is said to be _____ .

36. The _____ test is performed with the patient sitting with the forearms in supination and resting on the thighs. Palpate the radial pulse on the side to be tested, instructing the patient to extend the neck and turn the chin to the side to be tested.

37. The diagnosis of de Quervain's disease is confirmed when a tender nodule can be felt within one or both the tendons over the lateral aspect of the distal radius and when a positive _____ test is noted.

38. Reflex _____ bladder due to a transverse myelitis of the spinal cord, as in trauma,

characteristically produces a hyperactive bulbocavernosus reflex and saddle anesthesia.

39. The sign of inspiratory arrest (_____ sign) may be seen in the presence of acute cholecystitis.

40. _____ is the presence of pus in the anterior chamber of the eye, often with a horizontal fluid level.

41. Dyspnea precipitated by assuming the recumbent position is referred to as _____ .

42. An irritative lesion of a single dorsal _____ causes pain of a lancinating or burning character which is often precipitated or intensified by coughing or sneezing, sometimes by movements of the spine, and is associated with hyperesthesia and hyperalgesia over the full segmental distribution of the _____ .

43. _____ is the presence of blood in the anterior chamber of the eye.

Directions: For each of the following incomplete statements, select
 A. if the question is associated with A only
 B. if the question is associated with B only
 C. if the question is associated with both A and B
 D. if the question is associated with neither A nor B

44. Change in potassium metabolism may be reflected in
   A. increased excitability of neuromuscular tissue
   B. decreased excitability of neuromuscular tissue
   C. both
   D. neither

45. A very prominent, intermittent jugular pulse may indicate
   A. a situation of AV dissociation, where the atrium by chance is contracting against a closed AV valve

B. ventricular tachycardia until proven otherwise
C. both
D. neither

46. Left ventricular hypertrophy without significant dilatation may be

A. due to primary left ventricular disease, as in hypertrophic cardiomyopathy
B. secondary to systolic overload, as in aortic valvular stenosis
C. both
D. neither

47. Neurocirculatory asthenia

A. includes symptoms, especially general weakness on effort, that can be triggered by muscular exertion, emotion-provoking situations, and by a variety of life circumstances
B. the cause of this condition is unknown, and objective evidence of a significant "physical" or biochemical disorder has been lacking
C. both
D. neither

48. The diagnosis of a hemoglobin disorder

A. can be based solely on a hemoglobin pattern or a sickle cell preparation
B. may depend on the clinical picture and other factors
C. both
D. neither

49. Patients with primary alveoloar hypoventilation may have

A. normal pulmonary function tests
B. increased sensitivity to CO_2
C. both
D. neither

50. A dilated pupil in a comatose patient suggests which of the following principal locations(s) of the lesion?

A. at the junction of the carotid and posterior communicating artery, where an aneurysm may compress the third nerve as it passes toward the orbit
B. at the midbrain, where the third nerve may be involved by a variety of lesions within the midbrain or by compression from without; i.e., uncal herniation
C. both
D. neither

51. Patients with lactase deficiency often have

A. abdominal distress
B. constipation
C. both
D. neither

52. Dysmetria is a

A. disturbance of the power to control the range of movement in muscular action
B. sign of cerebellar dysfunction
C. both
D. neither

53. A radial nerve lesion may result in

A. wrist-drop
B. finger-drop
C. both
D. neither

54. In toxic adenoma,

A. radioiodine scan of the thyroid shows a "hot nodule" which is not suppressed by T_3 and the remainder of thyroid can be stimulated to take up iodine by thyroid-stimulating hormone (TSH)
B. both the clinical picture and the results of blood tests are unequivocal
C. both
D. neither

55. The finding of local inspiratory retraction of the intercostal spaces, indicating local bronchial obstruction, is diffuse in

A. asthma
B. emphysema
C. both
D. neither

56. Dyssynergia is

    A. a disturbance of muscular coordination
    B. not a sign of cerebellar dysfunction
    C. both
    D. neither

57. When bronchial breathing is heard over the upper anterior chest, the finding may be due to

    A. decreased transmission through consolidated lung
    B. normal tracheal breathing due to shift in tracheal position
    C. both
    D. neither

58. The cerebrospinal fluid is likely to contain red blood cells if a cerebral hemorrhage has ruptured into

    A. a ventricle
    B. the subarachnoid space
    C. both
    D. neither

Directions: Use the key below to answer questions 59 through 62. If the feature is characteristic of
  A. **conductive hearing loss**
  B. **perceptive hearing loss**

59. The patient often states that he hears but does not understand, which is indicative of poor discrimination.

60. The patient tends to speak loudly

61. The patient generally hears well on the telephone

62. The patient hears best in a noisy environment

Directions: Use the key below to answer questions 63 and 64. If the procedure is used to elicit
  A. **Trousseau's sign**
  B. **Chvostek's sign**

63. Temporarily interrupts the circulation to the forearm by applying a blood pressure cuff and inflating it above systolic pressure for at least 3 minutes

64. Tap over the facial nerve in front of the ear with the finger

Directions: Use the key below to answer questions 65 and 66. If the elevation of the testes
  A. **increases pain in this condition**
  B. **decreases pain in this condition**

65. Torsion of the spermatic cord

66. Epididymitis

Directions: Use the key below to answer questions 67 through 70. If the statement is characteristic of
  A. **myopic eyes**
  B. **hyperopia**
  C. **direct light reaction**
  D. **consensual light reaction**

67. The pupil of one eye constricts when the other eye is illuminated

68. The pupils are small

69. The pupils are large

70. The pupil constricts when illuminated

Directions: For each of the following multiple-choice questions, select the ONE CORRECT answer.

71. Evidence of hemolysis includes

    A. unconjugated hyperbilirubinemia
    B. increased free serum haptoglobin
    C. absence of reticulocytosis
    D. all of the above
    E. none of the above

72. In the comatose patient,

    A. the environment is not perceived
    B. even intense stimulation produces poor, primitive, or rudimentary motor responses (moderately deep coma) or no responses at all (deep coma)
    C. reflex reactions are entirely dependent on the location of the lesion
    D. all of the above
    E. none of the above

73. Pleural effusion includes

    A. empyema
    B. hemothorax
    C. chylothorax
    D. all of the above
    E. none of the above

74. Nystagmus due to disease of the labyrinth is usually

    A. horizontal
    B. vertical
    C. rotary
    D. all of the above
    E. none of the above

Directions: For each of the following incomplete statements, ONE or MORE of the numbered completions is correct. In each case, select
    A.   **if 1, 2, and 3 are correct**
    B.   **if 1 and 3 are correct**
    C.   **if 2 and 4 are correct**
    D.   **if only 4 is correct**
    E.   **if all statements are correct**

75. May cause great enlargement of the spleen (more than 8 cm of the splenic edge below the left costal margin on deep inspiration):

    1. chronic granulocytic leukemia
    2. chronic malaria
    3. congenital syphilis in the infant
    4. amyloidosis

76. Symptoms of cerebellar deficiency include

    1. muscular hypotonia
    2. static tremor
    3. ataxia or incoordination
    4. dysdiadochokinesis

77. Hemoptysis in a person with club fingers suggests the possibility of

    1. lung abscess
    2. cancer of the lung
    3. bronchiectasis
    4. emboli to the lungs in a person with subacute bacterial endocarditis

78. Target cells may be seen in

    1. Hb C disease

    2. thalassemia
    3. sickle cell anemia
    4. chronic liver disease

79. Angina pectoris, or cardiac pain mimicking angina pectoris without coronary heart disease, may occur in patients with

    1. arterial hypertension
    2. marked valvular disease
    3. congenital heart disease
    4. myocardiopathy

80. A roentgenographic cavitary lesion may indicate the presence of

    1. tuberculosis
    2. histoplasmosis, or other mycotic infection
    3. bronchiectasis
    4. neoplasm

81. Causes of central cyanosis include

    1. congenital heart diseases with right to left shunts
    2. pulmonary arteriovenous fistulae
    3. advanced pulmonary disease with cor pulmonale
    4. advanced pulmonary disease with incomplete oxygenation of the blood in the lungs

82. In papilledema,

    1. there is swelling of the optic disc
    2. in early stages, the disc is pinker than normal, and the veins appear somewhat full
    3. flame-shaped hemorrhages and white exudates may appear
    4. temporal edge of the disc becomes blurred before the nasal edge

83. A pleural fluid red blood cell count greater than 100,000/cu mm strongly suggests the possibility of

    1. malignant neoplasm
    2. pulmonary infarction
    3. trauma
    4. tuberculosis

84. Decorticate movement and postures

1. consist of flexion and adduction in the upper extremities (including the wrist and fingers) and extension of the lower extremities with internal rotation
2. are believed to be the result of a lesion of the pyramidal tract joint rostral to the midbrain, disconnecting the hemispheres from the brain stem
3. when present, suggest a large lesion usually involving the interior capsule or the nostral cerebral peduncle on the appropriate side
4. rarely involve the thalamus and its adjacent structures

85. Autonomous neurogenic bladder

1. is produced by a lesion affecting sacral segments 2, 3, and 4, such as occurs in myelomeningocele or myelodysplasia
2. results in a hyperactive bulbocavernosus reflex
3. can be associated with urine forced from the bladder by pressure in the suprapubic region
4. does not involve saddle anesthesia

Directions: Use the key below to answer the following questions.
   A. if choice A is greater than or more appropriate than B
   B. if choice B is greater or more appropriate than A
   C. if A and B are equal or approximately equal

86. The presence of a markedly hypotonic urine in patients at the time of hyponatremia suggests the diagnosis of

A. water intoxication
B. syndrome of inappropriate ADH secretion

87. The first symptoms of spinal cord compression are usually

A. sensory
B. motor

88. Disease of the larger bronchi results in

A. rhonchi
B. rales

89. In black populations, blood pressure and obesity are better correlated in

A. women
B. men

90. An S_4 gallop

A. most probably originates in the atrial chamber
B. is thought to result from a forceful voluminous atrial contraction injecting blood into a ventricle having a limited distensibility

91. Occurrence of hematuria is more frequently associated with

A. Hb SA
B. Hb SS

92. Status epilepticus is the first manifestation of cryptogenic epilepsy in

A. children
B. adults

93. Variable response of the pupils to light suggests

A. toxic or metabolic abnormalities
B. structural lesion of the brain stem

94. Increased total vital capacity when supine occurs in

A. patients with emphysema
B. cardiac patients

Directions: For each of the following multiple-choice questions, select the ONE INCORRECT answer.

95. Concerning eye signs of Graves' disease,

A. an infiltrative ophthalmopathy is characteristic of Graves' disease but not other types of hyperthyroidism
B. although both eyes are commonly affected, the changes can be unilateral or asymmetrical
C. if exophthalmos develops in a patient who is euthyroid, failure of triiodothyronine to suppress the uptake of radioactive iodine by the thyroid gland may reveal the associated

endocrine disorder, especially if the test is performed during active progression of the eye signs

D. the proptosis is linked with an increase in the orbital contents, principally fat, and this increase may be secondary to weakness of the extrinsic ocular muscles which allows the eyeball to come forward out of its socket

E. diplopia is an uncommon symptom

96. In spinal nerve root irritation,

A. the positive symptom is root pain, usually lancinating in character, and possessing the characteristic distribution of the affected root

B. the condition is often made worse by coughing, sneezing, and by changes in the position of the relevant area of the spine

C. affected dermatome may be hyperesthetic and hyperalgesic or anesthetic and analgesic

D. appreciation of passive movement is usually impaired after a single root lesion

97. Regarding transient ischemic attacks,

A. they must be distinguished from other paroxysmal disorders such as migraine, epilepsy, carotid sinus syncope and Meniere's syndrome

B. most patients have permanent neurological deficits

C. detection of bruits in the neck is one of the most important parts of clinical examination

D. a fundoscopic search for retinal microemboli should be made

E. the radial pulses and brachial blood pressure in the two arms should always be compared to detect subclavian stenosis

98. Decerebrate movement and postures

A. consist of adduction, extension, and pronation of all four extremities

B. when fully developed, the decerebrate state includes opisthotonos

C. are best thought of as an exaggerated posture of staring

D. are most commonly seen with lesions destroying or compressing the midbrain or with lesions affecting the upper pons

E. must be structural in nature, because they are not seen with metabolic disturbances such as hypoglycemia, intoxications, or anoxia

99. Regarding apathetic hyperthyroidism,

A. it is an atypical presentation of hyperthyroidism, which occurs in the young

B. prominent features are weight loss, myopathy, apathy, and depression with cardiac arrhythmias and possible congestive heart failure

C. there is danger of crisis if untreated

D. the thyroid may be impalpable and eye signs absent

E. the usual tests are diagnostic

100. Signs of hypercalcemia include

A. polyuria and polydipsia

B. abdominal pain

C. muscle hypotonicity

D. tachycardia

E. fatigue, depression, and confusion

101. In sarcoidosis, characteristic clinical features include

A. lymph node involvement (often a mass of enlarged mediastinal nodes) and a plasma protein abnormality (increased beta-globulin)

B. small skeletal cysts may be present, often in the fingers

C. the serum concentration of parathormone is usually low or undetectable

D. hypercalciuria is typically absent

E. hypercalcemia if present usually responds rapidly (within 7 to 10 days) to the administration of corticosteroids, a feature which may be helpful in diagnosis

102. In compression of the cauda equina,

    1. lumbar apophysial arthritis and thickened ligamenta flava may cause compression
    2. pain, in the lumbar or sacral regions, or referred to one or both lower limbs, is the earliest symptom
    3. atrophic paralysis, frequently below the knees, may occur
    4. sensory loss and later bladder and bowel symptoms may occur

103. Pulmonic systolic ejection murmurs

    1. occur with pulmonary valvular stenosis
    2. occur with pulmonary subvalvular stenosis
    3. are usually localized to the second and third intercostal spaces
    4. are not referred to the left upper chest

104. Criteria for the diagnosis of the syndrome of inappropriate secretion of ADH set down by Bartter include

    1. hyponatremia and hypoosmolality of extracellular fluids
    2. persistence of sodium in urine despite hyponatremia
    3. absence of signs of dehydration
    4. abnormal renal and adrenal function

105. Regarding RAI uptake,

    1. low uptakes may be obtained in patients with normal thyroid function (or even hyperthyroidism) who are concomitantly receiving iodides
    2. patients with high uptake may be euthyroid (iodine-deficient diet) or even hypothyroid (dyshormonogenesis)
    3. the normal range is 5 to 30% uptake of the administered dose in 24 hours
    4. administration of thyroid hormone will increase uptake

106. Water-hammer pulse is the basis for peripheral signs of aortic insufficiency, including

    1. "hopping carotids"
    2. "pistol-shot sounds"
    3. Duroziez's sign
    4. de Musset's sign

107. In diffuse acute bronchial obstruction,

    1. the patient is in extreme respiratory distress
    2. respiration is rapid
    3. the intercostal spaces retract on inspiration
    4. accessory respiratory muscles may be used

108. Complete paralysis of the third cranial nerve results in

    1. ptosis of the upper lid
    2. internal ophthalmoplegia
    3. a wide pupil which fails to react to light and accommodation
    4. paralysis of the superior, medial, and inferior recti, and the superior oblique

109. Enlargement of the gingivae may be seen in generalized form in conditions of

    1. chronic inflammation
    2. pregnancy
    3. endocrine disturbance
    4. sodium diphenylhydantoin (Dilantin) medication

110. Falsely low temperature readings may result from

    1. incomplete closure of the mouth
    2. breathing through the mouth
    3. leaving the thermometer in place for too short a time
    4. recent ingestion of cold substances

111. In pneumothorax,

    1. whether or not the patient is symptomatic depends on the extent, acuteness, and rapidity of progression of the pneumothorax
    2. percussion note is hyperresonant
    3. when hydropneumothorax is present, a succussion splash is frequently heard, and the dullness or flatness of the effusion shifts with change in position to a greater extent and more rapidly than in pleural effusion alone
    4. breath sounds are usually present

112. Diastolic murmurs may be divided into which of the following categories?

    1. high-pitched decrescendo murmurs of aortic insufficiency
    2. high-pitched decrescendo murmurs of mitral stenosis
    3. lower pitched murmurs of tricuspid stenosis
    4. lower pitched murmurs of pulmonic insufficiency

113. Fibrillation

    1. is the term applied to isolated spontaneous contraction of individual muscle fibers

    2. has the same significance as fasciculation
    3. indicates a lesion of the lower motor neuron
    4. is visible to the naked eye

114. Regarding lung consolidation,

    1. the patient is usually ill, depending upon the underlying condition
    2. breath sounds are loud and bronchovesicular or bronchial
    3. bronchophony and pectroriloquy may be present
    4. ventilation is usually shallow and slow

115. In pulmonary congestion,

    1. if the congestion is acute, the patient is in extreme distress; if partial or chronic, minimal dyspnea may be present
    2. the respiratory rate and use of accessory musculature depend upon the stage of the congestion
    3. breath sounds are of fair quality, and resonance is normal or only slightly impaired
    4. fine and medium rales that sound close to the ear and that do not shift after prolonged change of position are characteristic

Answers and Commentary

1. **False.** Nocturnal dyspnea is characteristic of asthma. (*Ann Intern Med*, 78:401, 1973)

2. **False.** If a drowsy patient responds to visual threat by blinking, but the response is asymmetric, this may indicate a homonymous field defect. When the response is absent, one cannot be certain whether this is due to decreased vision or depressed vision or depressed state of consciousness. (*Med Clin N Am*, 57:1363, 1973)

3. **True.** The physical signs of hemothorax are those of pleural effusion; these are diminished breath sounds at the base posteriorly on the involved side with dullness to percussion. The mediastinum may be shifted, and this may be detected by percussion and palpation of the trachea for shift. (2:313)

4. **True.** By far, the commonest cause of vertigo is a disturbance of function of the labyrinth. This may be the effect of unaccustomed stimuli acting upon normal labyrinths, as in rotation and motion-sickness. The commonest and therefore the most important form of vertigo arising in the labyrinth is Meniere's syndrome, causing recurrent aural vertigo. (1:65)

5. **False.** When nystagmus is due to disease of the labyrinth, it is usually associated with paroxysmal vertigo and deafness. (1:47)

6. **True.** In situations in which diabetic ketoacidosis is accompanied by lactic acidosis, a weakly positive nitroprusside reaction may not reflect the magnitude of ketonemia since the altered redox state favors conversion of acetoacetate to beta-hydroxybutyrate. (*N Engl J Med*, 290:130, 1974)

7. **True.** A classic attack of migraine begins with a visual disturbance which occurs within one pair of homonymous half-fields. For example, the patient notices that he cannot see clearly in a small area to one side of the fixation point. This area of defective vision may be described as misty or shimmering, and it may have an irregular, scintillating, and sometimes colored outline known as teichopsia, or fortification spectra. (1:191)

8. **True.** Certain wheezes due to extrabronchial compression or intrabronchial polypoid lesions appear only with change in position. (2:136)

9. **True.** A strong clue to the likelihood of analgesic nephropathy is renal papillary necrosis, with its usual symptoms of renal colic due to sloughed papilla passed down the ureter. (*Internist Observer*, p. 3, Oct – Nov 1973)

10. **False.** A low glucose concentration in pleural fluid may reflect the presence of malignancy. The primary tumor in such instances may be located in the lung or at some other site. (*Am J Respir Dis*, 103:427, 1971)

11. **True.** The character and location of any visible cardiac impulses should be noted during examination. Minor precordial movements can be amplified by observing during expiratory apnea. (2:146)

12. **True.** Serum chloride levels usually are elevated in hyperparathyroidism. They may also be elevated in instances of pseudohyperparathyroidism with production of a parathyroid hormone-like substance. (*Medicine*, 45:247, 1966)

13. **False.** Nystagmus is usually present in cerebellar disease. (1:46)

14. **True.** Eye signs may occur in the absence of active thyrotoxicosis (ophthalmic Graves' disease)

so that their presence and severity are not necessarily related to the thyroid state of the patient. (*Br Med J*, 2:399, 1972)

15. **False.** Among the neurologic findings associated with hypercalcemia are fatigue, muscle weakness, depressed tendon reflexes, disorientation, stupor, coma, and death.
(*Med Clin North Am*, 56:941, 1972)

16. **True.** As far as motor, sensory, and speech functions are concerned, symptoms of occlusion of the middle cerebral artery are indistinguishable from those of occlusion of the internal carotid artery. In doubtful cases, the diagnosis can be made only by angiography. (1:258)

17. **True.** The early symptoms of senile cataract may include visual blurring, especially involving distance. (2:73)

18. **True.** Small, contracted pupils which do not respond may be associated with midbrain damage. (2:310)

19. **False.** It has been pointed out that in patients with SIADH, the urine need not be hypertonic. What is necessary is that it be less than maximally dilute in the face of the serum hypotonicity that should lead to maximal urine dilution.
(*N Engl J Med*, 284:65, 1971)

20. **False.** Normal serum phosphorus levels may be found in hyperparathyroidism, and, in the presence of azotemia, one would expect phosphorus excretion to be impaired so that the serum phosphorus level might be higher than those found in patients with hyperparathyroidism in the absence of azotemia. (*Hosp Phys*, 1:71, 1971)

21. **True.** In appendicitis or other conditions secondarily affecting the psoas muscle, there may be flexion of the thigh due to contraction of the psoas muscle. (2:219)

22. **True.** Where an involved artery crosses a retinal vein, it may indent the vein and even cause evidence of back pressure in the vein distal to the crossing (A-V notching). The disappearance of the vein on both sides of the blood column representing the artery is a measure of thickening of the arteriolar wall. (2:77)

23. **True.** The patient with a trochlear palsy will complain of difficulty with vision in the lower field, as in reading, and if he has been able to maintain single binocular vision, his head will be tilted toward the shoulder opposite the side of the paralysis. It is useful to be able to test for intact trochlear function in the presence of a complete oculomotor paralysis, since in some conditions both nerves may be involved. (2:74)

24. **False.** Reduction in GFR alone is sufficient to account for the modest elevations of plasma amylase activity that may sometimes be encountered in renal failure.
(*N Engl J Med*, 290:785, 1974)

25. **C.** (2:195)

26. **G.** (2:196)

27. **B.** (2:195)

28. **A.** (2:195)

29. **F.** (2:196)

30. **D.** (2:196)

31. **E.** (2:196)

32. **Diaphragm, retrosternal.** In chronic obstructive pulmonary disease, the two most reliable radiologic signs of hyperinflation (best seen on a lateral film) are the flatness of the diaphragm and the depth of the retrosternal air space.
(*Mod Med*, 41:32, 1973)

33. **Hoffmann.** There are two basic pathologic reflexes, the Babinski and its variants, and the Hoffmann and its variants. (2:349)

34. **Causalgia.** Partial damage to a peripheral nerve may be followed by a characteristic type of pain termed causalgia. This may develop rapidly after injury or may require several days to make its appearance. It is characterized by constant, intense, burning pain. (2:319)

35. **Incarcerated.** When a hernia can no longer be reduced and the contents of the hernial sac cannot be returned to the peritoneal cavity, it is said to be incarcerated. (2:258)

36. **Adson.** The Adson test is performed with the patient sitting with the forearms in supination and resting on the thighs. Palpate the radial pulse on the side to be tested. Instruct the patient to extend the neck and turn the chin to the side to be tested. The transient disappearance of the radial pulse during inspiration signifies temporary occlusion of the subclavian artery as the anterior scalene muscle is tensed (by extension of the neck and rotation of the skull) while the "floor" of the thoracic outlet rises during inspiration. Compression of the brachial plexus in the supraclavicular fossa is suggested by intensification of pain and paresthesia in the arm as the Adson maneuver is performed, by tenderness to palpation over the brachial plexus, and by neurologic changes in arm and hand (particularly a decrease

in the ability to appreciate light touch over the fourth and fifth fingers of the hand). These signs may be intensified as the shoulder is abducted and externally rotated. (2:291–92)

37. **Finkelstein's.** The diagnosis of de Quervain's disease is confirmed when a tender nodule can be felt within one or both of the tendons over the lateral aspect of the distal radius and when a positive Finkelstein's test is noted. (2:295)

38. **Neurogenic.** Reflex neurogenic bladder due to a transverse myelitis of the spinal cord, as in trauma, characteristically produces a hyperactive bulbocavernosus reflex and saddle anesthesia. Associated neurologic findings due to the paraplegia facilitate this diagnosis. (2:250)

39. **Murphy's.** The sign of inspiratory arrest (Murphy's sign) may be seen in the presence of acute cholecystitis. This is elicited by having the patient take a deep breath while the examiner maintains pressure against the abdominal wall in the region of the gallbladder. As the liver descends with inspiration, the gallbladder comes in contact with the examining hand and the patient experiences a sharp pain and inspiration is arrested. (2:224)

40. **Hypopyon.** Hypopyon is the presence of pus in the anterior chamber of the eye, often with a horizontal fluid level. (2:61)

41. **Orthopnea.** Dyspnea precipitated by assuming the recumbent position is referred to as orthopnea. (2:164)

42. **Root, root.** An irritative lesion of a single dorsal root causes pain of a lancinating or burning character which is often precipitated or intensified by coughing or sneezing, sometimes by movements of the spine, and is associated with hyperesthesia and hyperalgesia over the full segmental distribution of the root. (1:336)

43. **Hyphemia.** Hyphemia is the presence of blood in the anterior chamber of the eye. (2:61)

44. **C.** Change in potassium metabolism may be reflected in increased or decreased excitability of neuromuscular tissue. The rate of change of potassium stores is of primary importance in the expression of clinical toxicity, for rapid increases or decreases in the serum potassium level may seriously alter membrane potential, resulting in either decreased or enhanced polarization. (*JAMA*, 231:631, 1975)

45. **C.** A very prominent, intermittent jugular pulse may indicate either of the disorders listed. (*Emerg Med*, 5:157, 1973)

46. **C.** Left ventricular hypertrophy without significant dilatation may be due to primary left ventricular disease, as in hypertrophic cardiomyopathy or secondary to systolic overload, as in aortic valvular stenosis. (*N Engl J Med*, 289:118, 1973)

47. **C.** Both statements are true of neurocirculatory asthenia. (*JAMA*, 229:847, 1974)

48. **B.** The diagnosis of a hemoglobin disorder cannot be based solely on a hemoglobin pattern or a sickle cell preparation but may depend on the clinical picture and other factors. (*Am Fam Physician*, 2:87, 1970)

49. **A.** Patients with primary alveolar hypoventilation may have normal pulmonary function tests and decreased sensitivity to CO_2. (*Mod Med*, 41:32, 1973)

50. **C.** A dilated pupil in a comatose patient may suggest either of the listed locations of the lesion. (*Med Clin North Am*, 57:1363, 1973)

51. **A.** Patients with lactase deficiency often have abdominal distress and diarrhea. (*N Engl J Med*, 281:1114, 1969)

52. **C.** Dysmetria is a disturbance of the power to control the range of movement in muscular action and is a sign of cerebellar dysfunction. (2:341)

53. **C.** A radial nerve lesion may result in wrist-drop and finger-drop. (1:355)

54. **A.** In toxic adenoma, both the clinical picture and the results of blood tests may be equivocal. (*Br Med J, 2*, 5810:337, 1972)

55. **C.** Local inspiratory retraction of the intercostal spaces means local bronchial obstruction; this finding is commonly diffuse in asthma and emphysema. (2:127–128)

56. **A.** Dyssynergia is a disturbance of muscular coordination and a sign of cerebellar dysfunction. (2:341)

57. **B.** When bronchial breathing is heard over the upper anterior chest, the finding may be due to increased transmission through consolidated lung or merely to normal tracheal breathing due to shift in tracheal position. (2:131)

58. **C.** The cerebrospinal fluid is likely to contain red blood cells if a cerebral hemorrhage has ruptured into a ventricle or the subarachnoid space. (1:271–72)

59. **B.** (2:101)

60. **B.** (2:101)

61. **A.** (2:101)

62. **A.** (2:101)

63. **A.** (2:50)

64. **B.** (2:50)

65. **A.** (2:251)

66. **B.** (2:251)

67. **D.** (2:67)

68. **B.** (2:67)

69. **A.** (2:67)

70. **C.** (2:67)

71. **A.** Evidence of hemolysis is associated with unconjugated hyperbilirubinemia, decreased or absent serum haptoglobin, and a significant reticulocytosis. (*Res Staff Phys*, 19:42, 1973)

72. **D.** All statements are true of the comatose patient. (*Med Clin North Am*, 57:1363, 1973)

73. **D.** Pleural effusion (fluid of any type in the pleural cavity) includes empyema, hemothorax, and chylothorax, which require thoracentesis for specific identification. (2:106)

74. **C.** Nystagmus due to disease of the labyrinth is usually rotary. (1:47)

75. **E.** All the diseases listed may cause great enlargement of the spleen. Additionally, agnogenic myeloid metaplasia and rare diseases such as Gaucher's disease, Niemann-Pick disease, kala-azar, or tropical eosinophilia may cause splenic enlargement. (2:237)

76. **E.** All the disorders listed, as well as nystagmus, are features of cerebellar deficiency. (1:96)

77. **E.** All the disorders listed may be associated with hemoptysis in a person with club fingers. (*Am Fam Physician*, 8:61, 1973)

78. **E.** Target cells may be seen in all the diseases listed. (*Res Staff Phys*, 19:24, 1973)

79. **E.** Angina pectoris or cardiac pain mimicking angina pectoris without coronary heart disease may occur in patients with arterial hypertension, marked valvular disease, congenital heart disease, myocardiopathy, or pericarditis. (*Circulation*, XLVII:1139, 1973)

80. **E.** A roentgenographic cavitary lesion may indicate the presence of any of the disorders listed. (*Lahey Clin Found Bull*, 20:129, 1971)

81. **E.** All the diseases listed may cause central cyanosis. (2:166)

82. **A.** In papilledema, the nasal edge of the disc becomes blurred; this blurring then extends to the temporal edge, and the physiological cup begins to fill with exudate. Later the swelling lifts the surface of the disc above the level of the surrounding retina. All other statements are correct. (1:28–29)

83. **A.** A pleural fluid red blood cell count greater than 100,000/cu mm strongly suggests malignant neoplasm, pulmonary infarction, or trauma. (*Arch Intern Med*, 132:854, 1973)

84. **A.** Often the thalamus and its adjacent structures may be involved during decorticate movement and postures. All other statements are correct. (*Med Clin North Am*, 57:1363, 1973)

85. **B.** In autonomous neurogenic bladder, there is no bulbocavernosus reflex and saddle anesthesia is present. All other statements are true. (2:249)

86. **A.** The syndrome of inappropriate ADH secretion is usually associated with hypertonic urine. (*Ann Intern Med*, 82:61, 1975)

87. **A.** The first symptoms of spinal cord compression are usually sensory, the commonest being pain radiating into the distribution of one or more spinal roots. (1:312)

88. **A.** Rhonchi imply disease of the larger bronchi, whereas moist medium and fine rales imply bronchiolar and alveolar disease. Rhonchi are usually heard earlier in inspiration than are rales, as sound is produced when the column of inspired air meets the exudate at its anatomic location. Sonorous rhonchi are low-pitched, as are coarse rales which are bubbling in quality. Both frequently clear with cough, while fine and medium rales due to inflammatory conditions are usually increased by cough. (2:132)

89. **A.** In black populations blood pressure and obesity are better correlated in women than men.
(*N Engl J Med*, 291:178, 1974)

90. **B.** An S₄ gallop most probably originates in the ventricular chamber, and although the exact mechanism of formation is not certain, it is thought to result from a forceful voluminous atrial contraction injecting blood into a ventricle having a limited distensibility.
(*N Engl J Med*, 284:85, 1971)

91. **A.** For reasons that are not clear, hematuria occurs more frequently in patients with Hb SA than in those with the more severe Hb SS.
(*Am Fam Physician*, 2:87, 1970)

92. **A.** Status epilepticus is rarely the first manifestation of cryptogenic epilepsy in adults, although it is often the first sign in children.
(*Mod Med*, 40:79, 1972)

93. **A.** Variable response of pupils to light suggests toxic or metabolic abnormality rather than structural lesion of the brain stem.
(*Med Clin North Am*, 57:1363, 1973)

94. **A.** In the absence of right heart failure, patients with the most severe emphysema can usually sleep flat, often on one side or the other, using only one pillow or none. Total vital capacity tends to be greater when the patient is supine than when standing; in contrast, the cardiac patient's total vital capacity when supine is significantly lower than when standing in many cases.
(*Hosp Med*, 9:8, 1973)

95. **E.** Diplopia is a common symptom of Graves' disease, and obvious impairment of eye movement is not rare. All other statements listed are true of Graves' disease. In addition, the earliest changes in the ocular muscles are the development of an inflammatory edema and an increase in the number of fibroblasts; the muscle structure becomes disorganized and later fibrosis and contracture may ensue. (*Lancet, 1*, 7856:491, 1974)

96. **D.** In lesions of spinal nerve roots, appreciation of passive movement is usually unimpaired after a single root lesion. All other statements are true of this disorder. (1:336)

97. **B.** Most patients do not have permanent neurological deficits in transient ischemic attacks. All other statements are true. In addition, x-ray films of the cervical spine should be included in the investigation of vertebrobasilar attacks because of their association with cervical spondylosis. Investigation is directed particularly towards finding atherosclerotic lesions in extracranial vessels that may be amenable to surgery.
(*Br Med J*, 1:91, 1972)

98. **E.** Decerebrate movement and postures need not be structural since decerebrate states may occur with metabolic disturbances such as hypoglycemia, intoxications, or anoxia. All other statements are correct. Also, if unilateral, the decerebrate postures are ipsilateral to the lesion and fragmentation of decerebrate postures has the same localizing significance as the fully developed decerebration.
(*Med Clin North Am*, 57:1363, 1973)

99. **A.** Apathetic hyperthyroidism is an atypical presentation of the disease which occurs in the elderly. All other statements are true.
(*Br Med J, 2*, 5810:337, 1972)

100. **D.** Bradycardia, rather than tachycardia, is usually seen in hypercalcemia. Most of the symptoms of hypercalcemia are nonspecific and, in addition to those listed, include constipation, nausea and vomiting, and anorexia. On occasion, coma and shock can be found.
(*Int Cons*, p. 44, 1972)

101. **D.** All features listed are characteristic of sarcoidosis with the exception that hypercalciuria is typically marked. Involvement of the liver and kidneys by the granulomatous process is common and may lead to increases in serum alkaline phosphatase and to azotemia, respectively. Nephrocalcinosis may result from hypercalcemia or hypercalciuria or both.
(*Med Clin North Am*, 56:941, 1972)

102. **E.** All statements are true of compression of the cauda equina, which may result from a tumor or displaced intervertebral disc. (1:319–20)

103. **A.** Pulmonic systolic ejection murmurs occur with pulmonary valvular and subvalvular stenosis, dilatation of the pulmonary artery, and increased pulmonary flow, as with atrial septal defect. They are usually localized to the second and third intercostal spaces and may be referred to the left upper chest. (2:186)

104. **A.** All of the findings listed may occur in the syndrome of inappropriate ADH secretion, as described by Bartter, with the exception that renal and adrenal functions are normal.
(*Ann Intern Med*, 82:811, 1975)

105. **A.** Administration of thyroid hormone will reduce RAI uptake. All other statements are correct.
(*Am Fam Physician*, 3:73, 1971) and (3:1698)

106. **E.** Water-hammer pulse is the basis for peripheral signs of aortic insufficiency including "hopping carotids," "pistol-shot sounds,"

Duroziez's sign, de Musset's sign and others. Although interesting, they are of little diagnostic importance. (2:171–72)

107. **E.** In diffuse acute bronchial obstruction, the patient is in extreme respiratory distress. With laryngeal obstruction crowing sounds are heard; with bronchial obstruction, wheezing is appreciated. Respiration is rapid. The intercostal spaces retract on inspiration. Accessory respiratory muscles may be used. Fremitus is decreased, but rhonchal fremitus may be present. The percussion note is normal or hyperresonant throughout. The breath sounds are diminished in intensity, although they may be extremely noisy because of rhonchi and coarse rales. Asthma, acute exacerbations of bronchitis, and foreign bodies produce this condition. (2:133)

108. **A.** Complete paralysis of the third cranial nerve results in paralysis of the superior, medial, and inferior recti, and the inferior oblique. All other statements are correct. (1:42)

109. **E.** Gingival swelling is a common sign of odontogenic infection, which may also produce sinus tracts draining dentoalveolar abscesses. Enlargement of the gingivae may be seen in generalized form in conditions of chronic inflammation, pregnancy, endocrine disturbance, Dilantin medication, blood dyscrasias, and as a familial tendency to gingival fibromatosis. (2:87)

110. **E.** Falsely low temperature levels may result from all the factors listed. (2:35)

111. **A.** In pneumothorax fremitus is absent and breath sounds are usually absent. All other statements are true. (2:135)

112. **B.** Diastolic murmurs may be divided into two categories: high-pitched decrescendo murmurs of aortic and pulmonic insufficiency, and the lower pitched murmurs of mitral and tricuspid stenosis. (2:188)

113. **A.** Fibrillation is the term applied to the isolated spontaneous contraction of individual muscle fibers. As the contraction of single fibers is not visible to the naked eye, it can only be recognized by electromyography. All other statements are correct. (1:89)

114. **A.** In lung consolidation, the patient is usually ill, depending upon the underlying condition. Ventilation is usually deep and rapid. Fremitus is increased; the percussion note is dull; the breath sounds are loud and bronchovesicular or bronchial. Fine and medium moist rales are heard which are consonating in quality. Bronchophony and pectoriloquy may be present. Consolidation occurs mainly in pulmonary infections and with large areas of pulmonary infarction. (2:135)

115. **A.** If the pulmonary congestion is acute, the patient is in extreme distress; if partial or chronic, minimal dyspnea may be present. The respiratory rate and use of accessory musculature depend upon this difference. Fremitus may be normal or slightly decreased. Associated signs of pleural effusion may be present at the base. Breath sounds are of fair quality, and resonance is normal or only slightly impaired. Fine and medium rales that do not sound close to the ear and that shift after prolonged change of position are characteristic. With marked pulmonary edema, bubbling coarse rales are also heard. (2:135–36)

Textbook References for Chapter 23

1. Bannister, Roger (1978): *Brain's Clinical Neurology*, Fifth Edition, Oxford Medical Publications, New York

2. Judge, R.D. and Zuidema, G.D., Editors (1974): *Physical Diagnosis: A Physiologic Approach to the Clinical Examination*, Little, Brown and Company, Boston.

3. Isselbacher, K.J., Editor (1980): *Harrison's Principles of Internal Medicine*, Ninth Edition, McGraw-Hill Book Company, New York.